Air Fryer Cookbook for Beginners

1001 Quick & Healthy Frying Recipes To Reduce Up To 75% The Fat Content Of Foods And The Risk Of An Instant Diabetes For You And Your Family

Elena Simmons

Toc

DESCRIPTION		16
INTRODUCTION		17
BREAKFAST		18
1.	Stuffed Portobello Mushrooms with Ground Beef	18
2.	Basil-Spinach Quiche	18
3.	Stuffed Chicken Roll with Mushrooms	18
4.	Eggs on Avocado Burgers	19
5.	Applesauce Mash with Sweet Potato	19
6.	Bacon and Kale Breakfast Salad	20
7.	Fish Fritatta	20
8.	Spinach Frittata	20
9.	Beef Balls with Sesame and Dill	21
10.	Zucchini Rounds with Ground Chicken	21
11.	Tomatoes with Chicken	22
12.	Meatball Breakfast Salad	22
13.	Cherry Tomatoes Fritatta	23
14.	Whisked Eggs with Ground Chicken	23
15.	Kale Quiche with Eggs	24
16.	Breakfast Bacon Hash	24
17.	Spaghetti Squash Casserole Cups	24
18.	Chopped Kale with Ground Beef	25
19.	Bacon Wrapped Chicken Fillet	25
20.	Egg Whites with Sliced Tomatoes	26
21.	Eggs in Avocado	26
22.	Maple Apple Quinoa	26
23.	Avocado Eggs Mix	27
24.	Turkey Tortillas	27
25.	Turkey and Peppers Bowls	27
26.	Potato Casserole	28
27.	Chives Quinoa Bowls	28
28.	Creamy Almond Rice	28
29.	Sweet Quinoa Mix	29
30.	Olives Rice Mix	29
31.	Eggplant and Sweet Potato Hash	29
32.	Sprouts, Avocado and Eggs	30
33.	Cheddar Sprouts Bowls	30
34.	Mozzarella Avocado Mix	30
35.	Salsa Omelet	31
36.	Salmon and Zucchini Salad	31
37.	Parsley Avocado Salad	31
38.	Bacon Omelet	31
39.	Spinach and Asparagus Frittata	32
40.	Asparagus Muffins	32
41.	Coconut Eggs Mix	33
42.	Eggplant and Avocado Salad	33
43.	Peppers, Coconut and Eggs Mix	33
44.	Yogurt Avocado Mix	34
45.	Asparagus, Shrimp and Avocado Salad	34
46.	Nutty Granola	34
47.	Fruit and Nut Keto Granola	35
48.	Strawberry and Nut Cereal	35
49.	Seedy Breakfast Granola	36
50.	Pepper Stuffed Spinach Parmesan Baked Eggs	36
51.	Pepper Stuffed Spinach and Feta Eggs	36
52.	Egg Stuffed Peppers and Cheese	37
53.	Bacon and Egg Stuffed Peppers	37
54.	Peppers and Eggs	37
55.	Pepper Stuffed Spinach Parmesan Baked Eggs	38
56.	Brussels Hash	38
57.	Zucchini Hash	39
58.	Vegetable Hash	39
59.	Ham, Cheese and Mushroom Melt	39
60.	Ham and Pepper Melt	40
61.	Veggie Melt	40
62.	Blueberry Breakfast Cake	41
63.	Red Pepper Breakfast Cake	41
64.	Zucchini Breakfast Cake	42
65.	Strawberry Breakfast Bread	42
66.	Raspberry Breakfast Cake	43
67.	Cheesy Bacon Pancake	43
68.	Cheesy Pancake	44
69.	Strawberry Feta Pancake	44
70.	Pepper Pancake	44

71.	Sausage Omelette	45
72.	Ham and Cheese Omelet	45
73.	Air fried Cheese Sandwich	46
74.	Green Beans Egg Bake	46
75.	Cod Corn Burritos	46
76.	Cheese and Ham Pockets	47
77.	Tuna Mayo Sandwiches	47
78.	Mint & Peas Omelet	48
79.	Vanilla Steel Cut Oats	48
80.	Pear Cinnamon Oatmeal	48
81.	Maple Rice Pudding	48
82.	Squash Mushroom Mix	49
83.	Tarragon Cheese Omelet	49
84.	Zucchini Chicken Burritos	49
85.	Kale & Pumpkin Seeds Sandwich	50
86.	Apple Cinnamon Pancakes	50
87.	Romanesco Tofu Quinoa	51
88.	Black Bean Cheese Burritos	51
89.	Mushroom Tofu Casserole	51
90.	Cinnamon Yam Pudding	52
91.	Tangy Cauliflower Hash	52
92.	Nutmeg Mushroom Fritters	53
93.	Tofu & Bell Peppers Medley	53
94.	Stuffed Feta Cheese Peppers	53
95.	Citrus Pepper Salad	54
96.	Spinach Egg Pie	54
97.	Eggplant & Zucchini Mix	54

MAINS   **56**

98.	Indian Chickpeas	56
99.	White Beans with Rosemary	56
100.	Squash Bowls	56
101.	Cauliflower Stew with Tomatoes and Green Chilies 57
102.	Simple Quinoa Stew	57
103.	Green Beans with Carrot	58
104.	Chickpeas and Lentils Mix	58
105.	Creamy Corn with Potatoes	58
106.	Spinach and Lentils Mix	59
107.	Cajun Mushrooms with Veggies and Beans	59
108.	Eggplant Stew	59
109.	Okra and Corn Mix	60
110.	Potato and Carrot with Vegan Cheese	60
111.	Winter Green Beans	60
112.	Spiced Green Beans with Veggies	61
113.	Chipotle Green Beans	61
114.	Tomato and Cranberry Beans Pasta	62
115.	Mexican Casserole	62
116.	Scallions and Endives with Rice	62
117.	Cabbage and Tomatoes	63
118.	Lemony Endive Mix	63
119.	Eggplant and Tomato Sauce	63
120.	Spiced Brown Rice with Mung Beans	64
121.	Lentils and Spinach Casserole	64
122.	Red Potatoes with Green Beans and Chutney	65
123.	Simple Italian Veggie Salad	65
124.	Roasted Cauliflower with Nuts & Raisins	65
125.	Spicy Herb Chicken Wings	66
126.	Lamb Meatballs	66
127.	Sweet & Sour Chicken Skewer	66
128.	Green Stuffed Peppers	67
129.	Beef Meatballs in Tomato Sauce	67
130.	Mustard Pork Balls	67
131.	Garlic Pork Chops	68
132.	Honey Ginger Salmon Steaks	68
133.	Rosemary & Lemon Salmon	68
134.	Fish with Capers & Herb Sauce	69
135.	Lemon Halibut	69
136.	Fried Cod & Spring Onion	69
137.	Medium-Rare Beef Steak	70
138.	Spicy Duck Legs	70
139.	Stuffed Turkey	70
140.	Turkey Breast with Maple Mustard Glaze	71
141.	Garlic Chicken Kebab	71
142.	Mozzarella & Parmesan Chicken Breasts	72
143.	Rotisserie Style Chicken	72
144.	Zucchini Manicotti	72
145.	Steamed Salmon with Dill Sauce	72
146.	Thai Roast Beef Salad with Nam Jim Dressing	73

#	Recipe	Page
147.	Air Fried Chicken Thighs	73
148.	Chicken Cheese Fillet	74
149.	Roasted Pepper Salad	74
150.	Pineapple Pizza	74
151.	Air Fryer Tortilla Pizza	75
152.	Air Fried Pork Apple Balls	75
153.	Stuffed Garlic Chicken	75
154.	Rosemary Citrus Chicken	76
155.	Air Fried Garlic Popcorn Chicken	76
156.	Macaroni Cheese Toast	76
157.	Cheese Burger Patties	77
158.	Grilled Cheese Corn	77
159.	Eggplant Fries	77
160.	Air Fried Pita Bread Pizza	77
161.	Light & Crispy Okra	78
162.	Chili Rellenos	78
163.	Persian Mushrooms	78
164.	Air Fried Chicken Cordon Bleu	79
165.	Chicken Noodles	79
166.	Mushroom & Herb Stuffed Pork Chops	80
167.	Roasted Lamb with Pumpkin	80
168.	Liver Curry	81
169.	Minced Beef Kebab Skewers	81
170.	Pomfret Fish Fry	81
171.	Cedar Planked Salmon	82
172.	Crested Halibut	82
173.	Creamy Halibut	82
174.	Air Fried Catfish	83
175.	Air Fried Spinach Fish	83
176.	Roly Poly Air Fried White Fish	83
177.	Air Fried Dragon Shrimp	84
178.	Lasagna Zucchini Cups	84
179.	Spinach Artichoke Stuffed Peppers	85
180.	Cauliflower Shepherd's Pie	85
181.	Coconut Lime Skirt Steak	86
182.	Spicy Chicken Enchilada Casserole	86
183.	Kale & Ground Beef Casserole	86
184.	Cauliflower-Cottage Pie	87
185.	Roasted Asian Shrimp & Brussels Sprouts	87
186.	Grilled Chicken with Garlic Sauce	88
187.	Bacon-Wrapped Stuffed Zucchini Boats	88
188.	Parmesan Chicken Wings	89
189.	Beef Burgers	89
190.	Bacon Wrapped Avocado	89
191.	Buffalo Chicken Meatballs	90
192.	Caprese Grilled Chicken with Balsamic Vinegar	90
193.	Philly Cheese Steak Stuffed Peppers	91
194.	Parmesan, Garlic, Lemon Roasted Zucchini	91
195.	Chicken Filet Stuffed with Sausage	91
196.	Bourbon Chicken	92
197.	Roasted Chicken Legs	92
198.	Mongolian Chicken	92
199.	Chicken Drumsticks with Spinach Sauce	93
200.	Parsley Meatballs	93
201.	Paprika Beef Short Ribs	94
202.	Lamb Burger	94
203.	Pesto Chicken	94
204.	Lemon Trout	95
205.	Stuffed Salmon Fillet with Tomatoes	95
206.	Tomato Beef Brisket	95
207.	Seafood Bowl	96
208.	Spicy Meat Bowl	96
209.	Stuffed Sweet Potato	97
210.	Basil Beef Shank	97
211.	Sesame Pork Cubes	98
212.	Thai Chicken	98
213.	Vegetable and Chicken Bowl	98
214.	Stuffed Cabbage	99
215.	Chili	99
216.	Lime Chicken with Pistachio	100
217.	Turkey Dill Meatballs	100
218.	Mango Turkey	100
219.	Turkey Burger with Jalapeno	101
220.	Fennel Fish Fillet	101
221.	Shrimp Chowder	102
222.	Ground Beef Bowl	102
223.	Turmeric Chicken Liver	102
224.	Chicken Burgers	103

225.	Zucchini Casserole	103
226.	Cherry Tuscan Pork Loin	104
227.	Ground Chicken and Ground Pork Mix	104
228.	Shrimp Salad with Greens and Avocado	105
229.	Cauliflower Fritters with Carrot	105
230.	Lamb Fillet with Tomato Gravy	106
231.	Chicken Strips with Orange Zest	106
232.	Broccoli Casserole	107
233.	Coconut Sour Shrimps with Greens	107
234.	Seafood Casserole	108
235.	Stuffed Chicken Breast with Avocado	108
236.	Spiralized Casserole	109
237.	Crunchy Chicken Fingers	109
238.	Egg Salad with Avocado	110
239.	Juicy Scallops	110
240.	Stuffed Pepper Halves with Ground Meat	110
241.	Pear Bowl with Nuts and Flax Seeds	111
242.	Sweet Potato Toasts	111
243.	Bacon Red Potato Halves	112
244.	Hash Brown	112
245.	Mixed Meat Sausages	113
246.	Asparagus with Chicken	113

SIDES — 115

247.	Grilled Pineapple with Cinnamon	115
248.	Bell Peppers with Potato Stuffing	115
249.	Chickpea & Zucchini Burgers	115
250.	36Spanish Style Spiced Potatoes	116
251.	Spicy Cheesy Breaded Mushrooms	116
252.	Broccoli with Cheese & Olives	116
253.	French Beans with Walnuts & Almonds	117
254.	Fried Zucchini, Squash, & Carrot Mix	117
255.	Hot Spicy Thyme Cherry Tomatoes	117
256.	Honey Roasted Carrots	118
257.	Spicy Mango Okra	118
258.	Parsley & Garlic Flavored Potatoes	118
259.	Turmeric & Garlic Roasted Carrots	118
260.	Paprika Chips	119
261.	Bacon & Veggie Mash	119
262.	Garlic & Parsley Roasted Mushrooms	120
263.	Ginger & Honey Cauliflower Bites	120
264.	Vegetable Fries	120
265.	Hot Pepper Pin Wheel	121
266.	Crab & Cheese Soufflé	121
267.	Lemon Courgette Caviar	121
268.	Chopped Liver with Eggs	122
269.	Baked Tomato & Egg	122
270.	Parmesan Asparagus Fries	122
271.	Spicy Mozzarella Stick	123
272.	Cheese Croquettes with Prosciutto	123
273.	Fried Garlic Calamari	123
274.	Crispy Cheese & Garlic Sticks	124
275.	Mushroom, Onion and Feta Frittata	124
276.	Bacon, Lettuce, Tempeh & Tomato Sandwiches	124
277.	Curried Cauliflower Florets	125
278.	Parsnip Fries	125
279.	Coconut Chips	125
280.	Sweet Potato Chips	126
281.	Vegetable Spring Rolls	126
282.	Onion Pakora	127
283.	Semolina Veggie Cutlets	127
284.	Charred Shishito Peppers	127
285.	Samosas	128
286.	Baked Tomatoes with Feta & Pesto	128
287.	Cumin, Chili & Squash	129
288.	Pineapple Sticks with Yogurt Dip	129
289.	Low-Carb Zucchini Roll-Ups	129
290.	Zucchini Fries & Roasted Garlic Aioli	129
291.	Zucchini, Carrots & Yellow Squash	130
292.	Roast Butternut Pumpkin with Nuts & Balsamic Vinaigrette	130
293.	Crispy Black-Eyed Peas	131
294.	Lemony Green Beans	131
295.	Roasted Orange Cauliflower	131
296.	Eggplant Parmesan Panini	132
297.	Spinach Samosa	132
298.	Avocado Fries	133
299.	Honey Roasted Carrots	133

#	Recipe	Page
300.	Crispy & Crunchy Baby Corn	133
301.	Tasty Tofu	134
302.	Crispy Herb Cauliflower Florets	134
303.	Roasted Corn	134
304.	Spicy Nuts	134
305.	Tawa Veggies	135
306.	Mediterranean Veggie Mix	135
SEAFOOD		**136**
307.	Ginger Salmon Mix	136
308.	Salmon Fillets and Green Olives	136
309.	Chervil Cod	136
310.	Honey Salmon	137
311.	Scallops Mix	137
312.	Shrimp and Cucumber Mix	137
313.	Shrimp and Potatoes	137
314.	Shrimp and Red Pepper Sauce	138
315.	Sage Shrimp	138
316.	Dill Sea Bass	138
317.	Baked Snapper	139
318.	Trout and Red Chili Mix	139
319.	Cilantro Shrimp and Apples Mix	139
320.	Saffron Salmon	140
321.	Salmon and Parsnips	140
322.	Spiced Cod	140
323.	Salmon and White Onions Mix	140
324.	Sherry Salmon Mix	141
325.	Sake Shrimp Mix	141
326.	Trout and Avocado Mix	141
327.	Shrimp and Sausage Mix	142
328.	Marjoram Shrimp	142
329.	Clams and Beer Sauce	142
330.	Oregano Clams	143
331.	Turmeric Trout and Beans	143
332.	Shrimp and Black Beans	143
333.	Salmon, Cauliflower and Red Quinoa	143
334.	Corn, Okra and Shrimp	144
335.	Tomato Clams	144
336.	Shrimp, Cod and Sauce	144
337.	Caraway Shrimp Mix	145
338.	Shrimp and Butternut Squash	145
339.	Calamari and Sauce	145
340.	Calamari Salsa Mix	146
341.	Maple Walnut Salmon	146
342.	Almond Crusted Salmon	146
343.	Maple Walnut Flounder	147
344.	Sesame Walnut Tuna	147
345.	Spicy Cod Fish Sticks	148
346.	Italian Fish Sticks	148
347.	Lemon Pepper Fish Sticks	149
348.	Salmon Fish Sticks	149
349.	Cajun Salmon Fish Sticks	150
350.	Bacon Wrapped Fish Sticks	150
351.	Keto Tuna Melt Cups	151
352.	Garlic Shrimp Bacon Bake	151
353.	Gruyere Shrimp Bacon Bake	151
354.	Cajun Shrimp Bacon Bake	152
355.	Garlic Shrimp Prosciutto Bake	152
356.	Garlic Shrimp Tuna Bake	153
357.	Jalapeno Tuna Melt Cups	153
358.	Herbed Tuna Melt Cups	153
359.	Cajun Tuna Melt Cups	154
360.	Cheddar Tuna Melt Cups	154
361.	Sesame Tuna Melt Cups	155
362.	Asian Style Crunchy Flounder	155
363.	Prosciutto Wrapped Cod	156
364.	Prosciutto Wrapped Salmon	156
365.	Fast Seared Scallops	157
366.	Lemon Scallops	157
367.	Dijon Baked Salmon	157
368.	Garlic Dijon Baked Salmon	158
369.	Crispy Salmon Fillets	158
370.	Tilapia and Tomato	158
371.	Cod and Spring Onions Sauce	159
372.	Sesame Crusted Tuna Steak	159
373.	Mustard Crusted Cod	159
374.	Italian Style Shrimp	160
375.	Rosemary Tomatoes and Shrimp	160

#	Title	Page
376.	Shrimp and Lemon Vinaigrette	160
377.	Shrimp and Chives	160
378.	Tilapia and Capers	161
379.	Pesto Almond Salmon	161
380.	Glazed Cod Fillets	161
381.	Lemongrass Sea Bass	162
382.	Baked Black Sea Bass	162
383.	Roasted Red Snapper	162
384.	Tuna Kabobs	163
385.	Catfish Fillet and Avocado	163
386.	Shrimp and Okra	163
387.	Chives Salmon	163
388.	Basil Swordfish Fillets	164
389.	Shrimp and Pesto	164

POULTRY — 165

#	Title	Page
390.	Chicken and Tabasco Sauce Mix	165
391.	Chicken, Leeks and Coriander Mix	165
392.	Turkey Stew	165
393.	Mozzarella Chicken Mix	166
394.	Chicken with Peppers and Zucchinis	166
395.	Maple Chicken Mix	166
396.	Whole Chicken Mix	167
397.	Chicken with Cauliflower Rice	167
398.	Chicken and Pineapple Mix	167
399.	Chicken and Veggies	167
400.	Chicken and Figs	168
401.	Pepper Chicken Mix	168
402.	Chicken and Pears Mix	168
403.	Chicken and Chili Sauce	169
404.	Chicken with Apples and Dates	169
405.	Chicken with Carrots and Celery	169
406.	Ginger Turkey and Yogurt mix	170
407.	Pesto Chicken Wings	170
408.	Spicy Tomato and Chicken Mix	170
409.	Turkey and Oyster Sauce	171
410.	Chicken Stew	171
411.	Parmesan Chicken	171
412.	Chicken, Sweet Potatoes and Radishes	172
413.	Balsamic Chicken and Beets	172
414.	Lemongrass Turkey	172
415.	Chicken and Coriander Sauce	173
416.	Turkey Chili	173
417.	Chicken and Chickpeas	173
418.	Turkey and Lentils	174
419.	Meatballs and Sauce	174
420.	Ground Turkey Mix	174
421.	Chicken and Bacon Mix	175
422.	Turkey and Mango Mix	175
423.	Herbed Turkey	175
424.	Chicken Wings and Sprouts	176
425.	Thyme Turkey	176
426.	Cumin Chicken	176
427.	Ground Chicken and Chilies	177
428.	Chopped Chicken Olive Tomato Sauce	177
429.	Chicken Thighs in Coconut Sauce, Nuts	177
430.	Forest Guinea Hen	178
431.	Fried and Crispy Chicken	178
432.	Orange Turkey Bites	179
433.	Chicken Thighs with Potatoes	179
434.	Chicken Blanquette With Soy	180
435.	Fish Sticks	180
436.	Vegetarian Curry with Pumpkin and Chickpeas	180
437.	Turkey Diced with Ginger, Apples and Vegetables	181
438.	Ligurian Rabbit	181
439.	Frozen Chicken Nuggets	181
440.	Chicken with Cacciatore (Chicken Hunter	182
441.	Devil Chicken	182
442.	Chicken with Pineapple	182
443.	Chicken Curry	183
444.	Chicken with Yogurt and Mustard	183
445.	Almond Chicken	184
446.	Mushroom Chicken	184
447.	Pepper Chicken	184
448.	Stuffed Chicken and Baked Potatoes	185
449.	Tandoori Chicken	185
450.	Crispy Chicken Fillets in Brine in Pickle Juice	185

#	Recipe	Page
451.	Turkey and Rosemary Butter	186
452.	Spiced Chicken Breasts	186
453.	Chicken and Pepperoni Pizza Bake	186
454.	Ginger Chicken Breasts	187
455.	Creamy Chicken Wings	187
456.	Jalapeño Popper Hasselback Chicken	187
457.	Thyme Duck Legs	188
458.	Chicken Enchiladas	188
459.	Crispy Chicken Tenders	189
460.	Chicken Cheese Sticks	189
461.	Marinated Drumsticks	189
462.	Mustard Turkey Bites	189
463.	Lemon Pepper Drumsticks	190
464.	Chives Chicken Tenders	190
465.	Cinnamon Duck Breasts	190
466.	Cheddar Turkey Bites	191
467.	Crispy Chicken Wings	191
468.	Mozzarella Chicken Breasts	191
469.	Smoked Chicken Wings	192
470.	Mediterranean Chicken	192
471.	Lemon-Oregano Chicken BBQ	192
472.	Chicken BBQ Recipe from Peru	193
473.	Turmeric and Lemongrass Chicken Roast	193
474.	Roast Chicken Recipe from Africa	193
475.	Shishito Pepper Rubbed Wings	194
476.	Grilled Chicken Recipe from Korea	194
477.	Lemon-Parsley Chicken Packets	194
478.	Grilled Chicken Wings with Curry-Yogurt Sauce	194
479.	Tomato, Eggplant 'n Chicken Skewers	195
480.	Garam Masala 'n Yogurt Marinated Chicken	195
481.	Grilled Chicken Pesto	196
482.	Quick 'n Easy Garlic Herb Wings	196
483.	Lemon-Aleppo Chicken	196
484.	Drunken Chicken Jerk Spiced	197
485.	Honey, Lime, And Garlic Chicken BBQ	197
486.	Chicken in Packets Southwest Style	197
487.	Cheese Stuffed Chicken	198
488.	Cilantro-Lime 'n Liquid Smoke Chicken Grill	198
489.	Chicken BBQ on Kale Salad	199
490.	Sriracha-vinegar Marinated Chicken	199
491.	Chicken BBQ Recipe from Italy	199
492.	Chili, Lime & Corn Chicken BBQ	200
493.	Honey-Balsamic Orange Chicken	200
494.	Salsa Verde Over Grilled Chicken	200
495.	Chicken Grill Recipe from California	201
496.	Grilled Thighs with Honey Balsamic Sauce	201
497.	Chicken Roast with Pineapple Salsa	202
498.	Sweet Lime 'n Chili Chicken Barbecue	202
499.	Sticky-Sweet Chicken BBQ	202

MEAT 204

#	Recipe	Page
500.	Lime Lamb Mix	204
501.	Lamb and Corn	204
502.	Herbed Beef and Squash	204
503.	Smoked Beef Mix	205
504.	Marjoram Pork Mix	205
505.	Nutmeg Lamb	205
506.	Greek Beef Mix	205
507.	Beef and Fennel	206
508.	Lamb and Eggplant Meatloaf	206
509.	Pork Chops with Olives and Corn	206
510.	Beef and Broccoli Mix	207
511.	Cajun Beef Mix	207
512.	Pork with Sprouts and Mushroom Mix	207
513.	Pork Chops and Yogurt Sauce	208
514.	Lamb and Macadamia Nuts Mix	208
515.	Beef, Cucumber and Eggplants	208
516.	Rosemary Pork and Artichokes	209
517.	Nutmeg Beef Mix	209
518.	Lamb and Asparagus Mix	209
519.	Paprika Lamb Chops	210
520.	Lamb and Mustard Sauce	210
521.	Beef with Apples and Plums	210
522.	Sage Beef	210
523.	Beef, Olives and Tomatoes	211
524.	Tarragon Beef	211
525.	Beef with Celery and Peas	211
526.	Lamb with Peas and Tomatoes	212

#	Title	Page
527.	Lamb with Zucchinis and Eggplants Mix	212
528.	Beef with Beans	212
529.	Mediterranean Lamb Meatballs	213
530.	Pork Rind	213
531.	Pork Trinoza Wrapped in Ham	214
532.	Homemade Flamingos	214
533.	North Carolina Style Pork Chops	214
534.	Beef with Sesame and Ginger	215
535.	Katsu Pork	215
536.	Pork on A Blanket	216
537.	Lamb Shawarma	216
538.	Stuffed Cabbage and Pork Loin Rolls	216
539.	Pork Head Chops with Vegetables	217
540.	Provencal Ribs	217
541.	Beef Scallops	218
542.	Potatoes with Loin and Cheese	218
543.	Potatoes with Loin and Cheese	219
544.	Russian Steaks with Nuts and Cheese	219
545.	Potatoes with Bacon, Onion and Cheese	219
546.	Pork Liver	220
547.	Marinated Loin Potatoes	220
548.	Pork Fritters	221
549.	Pork Tenderloin	221
550.	Cheesy Beef Paseíllo	222
551.	Beef Patty	222
552.	Roasted Pork	223
553.	Fried Pork Chops	223
554.	Crispy Pork Chops	223
555.	Pork Bondiola Chop	224
556.	Pork Taquitos	224
557.	Pork Knuckle	225

VEGETABLES — **226**

#	Title	Page
558.	Creamy Beets	226
559.	Chard and Olives	226
560.	Coconut Mushrooms Mix	226
561.	Kale and Tomatoes	227
562.	Brussels Sprouts and Tomatoes	227
563.	Italian Tomatoes	227
564.	Salsa Zucchini	227
565.	Green Beans and Olives	228
566.	Spicy Avocado Mix	228
567.	Spicy Black Beans	228
568.	Cajun Tomatoes and Peppers	229
569.	Olives and Sweet Potatoes	229
570.	Spinach and Sprouts	229
571.	Lemon Tomatoes	230
572.	Tomato and Green Beans	230
573.	Tomato and Onions Mix	230
574.	Kale Salad	231
575.	Garlic Carrots	231
576.	Creamy Green Beans and Walnuts	231
577.	Garlic Corn	232
578.	Green Beans Salad	232
579.	Red Cabbage and Tomatoes	232
580.	Savoy Cabbage Sauté	232
581.	Turmeric Kale	233
582.	Lemon Fennel	233
583.	Balsamic Kale	233
584.	Coriander Endives	234
585.	Cheesy Beets	234
586.	Frying Potatoes	234
587.	Avocado Fries	235
588.	Crispy French Fries	235
589.	Frying Potatoes with Butter	235
590.	Homemade French Fries	236
591.	Mini pepper/tomato/shallot/goat cheese tartlets 236	
592.	Almond Apples	236
593.	French fries without dry	237
594.	Bugnes Lyonnaises	237
595.	Green salad with roasted pepper	238
596.	Fat Free Crispy Fries	238
597.	Marinated Potatoes with Chimichurri Sauce	239
598.	Homemade Gluten Free Spicy Chips	239
599.	Funghetto Eggplant (Golden Neapolitan)	239
600.	Fried Bananas	240
601.	Sautéed air mushrooms and parsley	240

602.	Cauliflowers au gratin	241
603.	Peach Clafoutis	241
604.	Cauliflower Steak	241
605.	Chocolate Chip Pan Cookie	242
606.	Mustard Greens and Green Beans	242
607.	Artichoke Spinach Casserole	242
608.	Baked Egg and Veggies	243
609.	Mini Cheesecake	243
610.	Savoy Cabbage	244
611.	Spaghetti Squash Alfredo.	244
612.	Vanilla Pound Cake.	244
613.	Pumpkin Spice Pecans	245
614.	Cream Puffs	245
615.	Tomato and Asparagus	246
616.	Peanut Butter Cheesecake Brownies	246
617.	BBQ Pulled Mushrooms	246
618.	Blackberry Crisp	247
619.	Cheese Zucchini Boats	247
620.	Green Beans and Lime Sauce	248
621.	Roasted Broccoli Salad	248
622.	Quiche Stuffed Peppers	248
623.	Monkey Bread	249
624.	Broccoli Crust Pizza	249
625.	Cheesy Zoodle Bake	250
626.	Eggplant Stacks	250
627.	Roasted Garlic Zucchini Rolls	250
628.	Roasted Veggie Bowl	251
629.	Espresso Mini Cheesecake	251

SNACKS 253

630.	Bacon Snack	253
631.	Shrimp Snack	253
632.	Avocado Wraps	253
633.	Cheesy Meatballs	253
634.	Tuna Appetizer	254
635.	Cheese and Leeks Dip	254
636.	Cucumber Salsa	254
637.	Chicken Cubes	255
638.	Salmon Spread	255
639.	Crustless Pizza	255
640.	Olives and Zucchini Cakes	256
641.	Tomato Bites	256
642.	Spinach Rolls	256
643.	Ranch Roasted Almonds	257
644.	Pickled Snack	257
645.	Avocado Bites	257
646.	Asparagus Wraps	258
647.	Warm Tomato Salsa	258
648.	Zucchini Chips	258
649.	Parsley Meatballs	259
650.	Cheese Chips	259
651.	Sweet Pepper Poppers	259
652.	Bacon Wrapped Onion Rings.	259
653.	Zucchini Salsa	260
654.	Mushroom Platter	260
655.	Crab Balls	260
656.	Bacon Wrapped Brie	261
657.	Shrimp Balls	261

DESSERTS 262

658.	Awesome Chinese Doughnuts	262
659.	Crispy Bananas	262
660.	Air-Fried Banana and Walnuts Muffins	262
661.	Air-Fryer Blueberry Muffins	263
662.	Nutty Mix	263
663.	Vanilla Spiced Soufflé	263
664.	Apricot Blackberry Crumble	264
665.	Chocolate Cup cakes	264
666.	Stuffed Baked Apples	265
667.	Roasted Pineapples with Vanilla Zest	265
668.	Vanilla Coconut Pie	266
669.	Cookie Dough Ball	266
670.	Pumpkin Bread Cake	266
671.	Air Fried Beignets	267
672.	Chocolate Mayo Cake	267
673.	Homemade French Fries	268
674.	Sweet Potato Chips	268
675.	Cajun Style French Fries	269

#	Title	Page
676.	Fried Zucchini	269
677.	Fried Avocado	269
678.	Vegetables In air Fryer	270
679.	Crispy Rye Bread Snacks with Guacamole and Anchovies	270
680.	Mushrooms Stuffed with Tomato	271
681.	Spiced Potato Wedges	271
682.	Egg Stuffed Zucchini Balls	272
683.	Vegetables with Provolone	272
684.	Spicy Potatoes	272
685.	Scrambled Eggs with Beans, Zucchini, Potatoes and Onions	273
686.	French Toast	273
687.	Sweet Potato Salt and Pepper	274
688.	Potatoes with Provencal Herbs With Cheese	274
689.	Potato Wedges	275
690.	Onion Rings	275
691.	Onion Flower	276
692.	Hasselback Potatoes	276
693.	Roasted Potatoes	277
694.	Honey Roasted Carrots	277
695.	Roasted Broccoli with Garlic	277
696.	Roasted Cauliflower	278
697.	Roasted Corn	278
698.	Roasted Pumpkin	278
699.	Roasted Eggplant	279
700.	Corn And Cheese Cakes	279
701.	Olives, Bacon and Green beans	279
702.	Endives and Walnuts	280
703.	Asparagus and Yogurt Sauce	280
704.	Vinegar Broccoli	280
705.	Veggie Quesadilla	281
706.	Cajun Olives and Peppers	281
707.	Chili Broccoli	281
708.	Balsamic Kale	282
709.	Mustard Greens and Green Beans	282
710.	Olives and Cilantro Vinaigrette	282
711.	Broccoli and Tomatoes	282
712.	Kale and Mushrooms	283
713.	Spicy Olives and Avocado	283
714.	Lemon Endives	283
715.	Roasted Lemon Cauliflower	284
716.	Creamy Kale	284
717.	Mustard Asparagus	284
718.	Kale and Brussels Sprouts	285
719.	Butter Broccoli	285
720.	Oregano Kale	285
721.	Savoy Cabbage	285
722.	Broccoli and Tomato Sauce	286
723.	Italian Olives	286
724.	Kale and Olives	286
725.	Broccoli Casserole	286
726.	Cheesy Zoodle Bake	287
727.	Fennel and Collard Greens Sauté	287
728.	Tomato and Kale Salad	287
729.	Beef Stuffed Bell Peppers	288
730.	Crispy Leeks with Lemon	288
731.	Okra Salad with Tomato and Corn	289
732.	Cheesy Fennel	289
733.	Parmesan Swiss Chard with Sausage	289
734.	Beet, Red Onion and Tomato Mix with Goat Cheese	290
735.	Brussels Sprouts with Cherry Tomatoes and Green Onions	290
736.	Cheesy Radish Hash Browns	291
737.	Spinach Stuffed Spinach Pie	291
738.	Shrimp Stuffed Peppers	292
739.	Balsamic Cherry Tomatoes Salad	292
740.	Chinese Broccoli Salad	292
741.	Beet Salad with Parsley Dressing	293
742.	Eggplant and Garlic Sauce Recipe	293
743.	Cherry Tomatoes with Basil and Parmesan	294
744.	Lemony Eggplant and Zucchini Mix	294
745.	Mexican Style Stuffed Bell Peppers	294
746.	Balsamic Artichokes with Oregano	295
747.	Artichokes with Anchovy Sauce	295
748.	Beets and Arugula Salad with Cider Dressing	296
749.	Cheesy Artichokes	296

#	Title	Page
750.	Parmesan Brussels Sprouts	296
751.	Simple and Sweet Baby Carrots	297

SNACKS — 298

#	Title	Page
752.	Jackfruit Air-Fryer Fries	298
753.	Sweet & Sour Air-Fried Yam	298
754.	Air-Fried Sesame Tofu with Broccoli & Bell Pepper Salad	298
755.	Coconut Pumpkin Curry	299
756.	Tomato Vegetable Curry	299
757.	Crispy Air-Fried Gourd	300
758.	Air-Fried Vegan Noodles	300
759.	Sweet & Spicy Tofu with Steamed Spinach	300
760.	Air-Fried Walnuts & Green Beans	301
761.	Air-Fried Avocado & Yellow Pepper Salad	301
762.	Onion Strings	302
763.	Air-Fried Banana Turmeric Chips	302
764.	Spicy Air-Fried Eggplant	303
765.	Air-Fried Carrots with Lemon	303
766.	Air-Fried Radish Cake	303
767.	Air-Fried Roasted Potatoes with Rosemary	304
768.	Potato Fries with Bean Sprouts & Peanut Herb Salad	304
769.	Tuna with Roast Yams	304
770.	Air-Fried Ratatouille	305
771.	Toad in the Hole	305
772.	Glass Noodle & Tiger Shrimp Salad	305
773.	Air-Fried Fingerling Potatoes	306
774.	Parmesan Chicken Meatballs	306
775.	Meatballs with Mediterranean Dipping Sauce	307
776.	Mayo-Cheddar Jacket Potatoes	307
777.	Pork & Brie Meatballs	307
778.	Potato Chips & Tangy Dipping Sauce	308
779.	Beef Meatballs in Blueberry Chipotle Sauce	308
780.	Lemon Pepper Broccoli Crunch	308
781.	Sweet Broccoli Crunch	309
782.	Maple Broccoli Crunch	309
783.	Veggie Crunch	310
784.	Chili Lime Broccoli Crunch	310
785.	Zucchini Chips	311
786.	Cayenne Zucchini Chips	311
787.	Salt and Vinegar Zucchini Chips	311
788.	Smoked Zucchini Chips	312
789.	Yellow Zucchini Chips	312
790.	Soft Pretzels	312
791.	Soft Garlic Parmesan Pretzels	313
792.	Soft Cinnamon Pretzels	313
793.	Soft Pecan Pretzels	314
794.	Soft Cheesy Pretzels	315
795.	Sweet Zucchini Chips	315
796.	Cucumber Chips	315
797.	Dill and Onion Cucumber Chips	316
798.	Smokey Cucumber Chips	316
799.	Garlic Parmesan Cucumber Chips	317
800.	Sea Salt and Black Pepper Cucumber Chips	317
801.	Taco Cucumber Chips	317
802.	Dilly Almonds	318
803.	Garlic Almonds	318
804.	Sweet and Salty Almonds	319
805.	Cayenne Almonds	319
806.	Black Pepper Almonds	319
807.	Sweet Candied Pecans	320
808.	Garlicky Cauliflower Crunch	320
809.	Cajun Cauliflower Crunch	321
810.	Air Fried Red Cabbage, Garlic-flavored	321
811.	Healthy Italian Parmesan Mushrooms	321
812.	Sweet Tomatoes, Garlic-Herbed Dish	322
813.	Sweet Potato Chips	322
814.	Herbed Roasted Carrots	322
815.	Awesome Barley Risotto Recipe	322
816.	Healthy Cauliflower and Broccoli	323
817.	Garlic-Herbed Mayonnaise Brussels Sprouts Dish	323
818.	Unusual Risotto Recipe	323
819.	Lip-smacking Buttermilk-Biscuits	324
820.	Spicy Eggplant Dish	324
821.	Lip-smacking Mushroom Recipe	325
822.	Simple Creamy Fried Potato Dish	325
823.	Nice Veggie Fries Dish	325

#	Recipe	Page
824.	Enjoyable Green Beans Dish	326
825.	Healthy Cinnamon Roasted Pumpkin	326
826.	Cinnamon-Mayonnaise-Potato Fries	326
827.	Delicious Cauliflower Cakes	327
828.	Tasty Button Mushroom Dish Recipe	327
829.	Sweet Buttermilk-Tomatoes	327
830.	Delicious Garlic Potatoes	328
831.	Sweet Eggplant Dish with Garlic flavor	328
832.	Nice Cauliflower Healthy Dish	328
833.	Sweet Cauliflower Rice Dish	329
834.	Tasty Hassel-Back Potatoes	329
835.	Easy Buttered-Mushroom Cakes	329
836.	Delicious Beet Wedges Dish	330
837.	Tasty Roasted Peppers Dish	330
838.	Nice Vermouth-White Mushrooms Recipe	330
839.	Sweet Pumpkin Rice Dish	331
840.	Delicious Fried Creamy Cabbage	331
841.	Delicious Onion Rings Dish	331
842.	Pleasant Cajun Onion Wedges Dish	332
843.	Sweet Tortilla Chips	332
844.	Rice and Sausage Dish Recipe	332
845.	Coconut-Potatoes Recipes	333
846.	Sweet Glazed Beets Recipe	333
847.	Veggie Rice Recipe	333

DESSERTS — 334

#	Recipe	Page
848.	Ginger Cookies Cheesecake	334
849.	Winter Cherry Mix	334
850.	Carrot Pudding and Rum Sauce	334
851.	Lemon Pudding	335
852.	Strawberry and Chia Marmalade	335
853.	Lemon and Maple Syrup Pudding	335
854.	Sweet Corn Pudding	336
855.	Apricot Jam	336
856.	Banana Cake	337
857.	Pineapple Pudding	337
858.	Blueberry Jam	337
859.	Bread Pudding	337
860.	Coconut Cream and Cinnamon Pudding	338
861.	Plum Jam	338
862.	Cranberry Bread Pudding	339
863.	Apples and Pears Salad	339
864.	Blueberry and Coconut Sweet Bowls	339
865.	Coconut Pancake	340
866.	Apples and Red Grape Juice	340
867.	Strawberry Shortcakes	340
868.	Coconut and Avocado Pudding	341
869.	Cocoa and Milk Pudding	341
870.	Caramel Pudding	341
871.	Black Tea Cake	342
872.	Cinnamon Rolls	342
873.	Vegan Donuts	343
874.	Apple Cake	343
875.	Orange Lava Cake	344
876.	Cinnamon Apples	344
877.	Carrot and Pineapple Cinnamon Bread	344
878.	Cocoa and Coconut Bars	345
879.	Vanilla Cake	345
880.	Sweet Apple Cupcakes	346
881.	Orange Bread with Almonds	346
882.	Tangerine Cake	346
883.	Maple Tomato Bread	347
884.	Lemon Squares	347
885.	Dates and Cashew Sticks	347
886.	Grape Pudding	348
887.	Coconut and Pumpkin Seeds Bars	348
888.	Chocolate Cookies	349
889.	Cinnamon Bananas	349
890.	Coffee Pudding	349
891.	Almond and Cocoa Cake	350
892.	Blueberry Cake	350
893.	Peach Cinnamon Cobbler	351
894.	Easy Pears Dessert	351
895.	Strawberry Cheesecake	351
896.	Cherries and Rhubarb Bowls	352
897.	Chocolate Chips Cream	352
898.	Cinnamon Cream	352
899.	Pumpkin Bowls	353

xiii

#	Recipe	Page
900.	Mango and Pears Bowls	353
901.	Plums and Pineapple Cookies	353
902.	Apple Jam	353
903.	Pears Cake	354
904.	Yogurt and Pumpkin Cream	354
905.	Raisins Rice Mix	354
906.	Zucchini Bread	355
907.	Orange Bowls	355
908.	Maple Pears Mix	355
909.	Carrot and Zucchini Cake	356
910.	Apples Cheesecake	356
911.	Strawberry Jam	356
912.	Caramel Cream	357
913.	Cherry Squares	357
914.	Sweet Walnut Mix	357
915.	Creamy Blueberry Mix	357
916.	Butter Brownies	358
917.	Mandarin Cake	358
918.	White Chocolate Ramekins	358
919.	Rhubarb Jam	359
920.	Banana Cream	359
921.	Banana and Rice Bowls	359
922.	Lemon Mango Bowls	360
923.	Pear Stew	360
924.	Orange Jam	360
925.	Baked Apples and Pears	360
926.	Apricots Cream	361
927.	Ginger Cake	361
928.	Nutmeg Banana and Chia Bowls	361
929.	Chicken Dip	362
930.	Beet Salsa	362
931.	Carrot Chips	362
932.	Zucchini Cakes	363
933.	Rosemary Mushroom and Beets Salsa	363
934.	Mushroom Cakes	363
935.	Avocado Salsa	364
936.	Carrot Wraps	364
937.	Bacon Corn Mix	364
938.	Mayo Corn Spread	365
939.	Avocado Cakes	365
940.	Shrimp and Avocado Bowls	365
941.	Cashew Dip	365
942.	Smoked Salmon Salad	366
943.	Salmon Meatballs	366
944.	Chicken Meatballs	367
945.	Ginger Dip	367
946.	Asparagus and Olives Bowls	367
947.	Walnuts and Radish Bites	368
948.	Olives Spread	368
949.	Melon Salsa	368
950.	Shrimp Spread	369
951.	Pork Dip	369
952.	Spinach Dip	369
953.	Pork and Spinach Bowls	369
954.	Tomato and Radish Bowls	370
955.	Green Beans Bites	370
956.	Rosemary Shrimp Platter	370
957.	Chocolate Cake	371
958.	Peanut Butter Cake	371
959.	Hazelnut Cake	372
960.	Walnut Cake	373
961.	NY Keto Cheesecake	373
962.	Strawberry Cheesecake	374
963.	Blueberry Cheesecake	374
964.	Raspberry Cheesecake	375
965.	Cinnamon Cheesecake	375
966.	Chocolate Keto Cheesecake	376
967.	Chocolate Chip Cheesecake	376
968.	Pumpkin Spice Cheesecake	377
969.	Lemon Cheesecake	378
970.	Gingerbread Cheesecake	378
971.	Mascarpone Cheesecake	379
972.	Coconut Cheesecake	379
973.	Fudge Brownies	380
974.	Double Chocolate Brownies	380
975.	Chocolate Walnuts Brownies	381
976.	Peanut Butter Brownies	381
977.	Almond Brownies	382

978.	Chocolate Coconut Brownies	382
979.	Chocolate Mint Brownies	383
980.	Hazelnut Brownies	383
981.	Espresso Brownies	384
982.	Caramel Fudge Brownies	384
983.	Raspberry Brownies	385
984.	Cauliflower Rice and Plum Pudding	385
985.	Creamy Chia Seeds Pudding	386
986.	Ginger Cookies	386
987.	Spiced Avocado Pudding	386
988.	Coconut Bars	386
989.	Plum Cream	387
990.	Raspberry Muffins	387
991.	Cinnamon Plums	388
992.	Strawberry Cake	388
993.	Chocolate Pudding	388
994.	Cream Cheese Brownies	388
995.	Lemon Coconut Pie	389
996.	Almond Butter Cookies	389
997.	Avocado Granola	389
998.	Blackberry Chia Jam	390
999.	Lemon Bars	390
1000.	Strawberries Stew	390
1001.	Blueberries and Chocolate Cream	390
1002.	Cocoa Cake	391
1003.	Mini Lava Cakes	391
1004.	Avocado Brownies	391
1005.	Baked Plums	392
1006.	Lime Berry Pudding	392
1007.	Currant Pudding	392
1008.	Cocoa and Nuts Bombs	392
1009.	Blueberry Cream	393
1010.	Strawberry Jam	393
1011.	Butter Cookies	393
1012.	Cream Cheese and Zucchinis Bars	394
1013.	Coconut Cookies	394
1014.	Lemon Cookies	394
1015.	Delicious cheesecake	394
1016.	Macaroons	395
1017.	Orange cake	395
1018.	Amaretto and bread dough	395
1019.	Carrot cake	396
1020.	Banana bread	396
1021.	Granola	397
1022.	Espresso cream and pears	397
1023.	Banana cake	397
1024.	Fried banana	398
1025.	Coffee cheesecakes	398
1026.	Cinnamon rolls served with Cream cheese	398
1027.	Pumpkin cookies	399
1028.	Apple bread	399
1029.	Strawberry pie	400
1030.	Bread pudding	400
1031.	Pomegranate and chocolate bars	401
1032.	Crisp apples	401
1033.	Chocolate cookies	402

31-DAY MEAL PLAN   **403**

CONCLUSION   **405**

DESCRIPTION

The history of Air fryers dates back to a few years ago; exactly during the third quarter of the year 2010 and it was a completely revolutionary invention that was invented by Philips Electronics Company. Philips introduced the Air Fryer to the world and changed the conception of the culinary world all at once.

The Air Fryer is used as a substitute for your oven, stovetop, and deep fryer. It comes with various handy parts and other tools that you can buy to use your Air Fryer for different cooking styles, which include the following:
- Grilling. It provides the same heat to grill food ingredients without the need to flip them continuously. The hot air goes around the fryer, giving heating on all sides. The recipes include directions of how many times you ought to shake the pan during the cooking process.

To make the process of grilling faster, you can use a grill pan or a grill layer. They will soak the excess fat from the meat that you are cooking to give you delicious and healthy meals.

- Baking. The Air Fryer usually comes with a baking pan (or you can buy or use your ownto make treats that are typically done using an oven. You can bake goodies, such as cakes, bread, cupcakes, muffins, and brownies in your Air Fryer.
- Roasting. It roasts food ingredients, which include vegetables and meat, faster than when you do it in the oven.
- Frying is its primary purpose – to cook fried foods with little or no oil.

You can cook most food items in an Air Fryer. There are some foods that you should refrain from cooking in the fryer because they will taste better when cooked in the traditional ways — they include fried foods with batter and steamed veggies, such as beans and carrots.

Despite this, you will never run out of ingredients to cook using your Air Fryer – from veggies to seafood, chicken, egg, turkey, and a lot more. The most common component that is prepared using this appliance is potatoes.

The Air Fryer also comes with a separator, and this allows you to cook multiple dishes at the same time. You need to choose recipes that can be prepared at the same temperature setting.

This book covers the following topics:
- Breakfast
- Mains
- Sides
- Seafood
- Poultry
- Meat
- Vegetables
- Snacks
- Desserts and more!!!

INTRODUCTION

There are many kinds of foods that you can cook using an air fryer, but there are also certain types that are not suited for it. Avoid cooking ingredients, which can be steamed, like beans and carrots. You also cannot fry foods covered in heavy batter in this appliance.

Aside from the above mentioned, you can cook most kinds of ingredients using an air fryer. You can use it to cook foods covered in light flour or breadcrumbs. You can cook a variety of vegetables in the appliance, such as cauliflower, asparagus, zucchini, kale, peppers, and corn on the cob. You can also use it to cook frozen foods and home prepared meals by following a different set of instructions for these purposes.

An air fryer also comes with another useful feature - the separator. It allows you to cook multiple dishes at a time. Use the separator to divide ingredients in the pan or basket. You have to make sure that all ingredients have the same temperature setting so that everything will cook evenly at the same time.

The Benefits of Air fryer

It is important to note that air fried foods are still fried. Unless you've decided to eliminate the use of oils in cooking, you must still be cautious about the food you eat. Despite that, it clearly presents a better and healthier option than deep-frying. It helps you avoid unnecessary fats and oils, which makes it an ideal companion when you intend to lose weight. It offers a lot more benefits, which include the following:

- It is convenient and easy to use, plus, it's easy to clean.

- It doesn't give off unwanted smells when cooking.

- You can use it to prepare a variety of meals.

- It can withstand heavy cooking.

- It is durable and made of metal and high-grade plastic.

- Cooking using this appliance is not as messy as frying in a traditional way. You don't have to worry about greasy spills and stains in the kitchen.

DESCRIPTION

1. Stuffed Portobello Mushrooms with Ground Beef

Preparation time: 10 minutes

Cooking time: 13 minutes

Servings: 3

INGREDIENTS

- 3 Portobello mushrooms
- ½ cup ground beef
- 1 teaspoon minced garlic
- 1 oz onion, chopped
- 1 teaspoon olive oil
- ¾ teaspoon ground nutmeg
- ¾ teaspoon cilantro

DIRECTIONS

1. Put the ground beef in the mixing bowl.
2. Add minced garlic and chopped onion.
3. After this, add ground nutmeg and cilantro.
4. Mix the mixture up carefully.
5. Fill the mushrooms with the ground beef mixture.
6. Then sprinkle the mushrooms with the olive oil and wrap them in the foil.
7. Put the wrapped mushrooms in the air fryer basket and cook for 10 minutes at 380 F.
8. Then discard the foil from the mushrooms and cook them for 3 minutes more at 400 F.
9. Chill the cooked meal little and serve!

NUTRITION: Calories 42, Fat 1.8, Fiber 1.3, Carbs 4.5, Protein 3.3

2. Basil-Spinach Quiche

Preparation time: 10 minutes

Cooking time: 10 minutes

Servings: 4

INGREDIENTS

- ½ cup spinach
- 1 oz fresh basil, chopped
- 1 oz walnuts
- 3 eggs
- ¾ cup almond milk
- ½ teaspoon salt
- 1 tablespoon almond flour

DIRECTIONS

1. Chop the spinach and combine it together with the chopped basil.
2. Crush the walnuts and add them to the green mixture too.
3. After this, add the salt and almond flour.
4. Stir the mixture and place it in the air fryer basket.
5. Then beat the eggs in the separate bowl and whisk well.
6. Add almond milk and stir carefully.
7. Pour the egg mixture over the greens and cook it for 10 minutes at 375 F.
8. When the quiche is cooked – let it chill well and serve!

NUTRITION: Calories 237, Fat 21.8, Fiber 2.4, Carbs 5.3, Protein 8.7

3. Stuffed Chicken Roll with Mushrooms

Preparation time: 15 minutes

Cooking time: 23 minutes

Servings: 4

INGREDIENTS

- 13 oz chicken fillet
- 6 oz mushrooms
- 1 onion, chopped
- 1 garlic clove, chopped
- 1 teaspoon turmeric
- ½ teaspoon ground paprika
- ½ teaspoon oregano
- ¾ teaspoon chili pepper
- 1 teaspoon olive oil
- 1 teaspoon vinegar

DIRECTIONS

1. Beat the chicken fillet gently.
2. Then chop the mushrooms and put them in the air fryer.
3. Add turmeric, onion, garlic clove, ground paprika, oregano, chili pepper, and olive oil.
4. Stir the mixture and cook it for 8 minutes at 360 F.
5. Stir it every 2 minutes.
6. Then sprinkle the chicken fillets with the vinegar.
7. Place the cooked mushroom mixture on the chicken fillets and roll them.
8. Transfer the chicken rolls in the air fryer basket and cook for 15 minutes at 380 F.
9. You can stir the chicken rolls during cooking.
10. Then let the cooked chicken rolls chill little and serve them!

NUTRITION: Calories 210, Fat 8.3, Fiber 1.4, Carbs 5, Protein 28.5

4. **Eggs on Avocado Burgers**

Preparation time: 10 minutes

Cooking time: 15 minutes

Servings: 2

INGREDIENTS

- 1 avocado, pitted
- 2 eggs
- 1 tablespoon almond flour
- 1 oz onion, chopped
- ½ carrot, grated
- ½ teaspoon salt
- ¼ teaspoon ground black pepper

DIRECTIONS

1. Peel the avocado and mash it.
2. Add the almond flour and grated carrot in the mashed avocado mixture.
3. Then add salt and ground black pepper.
4. After this, mix the mixture until homogenous.
5. Make the small burgers from the mixture.
6. Pour the olive oil in the air fryer basket and add the avocado burgers.
7. Cook them for 8 minutes at 375 F. Flip them into another side after 4 minutes of cooking. Transfer the cooked burgers on the plates.
8. After this, beat the eggs in the air fryer basket and cook them for 7 minutes at 360 F or until you get cooked eggs.
9. Put the eggs over the avocado burgers and serve immediately!

NUTRITION: Calories 361, Fat 31, Fiber 9, Carbs 15, Protein 310.8

5. **Applesauce Mash with Sweet Potato**

Preparation time: 5 minutes

Cooking time: 7 minutes

Servings: 4

INGREDIENTS

- 1 sweet potato, peeled
- 2 apples
- ¾ teaspoon salt
- 1 teaspoon olive oil

DIRECTIONS

1. Grate the sweet potatoes and apples.
2. Place the grated ingredients in the air fryer basket.
3. Add salt and olive oil.
4. Stir the mixture with the help of the wooden spatula.
5. Cook the applesauce for 7 minutes at 390F.
6. When the applesauce is cooked- let it chill little and serve!

NUTRITION: Calories 94, Fat 1.4, Fiber 3.7, Carbs 21.3, Protein 0.9

6. Bacon and Kale Breakfast Salad

Preparation time: 10 minutes

Cooking time: 5 minutes

Servings: 6

INGREDIENTS

- 7 oz bacon, sliced
- 10 oz kale, chopped
- 1 teaspoon olive oil
- ¼ cup almonds, crushed
- ½ teaspoon paprika
- ½ teaspoon salt

DIRECTIONS

1. Place the bacon in the air fryer and sprinkle it with the paprika and salt.
2. Cook the bacon for 5 minutes at 400 F. Stir it after 3 minutes of cooking.
3. Meanwhile, place the kale in the salad bowl.
4. Add the olive oil and crushed almonds.
5. When the bacon is cooked – chop it roughly and add in the kale bowl.
6. Shake it gently and serve!

NUTRITION: Calories 232, Fat 16.6, Fiber 1.3, Carbs 6.4, Protein 14.5

7. Fish Fritatta

Preparation time: 10 minutes

Cooking time: 15 minutes

Servings: 3

INGREDIENTS

- 1 tablespoon fresh dill, chopped
- 1 tablespoon fresh parsley, chopped
- ¼ teaspoon ground nutmeg
- 2 tablespoons coconut milk
- 4 eggs
- 8 oz fillet chopped

DIRECTIONS

1. Beat the eggs in the mixing bowl and whisk well.
2. Add chopped salmon and fresh dill.
3. Add fresh parsley and ground nutmeg.
4. Stir the mixture gently and add coconut milk.
5. After this, pour the frittata mixture in the air fryer basket and cook for 15 minutes at 360 F.
6. When the meal is cooked – chill it little and serve!

NUTRITION: Calories 211, Fat 13, Fiber 0.4, Carbs 1.7, Protein 22.5

8. Spinach Frittata

Preparation time: 15 minutes

Cooking time: 15 minutes

Servings: 4

INGREDIENTS

- 4 eggs, beaten
- 1 cup spinach
- 1 tablespoon almond flour
- 1 teaspoon coconut flour
- 1/3 teaspoon ground paprika
- 1 teaspoon basil, dried
- ½ teaspoon salt
- 1 teaspoon olive oil

DIRECTIONS

1. Whisk the eggs.
2. Then place the spinach in the blender and blend well.
3. Add the spinach in the whisked eggs.
4. After this, add the almond flour and coconut flour.
5. Sprinkle the mixture with the ground paprika.
6. Add dried basil and salt.
7. Stir the mixture.
8. Pour the olive oil in the frittata molds.
9. Then add the frittata mixture and transfer the molds in the air fryer basket.
10. Cook the frittata for 15 minutes at 350 F.
11. Chill the cooked frittata to the room temperature and serve!

NUTRITION: Calories 118, Fat 9.2, Fiber 1.2, Carbs 2.6, Protein 7.4

9. Beef Balls with Sesame and Dill

Preparation time: 10 minutes

Cooking time: 10 minutes

Servings: 4

INGREDIENTS

- 1 teaspoon sesame seeds
- 1 tablespoon dill, dried
- 1 egg
- 10 oz ground beef
- 1 garlic clove, chopped
- ¾ teaspoon nutmeg
- 1 teaspoon olive oil
- 1 teaspoon almond flour

DIRECTIONS

1. Beat the egg in the bowl and whisk it.
2. Add dried dill and sesame seeds.
3. Stir gently and add chopped garlic clove and nutmeg.
4. Then add ground beef and almond flour.
5. Mix the mixture carefully with the help of the spoon.
6. Pour the olive oil in the air fryer basket.
7. Make the medium balls from the meat mixture and place them in the air fryer.
8. Cook the meatballs for 10 minutes at 380 F.
9. Stir the meatballs during the cooking with the help of the wooden spatula.
10. Transfer the cooked meatballs in the serving bowls.
11. Enjoy!

NUTRITION: Calories 207, Fat 10.7, Fiber 1.1, Carbs 2.7, Protein 24.7

10. Zucchini Rounds with Ground Chicken

Preparation time: 15 minutes

Cooking time: 8 minutes

Servings: 4

INGREDIENTS

- 8 oz ground chicken

- 1 zucchini
- 1 egg
- ¼ teaspoon ground black pepper
- ½ teaspoon salt
- 1 teaspoon paprika
- 1 teaspoon olive oil
- 1 teaspoon cilantro

DIRECTIONS

1. Beat the egg in the bowl and whisk well.
2. Add the ground black pepper, salt, paprika, and cilantro.
3. Add ground chicken and stir the mixture.
4. Cut zucchini into 4 rounds and remove the meat from them to make the zucchini circles.
5. Then place the zucchini circles in the air fryer basket.
6. Fill the zucchini with the ground chicken mixture.
7. Cook the breakfast for 8 minutes at 360 F.
8. When the meal is cooked – let it chill for 5 minutes and serve!

NUTRITION: Calories 143, Fat 6.6, Fiber 0.8, Carbs 2.1, Protein 18.5

11. Tomatoes with Chicken

Preparation time: 15 minutes

Cooking time: 10 minutes

Servings: 3

INGREDIENTS

- 3 tomatoes
- ½ cup ground chicken
- 1 teaspoon Paleo mayonnaise
- ¼ teaspoon turmeric
- ¾ teaspoon minced garlic
- 1 teaspoon chives

DIRECTIONS

1. Cut the "hats" in every tomato.
2. Then remove the meat from the tomatoes to get the tomato cups.
3. Mix up together the minced garlic, chives, turmeric, mayonnaise and ground chicken in the mixing bowl.
4. Stir the mixture.
5. After this, fill tomato cups with the ground chicken mixture and place them in the air fryer basket.
6. Cook the tomatoes for 10 minutes at 365 F.
7. When the time is over – check of the tomatoes is cooked and remove them from the air fryer.
8. Chill the tomatoes with chicken gently and serve!

NUTRITION: Calories 78, Fat 3.1, Fiber 1.5, Carbs 5.1, Protein 7.9

12. Meatball Breakfast Salad

Preparation time: 15 minutes

Cooking time: 10 minutes

Servings: 2

INGREDIENTS

- 1 cucumber, chopped
- 1 tomato, chopped
- 1 sweet red pepper, chopped
- ½ cup ground chicken
- 1 egg
- 1 tablespoon olive oil
- 2/3 teaspoon minced garlic
- ½ teaspoon ground black pepper

DIRECTIONS

1. Put the cucumber, tomato, and sweet red pepper in the mixing bowl.
2. Add olive oil and stir gently.

3. After this, mix up together the ground black pepper, minced garlic, and ground chicken.
4. Beat the egg in the chicken mixture and stir well. Make the medium meatballs.
5. After this, place the ground chicken meatballs in the air fryer basket and cook it for 10 minutes at 375 F.
6. Stir the ground chicken meatballs time to time.
7. Then chill the meatballs and add them in the salad.
8. Serve the breakfast immediately!

NUTRITION: Calories 208, Fat 12.2, Fiber 2.1, Carbs 12, Protein 14.9

13. Cherry Tomatoes Fritatta

Preparation time: 10 minutes

Cooking time: 15 minutes

Servings: 2

INGREDIENTS

- ¼ cup cherry tomatoes
- 1 tablespoon basil, chopped
- 3 eggs
- 2 tablespoon almond milk
- 1 teaspoon olive oil
- ¼ teaspoon turmeric
- 1 tablespoon almond flour

DIRECTIONS

1. Beat the eggs and whisk them well.
2. Add the chopped basil and almond milk.
3. Then add the almond flour and turmeric.
4. Stir the mixture well.
5. After this, cut the cherry tomatoes into the halves.
6. Pour the whisked egg mixture in the air fryer basket.
7. Add the cherry tomatoes.
8. Cook the frittata for 15 minutes at 355 F.
9. Then let the cooked frittata chill little.
10. Serve!

NUTRITION: Calories 234, Fat 19.6, Fiber 2.2, Carbs 5.4, Protein 11.9

14. Whisked Eggs with Ground Chicken

Preparation time: 10 minutes

Cooking time: 15 minutes

Servings: 4

INGREDIENTS

- 3 eggs, whisked
- 1 cup ground chicken
- ½ teaspoon salt
- 1 oz fresh parsley, chopped
- ½ teaspoon ground paprika
- ½ onion, chopped

DIRECTIONS

1. Put the ground chicken in the air fryer basket.
2. Add salt, chopped parsley, and ground paprika.
3. After this, add the chopped onion and stir the mixture with the help of the wooden spatula.
4. Cook the ground chicken mixture for 8 minutes at 375 F.
5. Stir it time to time.
6. Then pour the whisked eggs over the ground chicken mixture and cook it for 7 minutes more at 365 F.
7. When the meal is cooked – stir it carefully and transfer in the serving bowls.
8. Serve it immediately!

NUTRITION: Calories 122, Fat 6.6, Fiber 0.6, Carbs 2.1, Protein 14.7

15. Kale Quiche with Eggs

Preparation time: 10 minutes

Cooking time: 18 minutes

Servings: 6

INGREDIENTS

- 1 cup kale
- 3 eggs
- 2 oz bacon, chopped, cooked
- 1 sweet potato, grated
- ½ teaspoon thyme
- ½ teaspoon ground black pepper
- ½ teaspoon ground paprika
- ½ cup coconut milk
- 1 onion, chopped
- 1 teaspoon olive oil

DIRECTIONS

1. Chop the kale roughly and place it in the blender.
2. Blend it gently.
3. Then transfer the blended kale in the mixing bowl.
4. Add the grated potato and thyme.
5. Sprinkle the mixture with the ground black pepper and ground paprika.
6. Add coconut milk and chopped onion.
7. Pour the olive oil into the air fryer basket.
8. Then place the kale mixture in the air fryer basket,
9. Beat the eggs in the separate bowl and whisk well.
10. Pour the whisked eggs over the kale mixture. Add bacon.
11. Cook the quiche for 18 minutes at 350 F.
12. When the time is over – chill the quiche little and serve!

NUTRITION: Calories 166, Fat 11.8, Fiber 1.8, Carbs 8.5, Protein 7.7

16. Breakfast Bacon Hash

Preparation time: 10 minutes

Cooking time: 19 minutes

Servings: 2

INGREDIENTS

- 1 oz bacon, chopped
- 1 carrot
- 1 apple
- 1 teaspoon olive oil
- ½ teaspoon salt
- ¼ teaspoon thyme

DIRECTIONS

1. Put the chopped bacon in the air fryer basket.
2. Add salt and stir it gently.
3. Cook the bacon for 4 minutes at 365 F.
4. Peel the carrot and grate it.
5. Add the grated carrot.
6. Then grate the apple and add the carrot mixture too.
7. Stir it carefully.
8. Sprinkle the bacon hash with the thyme and stir gently again.
9. Cook the bacon hash for 15 minutes at 365 F.
10. Stir it carefully and serve!

NUTRITION: Calories 168, Fat 8.5, Fiber 3.5, Carbs 18.7, Protein 5.8

17. Spaghetti Squash Casserole Cups

Preparation time: 10 minutes

Cooking time: 15 minutes

Servings: 2

INGREDIENTS

- 12 oz spaghetti squash
- 1 carrot, grated
- 1 egg
- 1/3 teaspoon chili flakes
- 1 onion, chopped

DIRECTIONS

1. Peel the spaghetti squash and grate it.
2. Mix up together the spaghetti squash and carrot.
3. Beat the egg and stir it carefully.
4. After this, add the chili flakes and chopped onion.
5. Stir it.
6. Place the mixture in the air fryer basket and cook the casserole for 15 minutes at 365 F.
7. When the casserole is cooked – chill it till the room temperature.
8. Serve it!

NUTRITION: Calories 119, Fat 3.2, Fiber 1.9, Carbs 20.1, Protein 4.7

18. Chopped Kale with Ground Beef

Preparation time: 12 minutes

Cooking time: 16 minutes

Servings: 4

INGREDIENTS

- 12 oz kale
- 1 cup ground beef
- ½ teaspoon salt
- ½ onion, diced
- 1 teaspoon ground paprika
- ¼ teaspoon minced garlic
- 1 teaspoon dried dill
- 1 teaspoon olive oil
- 1 oz almonds, crushed

DIRECTIONS

1. Mix up together the salt, diced onion, ground paprika, minced garlic, and dried dill in the mixing bowl.
2. Add the olive oil and stir carefully.
3. After this, place the ground beef in the air fryer basket.
4. Add the olive oil mixture. Stir it carefully.
5. Cook the ground beef for 13 minutes at 370 F. Stir it time to time.
6. Meanwhile, chop the kale.
7. Add the kale and crushed almonds in the ground beef.
8. Stir it and cook for 3 minutes more at 350 F.
9. Then transfer the cooked meal in the serving bowls and serve!

NUTRITION: Calories 180, Fat 7.5, Fiber 2.7, Carbs 12.2, Protein 17.2

19. Bacon Wrapped Chicken Fillet

Preparation time: 15 minutes

Cooking time: 15 minutes

Servings: 6

INGREDIENTS

- 15 oz chicken fillet
- 6 oz bacon, sliced
- ½ teaspoon salt
- 1 teaspoon paprika
- 1 tablespoon olive oil
- 1 garlic clove, chopped

DIRECTIONS

1. Rub the chicken fillet with the salt, paprika, garlic clove and olive oil.
2. Wrap the rubbed chicken fillet in the bacon and secure gently with the toothpicks.

3. Place the chicken fillets in the air fryer basket.
4. Cook the chicken for 15 minutes at 380 F. Stir the chicken every 5 minutes.
5. Then slice the cooked chicken fillet and serve!

NUTRITION: Calories 310, Fat 19.5, Fiber 0.1, Carbs 0.8, Protein 31.1

20. Egg Whites with Sliced Tomatoes

Preparation time: 10 minutes

Cooking time: 15 minutes

Servings: 2

INGREDIENTS

- 1 tomato, sliced
- 2 egg whites
- ¼ teaspoon ground paprika
- ¼ teaspoon salt
- 1 teaspoon olive oil
- 1 teaspoon dried dill

DIRECTIONS

1. Pour the olive oil in the air fryer.
2. Then add the egg whites.
3. Sprinkle the egg whites with the salt, dried dill, and ground paprika.
4. Cook the egg whites for 15 minutes at 350 F.
5. When the egg whites are cooked – let them chill little.
6. Place the layer of the sliced tomatoes on the plate.
7. Then chop the egg whites roughly and place over the tomatoes.
8. Serve!

NUTRITION: Calories 45, Fat 2.5, Fiber 0.5, Carbs 1.9, Protein 4

21. Eggs in Avocado

Preparation time: 10 minutes

Cooking time: 7 minutes

Servings: 2

INGREDIENTS

- 1 avocado, pitted
- 2 eggs
- ½ ground black pepper
- ¾ teaspoon salt

DIRECTIONS

1. Cut the avocado into the halves.
2. Then sprinkle the avocado with the black pepper and salt.
3. Beat the eggs and place them in the avocado halve's wholes.
4. Place the avocado in the air fryer basket.
5. Cook the meal for 7 minutes at 380 F.
6. When the eggs are cooked – the meal is ready to eat.
7. Serve it immediately!

NUTRITION: Calories 268, Fat 24, Fiber 6.7, Carbs 9, Protein 7.5

22. Maple Apple Quinoa

Preparation time: 5 minutes

Cooking time: 20 minutes

Servings: 4

INGREDIENTS

- 1 cup quinoa
- 2 cups coconut milk
- 1 cup apples, cored, peeled and roughly chopped
- 3 tablespoons maple syrup
- 2 tablespoons butter, melted

- 1 teaspoon nutmeg, ground

DIRECTIONS

1. In your air fryer, mix the quinoa with the milk, apples and the other ingredients, toss, cover and cook at 370 degrees F for 20 minutes.
2. Divide into bowls and serve for breakfast.

NUTRITION: Calories 208, Fat 6, Fiber 9, Carbs 14, Protein 3

23. Avocado Eggs Mix

Preparation time: 5 minutes

Cooking time: 15 minutes

Servings: 4

INGREDIENTS

- 1 tablespoon avocado oil
- 1 cup avocado, peeled, pitted and mashed
- 8 eggs, whisked
- ½ teaspoon cumin, ground
- ½ teaspoon smoked paprika
- Salt and black pepper to the taste
- 1 tablespoon cilantro, chopped

DIRECTIONS

1. In a bowl, mix the eggs with the avocado and the other ingredients except the oil and whisk,
2. Heat up your air fryer with the oil at 360 degrees F, add the avocado mix, cover, cook for 15 minutes, divide between plates and serve.

NUTRITION: Calories 220, Fat 11, Fiber 3, Carbs 4, Protein 6

24. Turkey Tortillas

Preparation time: 5 minutes

Cooking time: 14 minutes

Servings: 4

INGREDIENTS

- 1 pound turkey breast, skinless, boneless, ground and browned
- 4 corn tortillas
- Cooking spray
- 1 cup cherry tomatoes, halved
- 1 cup kalamata olives, pitted and halved
- 1 cup corn
- 1 cup baby spinach
- 1 cup cheddar cheese, shredded
- Salt and black pepper to the taste

DIRECTIONS

1. Divide the meat, tomatoes and the other ingredients except the cooking spray on each tortilla, roll and grease them with the cooking spray
2. Preheat the air fryer at 350 degrees F, put the tortillas in the air fryer's basket, cook for 7 minutes on each side, divide between plates and serve for breakfast.

NUTRITION: Calories 244, Fat 11, Fiber 4, Carbs 5, Protein 7

25. Turkey and Peppers Bowls

Preparation time: 5 minutes

Cooking time: 20 minutes

Servings: 4

INGREDIENTS

- 1 red bell pepper, cut into strips
- 1-pound turkey breast, skinless, boneless, ground
- 4 eggs, whisked
- Salt and black pepper to the taste
- 1 cup corn

- 1 cup black olives, pitted and halved
- 1 cup mild salsa
- Cooking spray

DIRECTIONS

1. Heat up the air fryer at 350 degrees F, grease it with cooking spray, add the meat, peppers and the other ingredients, toss and cook for 20 minutes.
2. Divide into bowls and serve for breakfast.

NUTRITION: Calories 229, Fat 13, Fiber 3, Carbs 4, Protein 7

26. Potato Casserole

Preparation time: 5 minutes

Cooking time: 20 minutes

Servings: 4

INGREDIENTS

- 1 pound gold potatoes, peeled and cubed
- 4 eggs, whisked
- 1 teaspoon chili powder
- 1 cup carrots, peeled and sliced
- 1 cup black olives, pitted and halved
- 1 cup mozzarella, shredded
- 2 tablespoons butter, melted
- A pinch of salt and black pepper

DIRECTIONS

1. Heat up your air fryer at 320 degrees F, grease with the butter, and combine the potatoes with the eggs, chili and the other ingredients except the mozzarella and toss.
2. Sprinkle the mozzarella on top, cook for 20 minutes, divide between plates and serve for breakfast.

NUTRITION: Calories 240, Fat 9, Fiber 2, Carbs 4, Protein 8

27. Chives Quinoa Bowls

Preparation time: 5 minutes

Cooking time: 20 minutes

Servings: 4

INGREDIENTS

- 1 tablespoon olive oil
- 1 cup quinoa
- 2 cups almond milk
- 2 tablespoons chives, chopped
- ½ cup kalamata olives, pitted and halved
- ½ cup mozzarella, shredded
- ½ teaspoon turmeric powder
- Salt and black pepper to the taste

DIRECTIONS

1. Heat up the air fryer with the oil at 350 degrees F, combine the quinoa with the milk, chives and the other ingredients inside, cook for 20 minutes, divide into bowls and serve for breakfast.

NUTRITION: Calories 221, Fat 8, Fiber 3, Carbs 4, Protein 8

28. Creamy Almond Rice

Preparation time: 10 minutes

Cooking time: 20 minutes

Servings: 4

INGREDIENTS

- 2 cups almond milk
- 1 cup white rice
- ½ cup almonds, chopped
- ½ teaspoon vanilla extract
- ½ teaspoon almond extract
- ½ cup heavy cream
- Cooking spray

DIRECTIONS

1. Heat up your air fryer with the oil at 350 degrees F, grease it with the cooking spray, add the rice, milk and the other ingredients inside, toss, cook everything for 20 minutes, divide into bowls and serve.

NUTRITION: Calories 231, Fat 11, Fiber 3, Carbs 5, Protein 8

29. Sweet Quinoa Mix

Preparation time: 5 minutes

Cooking time: 20 minutes

Servings: 4

INGREDIENTS

- 1 cup quinoa
- 2 cups coconut milk
- 3 tablespoons sugar
- 2 tablespoons maple syrup
- Cooking spray
- Salt and black pepper to the taste

DIRECTIONS

1. Heat up the air fryer greased with the cooking spray at 350 degrees F, combine the quinoa with the milk and the other ingredients inside, cover and cook for 20 minutes.
2. Divide into bowls and serve.

NUTRITION: Calories 232, Fat 12, Fiber 4, Carbs 5, Protein 7

30. Olives Rice Mix

Preparation time: 5 minutes

Cooking time: 20 minutes

Servings: 4

INGREDIENTS

- 1 cup black olives, pitted and chopped
- 1 cup green olives, pitted and chopped
- 1 cup white rice
- 2 cups veggie stock
- ½ teaspoon turmeric powder
- ¼ teaspoon sweet paprika
- 1 tablespoon chives, chopped
- A pinch of salt and black pepper

DIRECTIONS

1. Heat up your air fryer at 350 degrees F, combine the rice with the olives and the ingredients inside, toss, cover and cook for 20 minutes.
2. Divide into bowls and serve for breakfast.

NUTRITION: Calories 240, Fat 14, Fiber 3, Carbs 5, Protein

31. Eggplant and Sweet Potato Hash

Preparation time: 5 minutes

Cooking time: 20 minutes

Servings: 4

INGREDIENTS

- 2 eggplants, cubed
- 2 sweet potatoes, peeled and roughly cubed
- 4 eggs, whisked
- 4 scallions, chopped
- Salt and black pepper to the taste
- 2 tablespoons chives, chopped
- 1 tablespoon olive oil
- 1 teaspoon chili powder

DIRECTIONS

1. Heat up the air fryer with the oil at 380 degrees F, combine the eggplants with

the potatoes and the other ingredients inside, cover and cook for 20 minutes.
2. Divide the hash into bowls and serve for breakfast.

NUTRITION: Calories 190, Fat 7, Fiber 3, Carbs 5, Protein 3

32. Sprouts, Avocado and Eggs

Preparation time: 5 minutes

Cooking time: 20 minutes

Servings: 4

INGREDIENTS

- 1 tablespoon olive oil
- 1 cup Brussels sprouts, trimmed and halved
- 1 cup avocado, peeled, pitted and cubed
- 8 eggs, whisked
- ½ cup heavy cream
- ½ teaspoon turmeric powder
- Salt and black pepper to the taste
- 1 tablespoon chives, chopped

DIRECTIONS

1. Preheat the Air Fryer with the oil at 360 degrees F, add the sprouts, avocado and the other ingredients, toss a bit and cook for 20 minutes.
2. Divide between plates and serve.

NUTRITION: Calories 242, Fat 12, Fiber 3, Carbs 5, Protein 9

33. Cheddar Sprouts Bowls

Preparation time: 5 minutes

Cooking time: 15 minutes

Servings: 4

INGREDIENTS

- 1 pound Brussels sprouts, trimmed and halved
- 1 cup cheddar cheese, grated
- 4 eggs, whisked
- 1 cup heavy cream
- 1 tablespoon cilantro, chopped
- Salt and black pepper to the taste

DIRECTIONS

1. Heat up the air fryer at 350 degrees F, add the sprouts, eggs and the other ingredients, toss, cook for 15 minutes, divide into bowls and serve for breakfast.

NUTRITION: Calories 214, Fat 14, Fiber 2, Carbs 4, Protein 9

34. Mozzarella Avocado Mix

Preparation time: 5 minutes

Cooking time: 10 minutes

Servings: 4

INGREDIENTS

- 2 tablespoons butter, melted
- 1 cup avocado, peeled, pitted and cubed
- 1 cup black olives, pitted and sliced
- 1 cup mozzarella cheese, grated
- 1 tablespoon basil, chopped
- ½ teaspoon chili powder
- A pinch of salt and black pepper

DIRECTIONS

1. Preheat your Air Fryer at 360 degrees F, grease with the butter, add the avocado, olives and the other ingredients, toss, cook for 10 minutes, divide into bowls and serve for breakfast.

NUTRITION: Calories 207, Fat 14, Fiber 3, Carbs 4, Protein 8

35. Salsa Omelet

Preparation time: 5 minutes

Cooking time: 20 minutes

Servings: 4

INGREDIENTS

- 8 eggs, whisked
- 1 cup mild salsa
- 4 scallions, chopped
- 1 tablespoon parsley, chopped
- Cooking spray
- ¼ cup mozzarella, shredded
- Salt and black pepper to the taste

DIRECTIONS

1. Heat up the air fryer at 360 degrees F, grease it with the cooking spray, add the eggs mixed with the salsa and the other ingredients, spread, cook for 20 minutes, divide between plates and serve.

NUTRITION: Calories 230, Fat 14, Fiber 3, Carbs 5, Protein 11

36. Salmon and Zucchini Salad

Preparation time: 5 minutes

Cooking time: 15 minutes

Servings: 4

INGREDIENTS

- 1 cup zucchinis, roughly cubed
- 1 pound salmon fillets, boneless and cubed
- 1 tablespoon olive oil
- 1 cup baby spinach
- 1 cup cherry tomatoes
- ½ teaspoon chili powder
- 1 tablespoon chives, chopped
- Salt and black pepper to the taste

DIRECTIONS

1. Heat up the Air Fryer with the oil at 360 degrees F, add the salmon and chili powder and cook for 5 minutes.
2. Add the rest of the ingredients, toss, and cook for 10 more minutes, divide into bowls and serve for breakfast.

NUTRITION: Calories 240, Fat 14, Fiber 2, Carbs 5, Protein 11

37. Parsley Avocado Salad

Preparation time: 5 minute

Cooking time: 8 minutes

Servings: 4

INGREDIENTS

- 1 cup avocado, peeled, pitted and roughly cubed
- 1 tablespoon lime juice
- 1 cup baby spinach
- 1 cup cucumber, roughly cubed
- 1 cup cherry tomatoes, halved
- 1 tablespoon parsley, chopped
- Cooking spray

DIRECTIONS

1. Grease the Air Fryer with the cooking spray, add the avocado, spinach and the other ingredients inside, and cook at 330 degrees F for 8 minutes.
2. Divide the salad into bowls and serve for breakfast.

NUTRITION: Calories 240, Fat 13, Fiber 4, Carbs 6, Protein 9

38. Bacon Omelet

Preparation time: 5 minutes

Cooking time: 20 minutes

Servings: 4

INGREDIENTS

- 2 tablespoons butter, melted
- 1 cup bacon, chopped
- 1 yellow onion, chopped
- 8 eggs, whisked
- ½ teaspoon turmeric powder
- ½ teaspoon sweet paprika
- 1 tablespoon chives, chopped
- Salt and black pepper to the taste

DIRECTIONS

1. Heat up the air fryer with the butter at 370 degrees F, add the bacon and cook for 5 minutes.
2. Add the eggs and the other ingredients, spread into the machine, toss, cook for 15 minutes more, divide the omelet between plates and serve.

NUTRITION: Calories 200, Fat 4, Fiber 2, Carbs 4, Protein 4

39. Spinach and Asparagus Frittata

Preparation time: 5 minutes

Cooking time: 20 minutes

Servings: 4

INGREDIENTS

- 1 tablespoon olive oil
- 1 cup baby spinach
- 1 cup asparagus, trimmed and sliced
- 8 eggs, whisked
- ½ teaspoon sweet paprika
- ½ cup heavy cream
- Salt and black pepper to the taste

DIRECTIONS

1. In a bowl, combine the eggs with the spinach and the other ingredients except the oil and whisk.
2. Grease the air fryer's pan with the oil, pour the frittata mix, spread, put the pan in the machine, cook at 380 degrees F for 20 minutes, divide between plates and serve for Breakfast.

NUTRITION: Calories 240, Fat 8, Fiber 3, Carbs 6, Protein 12

40. Asparagus Muffins

Preparation time: 5 minutes

Cooking time: 15 minutes

Servings: 4

INGREDIENTS

- 3 eggs, whisked
- 1 cup asparagus, chopped
- Cooking spray
- 2 cups almond milk
- 1 cup almond flour
- 1 teaspoon baking soda
- 1 teaspoon baking powder
- 1 tablespoon cheddar, grated

DIRECTIONS

1. In a bowl, combine the asparagus with the eggs and the other ingredients except the cooking spray and whisk.
2. Grease a muffin pan that fits your air fryer with the cooking spray, divide the asparagus mix inside, put the pan in the air fryer, cook at 380 degrees F for 15 minutes, divide the muffins between plates and serve.

NUTRITION: Calories 210, Fat 12, Fiber 3, Carbs 5, Protein 8

41. Coconut Eggs Mix

Preparation time: 5 minutes

Cooking time: 20 minutes

Servings: 4

INGREDIENTS

- 1 cup coconut cream
- 8 eggs, whisked
- ½ cup coconut flesh, shredded
- ½ teaspoon turmeric powder
- 2 tablespoons chives, chopped
- A pinch of salt and black pepper
- 1 tablespoon mozzarella, shredded

DIRECTIONS

1. In a bowl, combine the eggs with the cream, coconut flesh and the other ingredients and whisk
2. Heat up the air fryer at 360 degrees F, add the eggs mix, stir, cook for 20 minutes shaking the machine halfway, divide between plates and serve for breakfast.

NUTRITION: Calories 220, Fat 14, Fiber 2, Carbs 5, Protein 11

42. Eggplant and Avocado Salad

Preparation time: 10 minutes

Cooking time: 10 minutes

Servings: 4

INGREDIENTS

- 1 pound eggplant, cubed
- 1 cup avocado, peeled, pitted and cubed
- 1 cup cherry tomatoes, halved
- 1 cup kalamata olives, pitted and cubed
- 4 eggs, whisked
- 1 tablespoon cilantro, chopped
- Salt and black pepper to the taste
- 1 tablespoon chives, chopped

DIRECTIONS

1. Heat up the air fryer with the cooking spray at 350 degrees F, add the eggplant, avocado and the other ingredients and cook for 10 minutes.
2. Divide the mix into bowls and serve for breakfast.

NUTRITION: Calories 241, Fat 11, Fiber 4, Carbs 5, Protein 12

43. Peppers, Coconut and Eggs Mix

Preparation time: 5 minutes

Cooking time: 20 minutes

Servings: 4

INGREDIENTS

- Cooking spray
- 1 cup green bell peppers, cut into strips
- 1 cup coconut flesh, shredded
- 8 eggs, whisked
- 2 spring onions, chopped
- 1 teaspoon oregano, dried
- Salt and black pepper to the taste
- 1 cup coconut cream

DIRECTIONS

1. In a bowl, combine the peppers with the coconut, eggs and the other ingredients except the cooking spray and whisk well.
2. Grease the air fryer's pan with the cooking spray, add the peppers mix, put the pan in the machine and cook at 350 degrees F for 20 minutes.
3. Divide between plates and serve for breakfast.

NUTRITION: Calories 251, Fat 16, Fiber 3, Carbs 6, Protein 11

44. Yogurt Avocado Mix

Preparation time: 5 minutes

Cooking time: 20 minutes

Servings: 4

INGREDIENTS

- Salt and black pepper to the taste
- 2 cups Greek yogurt
- 1 cup avocado, peeled, pitted and cubed
- 4 eggs, whisked
- 1 tablespoon chives, chopped
- ½ teaspoon chili powder

DIRECTIONS

1. In a bowl, mix all the ingredients except the cooking spray and whisk well.
2. Grease the air fryer's pan with the cooking spray, pour the avocado and yogurt mix, toss, and cook at 360 degrees F for 20 minutes.
3. Divide between plates and serve for breakfast.

NUTRITION: Calories 221, Fat 14, Fiber 4, Carbs 6, Protein 11

45. Asparagus, Shrimp and Avocado Salad

Preparation time: 5 minutes

Cooking time: 10 minutes

Servings: 4

INGREDIENTS

- 1 bunch asparagus, trimmed and halved
- ½ pound shrimp, peeled and deveined
- 1 cup avocado, peeled, pitted and cubed
- 1 tablespoon olive oil
- 1 tablespoon lime juice
- ½ cup mild salsa
- A pinch of salt and black pepper

DIRECTIONS

1. In the air fryer, combine the asparagus with the shrimp and the other ingredients, toss and cook at 360 degrees F for 10 minutes.
2. Divide into bowls and serve for breakfast.

NUTRITION: Calories 200, Fat 5, Fiber 1, Carbs 4, Protein 5

46. Nutty Granola

Preparation time: 10 minutes

Cooking time: 18 minutes

Servings: 12

INGREDIENTS

- 1 cup almonds, chopped finely
- ½ cup walnuts, chopped finely
- ½ cup hazelnuts, peeled, chopped finely
- 1 cup pecans, chopped finely
- 1/3 cup pumpkin seeds
- 1/3 cup hemp seeds
- ½ cup ground flaxseeds
- 1 tsp vanilla
- 1 egg white, whisked
- ¼ cup butter, melted

DIRECTIONS:

1. Preheat your air fryer to 325 degrees F.
2. Line your air fryer basket with parchment.
3. Place the chopped nuts in a large bowl and then add the pumpkin seeds, hemp seeds and flaxseed. Toss well.
4. Add the remaining ingredients and toss well.
5. Pour the nut mix into the air fryer basket and bake for 18 minutes, tossing halfway through to bake evenly.

6. Empty the granola onto a try and let cool completely. Enjoy with milk or own its own.

NUTRITION: Calories 278, Total Fat 26, Saturated Fat 18g, Total Carbs 7g, Net Carbs 2g, Protein 7g, Sugar 1g, Fiber 5g, Sodium 187mg, Potassium 54g

47. Fruit and Nut Keto Granola

Preparation time: 10 minutes

Cooking time: 18 minutes

Servings: 12

INGREDIENTS

- 1 cup almonds, chopped finely
- ½ cup walnuts, chopped finely
- ½ cup hazelnuts, peeled, chopped finely
- ½ cup dried blueberries
- 1/3 cup pumpkin seeds
- 1/3 cup hemp seeds
- ½ cup ground flaxseeds
- 1 tsp vanilla
- 1 egg white, whisked
- ¼ cup butter, melted

DIRECTIONS:

1. Preheat your air fryer to 325 degrees F.
2. Line your air fryer basket with parchment.
3. Place the chopped nuts in a large bowl and then add the pumpkin seeds, hemp seeds, dried blueberries and flaxseed. Toss well.
4. Add the remaining ingredients and toss well.
5. Pour the nut mix into the air fryer basket and bake for 18 minutes, tossing halfway through to bake evenly.
6. Empty the granola onto a try and let cool completely. Enjoy with milk or own its own.

NUTRITION: Calories 328, Total Fat 26, Saturated Fat 18g, Total Carbs 13g, Net Carbs 8g, Protein 7g, Sugar 3g, Fiber 5g, Sodium 187mg, Potassium 54g

48. Strawberry and Nut Cereal

Preparation time: 10 minutes

Cooking time: 12 minutes

Servings: 12

INGREDIENTS

- 1 cup almonds, chopped finely
- ½ cup walnuts, chopped finely
- ½ cup dried strawberries
- 1 cup pecans, chopped finely
- 1/3 cup pumpkin seeds
- 1/3 cup hemp seeds
- ½ cup ground flaxseeds
- 1 tsp vanilla
- 1 egg white, whisked
- ¼ cup butter, melted

DIRECTIONS:

1. Preheat your air fryer to 325 degrees F.
2. Line your air fryer basket with parchment.
3. Place the chopped nuts in a large bowl and then add the pumpkin seeds, hemp seeds and flaxseed. Toss well.
4. Add the remaining ingredients and toss well.
5. Pour the nut mix into the air fryer basket and bake for 18 minutes, tossing halfway through to bake evenly.
6. Empty the granola onto a try and let cool completely. Enjoy with milk or own its own.

NUTRITION: Calories 298, Total Fat 27, Saturated Fat 18g, Total Carbs 11g, Net Carbs 6g, Protein 7g, Sugar 3g, Fiber 5g, Sodium 187mg, Potassium 54g

49. Seedy Breakfast Granola

Preparation time: 10 minutes

Cooking time: 18 minutes

Servings: 12

INGREDIENTS

- 1 cup almonds, chopped finely
- ½ cup walnuts, chopped finely
- ½ cup hazelnuts, peeled, chopped finely
- 1 cup pecans, chopped finely
- 1/3 cup pumpkin seeds
- 1/3 cup hemp seeds
- 1/3 cup chia seeds
- ½ cup ground flaxseeds
- 1 tsp vanilla
- 1 egg white, whisked
- ¼ cup butter, melted

DIRECTIONS:

1. Preheat your air fryer to 325 degrees F.
2. Line your air fryer basket with parchment.
3. Place the chopped nuts in a large bowl and then add the pumpkin seeds, hemp seeds, chia seeds and flaxseed. Toss well.
4. Add the remaining ingredients and toss well.
5. Pour the nut mix into the air fryer basket and bake for 18 minutes, tossing halfway through to bake evenly.
6. Empty the granola onto a try and let cool completely. Enjoy with milk or own its own.

NUTRITION: Calories 342, Total Fat 32, Saturated Fat 22g, Total Carbs 7g, Net Carbs 2g, Protein 9g, Sugar 1g, Fiber 5g, Sodium 187mg, Potassium 54g

50. Pepper Stuffed Spinach Parmesan Baked Eggs

Preparation time: 5 minutes

Cooking time: 14 minutes

Servings: 2

INGREDIENTS

- 4 eggs
- 2 Tbsp heavy cream
- 2 Tbsp frozen, chopped spinach, thawed
- 2 Tbsp grated parmesan cheese
- ½ tsp salt
- 1/8 tsp ground black pepper
- 1 large red pepper, cut in half vertically, seeds removed

DIRECTIONS:

1. Preheat your air fryer to 330 degrees F.
2. Place red pepper halves in the air fryer basket and cook for 5 minutes.
3. In a small bowl, whisk together all the ingredients
4. Pour the eggs into the partially cooked peppers and bake for 7 minutes.
5. Enjoy straight out of the baking cup!

NUTRITION: Calories 189, Total Fat 11g, Saturated Fat 4g, Total Carbs 5g, Net Carbs 3g, Protein 14g, Sugar 2g, Fiber 2g, Sodium 134mg, Potassium 148g

51. Pepper Stuffed Spinach and Feta Eggs

Preparation time: 5 minutes

Cooking time: 14 minutes

Servings: 2

INGREDIENTS

- 4 eggs
- 2 Tbsp heavy cream
- 2 Tbsp frozen, chopped spinach, thawed
- ¼ cup feta crumbles
- ½ tsp salt
- 1/8 tsp ground black pepper

- 1 large red pepper, cut in half vertically, seeds removed

DIRECTIONS:

1. Preheat your air fryer to 330 degrees F.
2. Place red pepper halves in the air fryer basket and cook for 5 minutes.
3. In a small bowl, whisk together all the ingredients
4. Pour the eggs into the partially cooked peppers and bake for 7 minutes.
5. Enjoy straight out of the baking cup!

NUTRITION: Calories 192, Total Fat 11g, Saturated Fat 6g, Total Carbs 5g, Net Carbs 3g, Protein 14g, Sugar 2g, Fiber 2g, Sodium 156mg, Potassium 148g

52. Egg Stuffed Peppers and Cheese

Preparation time: 5 minutes

Cooking time: 14 minutes

Servings: 2

INGREDIENTS

- 4 eggs
- 2 Tbsp heavy cream
- 2 Tbsp grated cheddar cheese
- 2 Tbsp grated parmesan cheese
- ½ tsp salt
- 1/8 tsp ground black pepper
- 1 large red pepper, cut in half vertically, seeds removed

DIRECTIONS:

1. Preheat your air fryer to 330 degrees F.
2. Place red pepper halves in the air fryer basket and cook for 5 minutes.
3. In a small bowl, whisk together all the ingredients
4. Pour the eggs into the partially cooked peppers and bake for 7 minutes.
5. Enjoy straight out of the baking cup!

NUTRITION: Calories 178, Total Fat 16g, Saturated Fat 8g, Total Carbs 5g, Net Carbs 3g, Protein 10g, Sugar 2g, Fiber 2g, Sodium 134mg, Potassium 148g

53. Bacon and Egg Stuffed Peppers

Preparation time: 5 minutes

Cooking time: 14 minutes

Servings: 2

INGREDIENTS

- 4 eggs
- 2 Tbsp heavy cream
- 2 Tbsp chopped cooked bacon
- 2 Tbsp grated cheddar cheese
- ½ tsp salt
- 1/8 tsp ground black pepper
- 1 large red pepper, cut in half vertically, seeds removed

DIRECTIONS:

1. Preheat your air fryer to 330 degrees F.
2. Place red pepper halves in the air fryer basket and cook for 5 minutes.
3. In a small bowl, whisk together all the ingredients
4. Pour the eggs into the partially cooked peppers and bake for 7 minutes.
5. Enjoy straight out of the baking cup!

NUTRITION: Calories 210, Total Fat 19g, Saturated Fat 9, Total Carbs 9g, Net Carbs 4g, Protein 14g, Sugar 2g, Fiber 5g, Sodium 198mg, Potassium 148g

54. Peppers and Eggs

Preparation time: 5 minutes

Cooking time: 14 minutes

Servings: 2

INGREDIENTS

- 4 eggs
- 2 Tbsp heavy cream
- 1 jalapeno, sliced
- 2 Tbsp grated cheddar cheese
- ½ tsp salt
- 1/8 tsp ground black pepper
- 1 large red pepper, cut in half vertically, seeds removed

DIRECTIONS:

1. Preheat your air fryer to 330 degrees F.
2. Place red pepper halves in the air fryer basket and cook for 5 minutes.
3. In a small bowl, whisk together all the ingredients
4. Pour the eggs into the partially cooked peppers and bake for 7 minutes.
5. Enjoy straight out of the baking cup!

NUTRITION: Calories 154, Total Fat 11g, Saturated Fat 4g, Total Carbs 5g, Net Carbs 3g, Protein 9g, Sugar 2g, Fiber 2g, Sodium 126mg, Potassium 154g

55. Pepper Stuffed Spinach Parmesan Baked Eggs

Preparation time: 5 minutes

Cooking time: 14 minutes

Servings: 2

INGREDIENTS

- 4 eggs
- 2 Tbsp heavy cream
- ¼ zucchini, sliced and chopped thinly
- 2 Tbsp grated parmesan cheese
- ½ tsp salt
- 1/8 tsp ground black pepper
- 1 large red pepper, cut in half vertically, seeds removed

DIRECTIONS:

1. Preheat your air fryer to 330 degrees F.
2. Place red pepper halves in the air fryer basket and cook for 5 minutes.
3. In a small bowl, whisk together all the ingredients
4. Pour the eggs into the partially cooked peppers and bake for 7 minutes.
5. Enjoy straight out of the baking cup!

NUTRITION: Calories 172, Total Fat 7g, Saturated Fat 3g, Total Carbs 8g, Net Carbs 4g, Protein 14g, Sugar 2g, Fiber 4g, Sodium 117mg, Potassium 154g

56. Brussels Hash

Preparation time: 10 minutes

Cooking time: 25 minutes

Servings: 4

INGREDIENTS

- 6 slices bacon, chopped, cooked
- ½ cup chopped white onion
- 1 pound Brussel sprouts, sliced in quarters
- ½ tsp salt
- ½ tsp ground black pepper
- 2 cloves garlic, minced
- 4 eggs, whisked

DIRECTIONS:

1. Preheat your air fryer to 350 degrees F.
2. Toss the bacon, onion, Brussels, salt, pepper and garlic together in a large bowl.
3. Pour the mix into a seven inch pan that will fit in your air fryer basket.
4. Place in the air fryer and cook for 15 minutes.
5. Pour the whisked eggs in the basket and return the pan to the air fryer to cook for 10 more minutes.

6. Mix well to break up the hash and enjoy while hot.

NUTRITION: Calories 238, Total Fat 12g, Saturated Fat 7g, Total Carbs 6g, Net Carbs 3g, Protein 12g, Sugar 1g, Fiber 3g, Sodium 189mg, Potassium 217g

57. Zucchini Hash

Preparation time: 10 minutes

Cooking time: 25 minutes

Servings: 4

INGREDIENTS

- 6 slices bacon, chopped, cooked
- ½ cup chopped white onion
- 1 pound shredded zucchini, water squeezed out
- ½ tsp salt
- ½ tsp ground black pepper
- 2 cloves garlic, minced
- 4 eggs, whisked

DIRECTIONS:

1. Preheat your air fryer to 350 degrees F.
2. Toss the bacon, onion, zucchini, salt, pepper and garlic together in a large bowl.
3. Pour the mix into a seven inch pan that will fit in your air fryer basket.
4. Place in the air fryer and cook for 15 minutes.
5. Pour the whisked eggs in the basket and return the pan to the air fryer to cook for 10 more minutes.
6. Mix well to break up the hash and enjoy while hot.

NUTRITION: Calories 215, Total Fat 11g, Saturated Fat 7g, Total Carbs 8g, Net Carbs 5g, Protein 10g, Sugar 3g, Fiber 3g, Sodium 189mg, Potassium 211g

58. Vegetable Hash

Preparation time: 10 minutes

Cooking time: 25 minutes

Servings: 4

INGREDIENTS

- 6 slices bacon, chopped, cooked
- ½ cup chopped white onion
- 2 cups Brussel sprouts, sliced in quarters
- 2 cups diced green bell peppers
- ½ tsp salt
- ½ tsp ground black pepper
- 2 cloves garlic, minced
- 4 eggs, whisked

DIRECTIONS:

1. Preheat your air fryer to 350 degrees F.
2. Toss the bacon, onion, Brussels, bell peppers, salt, pepper and garlic together in a large bowl.
3. Pour the mix into a seven inch pan that will fit in your air fryer basket.
4. Place in the air fryer and cook for 15 minutes.
5. Pour the whisked eggs in the basket and return the pan to the air fryer to cook for 10 more minutes.
6. Mix well to break up the hash and enjoy while hot.

NUTRITION: Calories 238, Total Fat 12g, Saturated Fat 7g, Total Carbs 6g, Net Carbs 3g, Protein 12g, Sugar 1g, Fiber 3g, Sodium 189mg, Potassium 217g

59. Ham, Cheese and Mushroom Melt

Preparation time: 12 minutes

Cooking time: 18 minutes

Servings: 4

INGREDIENTS

- 2 Tbsp butter
- ½ pound sliced mushrooms
- 1 clove garlic, minced
- ¼ cup white onion, diced
- 1-16 oz ham steak, cooked
- ¼ cup cooked, crumbled bacon
- 1 Tbsp fresh parsley, chopped
- 1 cup grated gruyere cheese

DIRECTIONS:

1. Preheat your air fryer to 350 degrees F.
2. In a pan that will fit inside your air fryer, combine the butter and diced onion. Place in the preheated air fryer and cook for 5 minutes.
3. Remove the pan from the air fryer and stir in the garlic and mushrooms. Return to the air fryer for another 5 minutes.
4. Remove the pan again and add the ham steak, pushing it toward the bottom of the pan. Top with the bacon and grated cheese and place in the air fryer for another 8 minutes.
5. Move the ham steak and pan contents to a plate, garnish with the parsley and serve while hot.

NUTRITION: Calories 352, Total Fat 22g, Saturated Fat 11g, Total Carbs 5g, Net Carbs 4g, Protein 34g, Sugar 2g, Fiber 1g, Sodium 1576mg, Potassium 387g

60. Ham and Pepper Melt

Preparation time: 10 minutes

Cooking time: 18 minutes

Servings: 4

INGREDIENTS

- 2 Tbsp butter
- 1 cup diced red peppers
- 1 clove garlic, minced
- ¼ cup white onion, diced
- 1-16 oz ham steak, cooked
- ¼ cup cooked, crumbled bacon
- 1 Tbsp fresh parsley, chopped
- 1 cup blue cheese

DIRECTIONS:

1. Preheat your air fryer to 350 degrees F.
2. In a pan that will fit inside your air fryer, combine the butter, bell peppers and diced onion. Place in the preheated air fryer and cook for 5 minutes.
3. Remove the pan from the air fryer and stir in the garlic and mushrooms. Return to the air fryer for another 5 minutes.
4. Remove the pan again and add the ham steak, pushing it toward the bottom of the pan. Top with the bacon and blue cheese and place in the air fryer for another 8 minutes.
5. Move the ham steak and pan contents to a plate, garnish with the parsley and serve while hot.

NUTRITION: Calories 382, Total Fat 25g, Saturated Fat 13g, Total Carbs 5g, Net Carbs 4g, Protein 35g, Sugar 2g, Fiber 1g, Sodium 1576mg, Potassium 387g

61. Veggie Melt

Preparation time: 10 minutes

Cooking time: 14 minutes

Servings: 4

INGREDIENTS

- 2 Tbsp butter
- ½ pound sliced mushrooms
- 1 clove garlic, minced
- ¼ cup white onion, diced
- 1 cup diced green bell peppers
- 1 cup diced zucchini
- 1 cup chopped baby spinach

- 1 Tbsp fresh parsley, chopped
- 1 cup grated gruyere cheese

DIRECTIONS:

1. Preheat your air fryer to 350 degrees F.
2. In a pan that will fit inside your air fryer, combine the butter, bell pepper and diced onion. Place in the preheated air fryer and cook for 5 minutes.
3. Remove the pan from the air fryer and stir in the garlic, zucchini and mushrooms. Return to the air fryer for another 5 minutes.
4. Remove the pan again and add the baby spinach and grated cheese and place in the air fryer for another 4 minutes.
5. Move the ham steak and pan contents to a plate, garnish with the parsley and serve while hot.

NUTRITION: Calories 268, Total Fat 11g, Saturated Fat 7g, Total Carbs 8g, Net Carbs 5g, Protein 34g, Sugar 2g, Fiber 3g, Sodium 452mg, Potassium 254g

62. Blueberry Breakfast Cake

Preparation time: 10 minutes

Cooking time: 24 minutes

Servings: 12

INGREDIENTS

- 1 cup almond flour
- 1 Tbsp powdered stevia
- ¼ cup whole milk
- 1 egg
- ¼ tsp salt
- ¼ tsp ground cinnamon
- 2 tsp baking powder
- ½ cup frozen or fresh blueberries

DIRECTIONS:

1. Preheat your air fryer to 350 degrees F.
2. Spray a cake pan lightly with cooking spray. A seven inch pan will fit in most air fryers.
3. In a large bowl, stir together the almond flour, stevia, salt, cinnamon, and baking powder.
4. Add the eggs and milk and stir well.
5. Fold in the blueberries.
6. Pour the batter into the prepared pan and place into the air fryer basket and cook for 24 minutes or until a toothpick comes out cleanly when inserted into the center.
7. Remove from the air fryer and let cool.
8. Serve and enjoy!

NUTRITION: Calories 42, Total Fat 3g, Saturated Fat 1g, Total Carbs 3g, Net Carbs 2g, Protein 2g, Sugar 0g, Fiber 1g, Sodium 36mg, Potassium 68g

63. Red Pepper Breakfast Cake

Preparation time: 10 minutes

Cooking time: 24 minutes

Servings: 12

INGREDIENTS

- 1 cup almond flour
- 1 Tbsp powdered stevia
- ¼ cup whole milk
- 1 egg
- ¼ tsp salt
- ¼ tsp ground cayenne
- 2 tsp baking powder
- ½ cup sauted red peppers, diced

DIRECTIONS:

1. Preheat your air fryer to 350 degrees F.
2. Spray a cake pan lightly with cooking spray. A seven inch pan will fit in most air fryers.
3. In a large bowl, stir together the almond flour, stevia, salt, cayenne, and baking powder.

4. Add the eggs and milk and stir well.
5. Fold in the red peppers.
6. Pour the batter into the prepared pan and place into the air fryer basket and cook for 24 minutes or until a toothpick comes out cleanly when inserted into the center.
7. Remove from the air fryer and let cool.
8. Serve and enjoy!

NUTRITION: Calories 32, Total Fat 3g, Saturated Fat 1g, Total Carbs 2g, Net Carbs 2g, Protein 2g, Sugar 0g, Fiber 1g, Sodium 36mg, Potassium 68g

64. Zucchini Breakfast Cake

Preparation time: 10 minutes

Cooking time: 28 minutes

Servings: 12

INGREDIENTS

- 1 cup almond flour
- 1 Tbsp powdered stevia
- ¼ cup whole milk
- 1 egg
- ¼ tsp salt
- ¼ tsp ground cinnamon
- 2 tsp baking powder
- ½ cup shredded zucchini, water squeezed out

DIRECTIONS:

1. Preheat your air fryer to 350 degrees F.
2. Spray a cake pan lightly with cooking spray. A seven inch pan will fit in most air fryers.
3. In a large bowl, stir together the almond flour, stevia, salt, cinnamon, and baking powder.
4. Add the eggs and milk and stir well.
5. Fold in the zucchini.
6. Pour the batter into the prepared pan and place into the air fryer basket and cook for 24 minutes or until a toothpick comes out cleanly when inserted into the center.
7. Remove from the air fryer and let cool.
8. Serve and enjoy!

NUTRITION: Calories 42, Total Fat 3g, Saturated Fat 1g, Total Carbs 3g, Net Carbs 2g, Protein 2g, Sugar 0g, Fiber 1g, Sodium 36mg, Potassium 68g

65. Strawberry Breakfast Bread

Preparation time: 10 minutes

Cooking time: 24 minutes

Servings: 12

INGREDIENTS

- 1 cup almond flour
- 1 Tbsp powdered stevia
- ¼ cup whole milk
- 1 egg
- ¼ tsp salt
- ¼ tsp ground cinnamon
- 2 tsp baking powder
- ½ cup chopped fresh strawberries

DIRECTIONS:

1. Preheat your air fryer to 350 degrees F.
2. Spray a cake pan lightly with cooking spray. A seven inch pan will fit in most air fryers.
3. In a large bowl, stir together the almond flour, stevia, salt, cinnamon, and baking powder.
4. Add the eggs and milk and stir well.
5. Fold in the strawberries.
6. Pour the batter into the prepared pan and place into the air fryer basket and cook for 24 minutes or until a toothpick comes out cleanly when inserted into the center.
7. Remove from the air fryer and let cool.
8. Serve and enjoy!

NUTRITION: Calories 42, Total Fat 3g, Saturated Fat 1g, Total Carbs 3g, Net Carbs 2g, Protein 2g, Sugar 0g, Fiber 1g, Sodium 36mg, Potassium 68g

66. Raspberry Breakfast Cake

Preparation time: 10 minutes

Cooking time: 24 minutes

Servings: 12

INGREDIENTS

- 1 cup almond flour
- 1 Tbsp powdered stevia
- ¼ cup whole milk
- 1 egg
- ¼ tsp salt
- ¼ tsp ground cinnamon
- 2 tsp baking powder
- ½ cup frozen or fresh raspberries

DIRECTIONS:

1. Preheat your air fryer to 350 degrees F.
2. Spray a cake pan lightly with cooking spray. A seven inch pan will fit in most air fryers.
3. In a large bowl, stir together the almond flour, stevia, salt, cinnamon, and baking powder.
4. Add the eggs and milk and stir well.
5. Fold in the raspberries.
6. Pour the batter into the prepared pan and place into the air fryer basket and cook for 24 minutes or until a toothpick comes out cleanly when inserted into the center.
7. Remove from the air fryer and let cool.
8. Serve and enjoy!

NUTRITION: Calories 42, Total Fat 3g, Saturated Fat 1g, Total Carbs 7g, Net Carbs 4g, Protein 2g, Sugar 4g, Fiber 3g, Sodium 36mg, Potassium 68g

67. Cheesy Bacon Pancake

Preparation time: 10 minutes

Cooking time: 9 minutes

Servings: 2

INGREDIENTS

- 2 eggs
- ½ cup whole milk
- 2 Tbsp butter, melted
- 1 tsp vanilla extract
- 1 ¼ cup almond flour
- 2 Tbsp granulated erythritol
- 1 tsp baking powder
- 1/8 tsp salt
- ½ cup crumbled, cooked bacon
- ¼ cup grated cheddar cheese

DIRECTIONS:

1. Preheat your air fryer to 400 degrees F and line a baking pan with parchment paper. Be sure the pan will fit in your air fryer- typically a seven inch round pan will work perfectly.
2. Place the eggs, milk, butter and vanilla extract in a blender and puree for about thirty seconds.
3. Add the remaining ingredients to the blender and puree until smooth.
4. Pour the pancake batter into the prepared pan and stir in the cheese and bacon.
5. Place in the air fryer.
6. Cook for 9 minutes or until the pancake is puffed and the top is golden brown.
7. Slice and serve with keto, sugar free syrup!

NUTRITION: Calories 278, Total Fat 28g, Saturated Fat 12g, Total Carbs 15g, Net Carbs 10g, Protein 15g, Sugar 3g, Fiber 5g, Sodium 125mg, Potassium 111g

68. Cheesy Pancake

Preparation time: 10 minutes

Cooking time: 9 minutes

Servings: 2

INGREDIENTS

- 2 eggs
- ½ cup whole milk
- 2 Tbsp butter, melted
- 1 tsp vanilla extract
- 1 ¼ cup almond flour
- 2 Tbsp granulated erythritol
- 1 tsp baking powder
- 1/8 tsp salt
- ½ cup grated cheddar cheese

DIRECTIONS:

1. Preheat your air fryer to 400 degrees F and line a baking pan with parchment paper. Be sure the pan will fit in your air fryer- typically a seven inch round pan will work perfectly.
2. Place the eggs, milk, butter and vanilla extract in a blender and puree for about thirty seconds.
3. Add the remaining ingredients to the blender and puree until smooth.
4. Pour the pancake batter into the prepared pan and stir in the cheese.
5. Place in the air fryer.
6. Cook for 9 minutes or until the pancake is puffed and the top is golden brown.
7. Slice and serve with keto, sugar free syrup!

NUTRITION: Calories 261, Total Fat 28g, Saturated Fat 12g, Total Carbs 12g, Net Carbs 9g, Protein 9g, Sugar 3g, Fiber 5g, Sodium 125mg, Potassium 111g

69. Strawberry Feta Pancake

Preparation time: 10 minutes

Cooking time: 9 minutes

Servings: 2

INGREDIENTS

- 2 eggs
- ½ cup whole milk
- 2 Tbsp butter, melted
- 1 tsp vanilla extract
- 1 ¼ cup almond flour
- 2 Tbsp granulated erythritol
- 1 tsp baking powder
- 1/8 tsp salt
- ¼ cup chopped strawberries
- ¼ cup feta cheese

DIRECTIONS:

1. Preheat your air fryer to 400 degrees F and line a baking pan with parchment paper. Be sure the pan will fit in your air fryer- typically a seven inch round pan will work perfectly.
2. Place the eggs, milk, butter and vanilla extract in a blender and puree for about thirty seconds.
3. Add the remaining ingredients to the blender and puree until smooth.
4. Pour the pancake batter into the prepared pan and stir in the feta and strawberries.
5. Place in the air fryer.
6. Cook for 9 minutes or until the pancake is puffed and the top is golden brown.
7. Slice and serve with keto, sugar free syrup!

NUTRITION: Calories 262, Total Fat 22g, Saturated Fat 10g, Total Carbs 15g, Net Carbs 10g, Protein 15g, Sugar 3g, Fiber 5g, Sodium 145mg, Potassium 109g

70. Pepper Pancake

Preparation time: 10 minutes

Cooking time: 9 minutes

Servings: 2

INGREDIENTS

- 2 eggs
- ½ cup whole milk
- 2 Tbsp butter, melted
- 1 tsp vanilla extract
- 1 ¼ cup almond flour
- 2 Tbsp granulated erythritol
- 1 tsp baking powder
- 1/8 tsp salt
- ½ cup diced bell pepper

DIRECTIONS:

1. Preheat your air fryer to 400 degrees F and line a baking pan with parchment paper. Be sure the pan will fit in your air fryer- typically a seven inch round pan will work perfectly.
2. Place the eggs, milk, butter and vanilla extract in a blender and puree for about thirty seconds.
3. Add the remaining ingredients to the blender and puree until smooth.
4. Pour the pancake batter into the prepared pan and stir in the bell pepper.
5. Place in the air fryer.
6. Cook for 9 minutes or until the pancake is puffed and the top is golden brown.
7. Slice and serve with keto, sugar free syrup!

NUTRITION: Calories 189, Total Fat 16g, Saturated Fat 8g, Total Carbs 12g, Net Carbs 7g, Protein 9g, Sugar 3g, Fiber 5g, Sodium 125mg, Potassium 111g

71. Sausage Omelette

Preparation time: 5 minutes

Cook time: 11 minutes

Servings: 4

INGREDIENTS

- 4 eggs
- 3 Tbsp heavy whipping cream
- ¼ cup cheddar cheese, grated
- ½ cup cooked, chopped sausage
- ½ tsp salt
- ¼ tsp ground black pepper

DIRECTIONS:

1. Preheat your air fryer to 350 degrees F and line a baking pan with parchment paper. Be sure the pan will fit in your air fryer- typically a seven inch round pan will work perfectly.
2. In a small bowl, whisk together the eggs, cream, salt and pepper. Stir in the sausage.
3. Pour the mix into the prepared baking pan and then place the pan in your preheated air fryer.
4. Cook for about 10 minutes or until the eggs are completely set.
5. Sprinkle the cheese across the cooked eggs and return the pan to the air fryer for another minute to melt the cheese.
6. Fold the omelet in half.
7. Slice into wedges and serve while hot.

NUTRITION: Calories 210, Total Fat 22g, Saturated Fat 14g, Total Carbs 6g, Net Carbs 3g, Protein 7g, Sugar 1g, Fiber 3g, Sodium 863mg, Potassium 125g

72. Ham and Cheese Omelet

Preparation time: 5 minutes

Cook time: 11 minutes

Servings: 4

INGREDIENTS

- 4 eggs
- 3 Tbsp heavy whipping cream
- ¼ cup cheddar cheese, grated

- ½ cup chopped, cooked ham
- ½ tsp salt
- ¼ tsp ground black pepper

DIRECTIONS:

1. Preheat your air fryer to 350 degrees F and line a baking pan with parchment paper. Be sure the pan will fit in your air fryer- typically a seven inch round pan will work perfectly.
2. In a small bowl, whisk together the eggs, cream, salt and pepper. Stir in the ham.
3. Pour the mix into the prepared baking pan and then place the pan in your preheated air fryer.
4. Cook for about 10 minutes or until the eggs are completely set.
5. Sprinkle the cheese across the cooked eggs and return the pan to the air fryer for another minute to melt the cheese.
6. Fold the omelet in half.
7. Slice into wedges and serve while hot.

NUTRITION: Calories 218, Total Fat 19g, Saturated Fat 9g, Total Carbs 6g, Net Carbs 2g, Protein 7g, Sugar 1g, Fiber 4g, Sodium 890mg, Potassium 343g

73. Air fried Cheese Sandwich

Preparation Time: 13 Minutes

Servings: 2

INGREDIENTS

1. Bread slices-4
2. Butter softened -4 tsp.
3. Cheddar cheese slices -4
4. Directions:
5. Layer the top of bread slices with butter.
6. Place two cheese slices each on 2 slices of bread.
7. Cover it with remaining two slices of bread then cut in half diagonally.
8. Place the sandwiches in the Air fryer basket and seal it.
9. Cook for 8 minutes at 370 o F on Air fryer mode.
10. Serve fresh.

NUTRITION: Calories: 200, Fat: 3g, Fiber: 5g, Carbs: 12g, Protein: 4g

74. Green Beans Egg Bake

Preparation Time: 15 Minutes

Servings: 4

INGREDIENTS

- Eggs, whisked-4
- Soy sauce -1 tbsp.
- Olive oil-1 tbsp.
- Garlic cloves, minced-4
- Green beans, trimmed and halved-3 ounces
- Salt and black pepper -to taste

DIRECTIONS

1. Whisk everything in a bowl except oil and beans.
2. Let your Air fryer preheat and grease its pan with oil.
3. Add beans to the pan and sauté for 3 minutes.
4. Pour the prepared mixture over then seal the Fryer.
5. Cook for 8 minutes at the same temperature on Air fryer mode.
6. Slice and serve to enjoy.

NUTRITION: Calories: 212, Fat: 8g, Fiber: 6g, Carbs: 8g, Protein: 6g

75. Cod Corn Burritos

Preparation Time: 27 Minutes

Servings: 4

INGREDIENTS

- Tortillas -4
- Olive oil- a drizzle
- Green bell pepper, chopped-1
- Red onion, chopped -1
- Corn -1 cup
- Cod fillets, skinless and boneless -4
- Salsa -½ cup
- Baby spinach - a handful
- Parmesan cheese, grated -4 tbsp.

DIRECTIONS

1. Place the fish in the Air fryer's basket.
2. Secure the Fryer and cook for 6 minutes at 350 o F on Air fryer mode.
3. Meanwhile, preheat a pan with oil and sauté bell peppers, corn, and onions in it.
4. After 5 minutes put off the heat.
5. Spread the tortillas on a working surface then divide the fish, salsa, spinach, sautéed veggies and parmesan over each tortilla.
6. Roll them into a burrito then place them in the Air fryer basket.
7. Seal it and cook for 6 minutes at 350 o F on Air fryer mode.
8. Serve warm.

NUTRITION: Calories: 230, Fat: 12g, Fiber: 7g, Carbs: 14g, Protein: 5g

76. Cheese and Ham Pockets

Preparation Time: 20 Minutes

Servings: 4

INGREDIENTS

- Puff pastry sheet -1
- Mozzarella cheese, grated -4 handfuls
- Mustard -4 tsp.
- Ham slices, chopped-8

DIRECTIONS

1. Spread the puff pastry on a working surface and slice it into 12 squares.
2. Top the half of the pieces with an equal amount of cheese, mustard, and ham.
3. Place the remaining halves on top and seal their edges.
4. Place these pockets in the Air fryer's basket then seal the Fryer.
5. Cook for 10 minutes at 370 o F on Air fryer mode.
6. Serve warm and fresh.

NUTRITION: Calories: 212, Fat: 12g, Fiber: 7g, Carbs: 14g, Protein: 8g

77. Tuna Mayo Sandwiches

Preparation Time: 14 Minutes

Servings: 4

INGREDIENTS

- Canned tuna, drained-16 ounces
- Mayonnaise -¼ cup
- Mustard -2 tbsp.
- Lime juice -1 tbsp.
- Spring onions, chopped -2
- Bread slices -6
- Butter, melted-3 tbsp.
- Provolone cheese slices -6

DIRECTIONS

1. Toss tuna with lime juice, mayo, spring onions and mustard in a bowl.
2. Layer the bread slices with butter then place them in the Air fryer basket.
3. Seal the fryer and cook for 5 minutes at 350 o F on Air fryer.
4. Top the half of the bread slices with tuna mixture and cheese.
5. Place the remaining slices on top and place the sandwich in the Air fryer basket.
6. Seal the fryer and cook for 4 minutes at Air fryer mode at 350 o F.

7. Serve warm.

NUTRITION: Calories: 212, Fat: 8g, Fiber: 7g, Carbs: 8g, Protein: 6g

78. Mint & Peas Omelet

Preparation Time: 15 Minutes

Servings: 8

INGREDIENTS

- Baby peas-½ pound
- Avocado oil-3 tbsp.
- Yogurt -1½ cups
- Eggs, whisked-8
- Mint, chopped -½ cup
- Salt and black pepper -to taste

DIRECTIONS

1. Add oil to a pan, suitable to fit the Air fryer and place it over medium heat.
2. Add peas and sauté for 4 minutes.
3. Whisk yogurt with mint, eggs, pepper, and salt in a bowl.
4. Add the mixture over the peas and toss well.
5. Place this pea pan in the Air fryer and seal the fryer.
6. Cook for 7 minutes at 350 o F on Air fryer mode.
7. Slice and serve.

NUTRITION: Calories: 212, Fat: 9g, Fiber: 4g, Carbs: 13g, Protein: 7g

79. Vanilla Steel Cut Oats

Preparation Time: 22 Minutes

Servings: 4

INGREDIENTS

- Milk -1 cup
- Steel cut oats -1 cup
- Water -2½ cups
- Brown sugar -2 tbsp.
- Vanilla extract -2 tsp.

DIRECTIONS

1. Take a pan, suitable to fit the Air Fryer.
2. Add everything to this pan and mix well.
3. Place this pan in the Air fryer and seal it.
4. Cook for 17 minutes at 360 o F on Air fryer mode.
5. Serve fresh.
6. Enjoy!

NUTRITION: Calories: 161, Fat: 7g, Fiber: 6g, Carbs: 9g, Protein: 6g

80. Pear Cinnamon Oatmeal

Preparation Time: 17 Minutes

Servings: 4

INGREDIENTS

- Milk -1 cup
- Butter, softened -1 tbsp.
- Brown sugar -¼ cups
- Cinnamon powder -½ tbsp.
- Old fashioned oats -1 cup
- Walnuts, chopped-½ cup
- Pear, peeled and chopped-2 cups

DIRECTIONS

1. Take a pan, suitable to fit the Air Fryer.
2. Add everything to the pan and mix well.
3. Place this pan in the Air fryer and seal it.
4. Cook for 12 minutes at 360 o F on Air fryer mode.
5. Serve right away.

NUTRITION: Calories: 210, Fat: 9g, Fiber: 11g, Carbs: 12g, Protein: 5g

81. Maple Rice Pudding

Preparation Time: 25 Minutes

Servings: 4

INGREDIENTS

- Brown rice-1 cup
- Coconut, shredded-½ cup
- Almond milk-3 cups
- Maple syrup -½ cup
- Almonds, chopped -½ cup

DIRECTIONS

1. Add rice to a pan, suitable to the Air Fryer.
2. Stir in remaining things and toss them well.
3. Place this pan in the Air fryer basket and seal it.
4. Cook at 360 o F for 20 minutes on Air fryer mode.
5. Serve right away.

NUTRITION: Calories: 201, Fat: 6, Fiber: 8, Carbs: 19, Protein: 6

82. Squash Mushroom Mix

Preparation Time: 15 Minutes

Servings: 4

INGREDIENTS

- Red bell pepper, roughly chopped-1
- White mushrooms, sliced-1 cup
- Yellow squash, cubed -1
- Green onions, sliced-2
- Butter, softened-2 tbsp.
- Feta cheese, crumbled-½ cup

DIRECTIONS

1. Add everything to a bowl except feta cheese.
2. Spread this mixture in the Air fryer pan then seal it.
3. Cook for 10 minutes at 350 o F on Air fryer mode.
4. Garnish with feta cheese.
5. Serve fresh.

NUTRITION: Calories: 202, Fat: 12g, Fiber: 4g, Carbs: 7g, Protein: 2g

83. Tarragon Cheese Omelet

Preparation Time: 20 Minutes

Servings: 4

INGREDIENTS

- Eggs, whisked-6
- Parsley, a chopped-1 tbsp.
- Tarragon, chopped -1 tbsp.
- Chives, chopped-2 tbsp.
- Salt and black pepper -to taste
- Parmesan cheese, grated-2 tbsp.
- Heavy cream-4 tbsp.

DIRECTIONS

1. Mix everything in a bowl except parmesan.
2. Add this mixture to a pan, suitable to fit in the Air fryer basket.
3. Seal it and cook for 15 minutes at 350 o F on Air fryer mode.
4. Slice and serve with parmesan cheese on top.
5. Enjoy.

NUTRITION: Calories: 251, Fat: 8g, Fiber: 4g, Carbs: 15g, Protein: 4g

84. Zucchini Chicken Burritos

Preparation Time: 12 Minutes

Servings: 4

INGREDIENTS

- Tortillas -4
- Butter softened -4 tbsp.

- Rotisserie chicken, cooked and shredded- 6 ounces
- Zucchini, shredded-1 cup
- Mayonnaise-⅓ cup
- Mustard -2 tbsp.
- Parmesan cheese, grated-1 cup

DIRECTIONS

1. Layer the tortillas with butter then place then in the Air fryer's basket.
2. Seal it and cook for 3 minutes at 400 o F on Air fryer mode.
3. Toss chicken with mustard, mayo, and zucchini in a bowl.
4. Divide this prepared mixture in the tortillas and top them with cheese.
5. Roll each tortilla and place them in the Air fryer basket.
6. Seal it and cook for 4 minutes at 400 o F on Air fryer mode.
7. Serve.

NUTRITION: Calories: 212, Fat: 8g, Fiber: 8g, Carbs: 9g, Protein: 4g

85. Kale & Pumpkin Seeds Sandwich

Preparation Time: 11 Minutes

Servings: 1

INGREDIENTS

- Olive oil-1 tbsp.
- Kale, torn-2 cups
- Salt and black pepper - a pinch
- Pumpkin seeds-2 tbsp.
- Small shallot, chopped-1
- Mayonnaise-1½ tbsp.
- Avocado slice -1
- English muffin, halved-1

DIRECTIONS

1. Let you Air fryer preheat at 360 o F with its pan greased with oil.
2. Add salt, pepper, kale, shallots and pumpkin seeds.
3. Toss well then seal the fryer and cook for 6 minutes at Air fryer mode.
4. Shake it well once cooked half way through.
5. Layer the English muffin halves with mayo.
6. Top the half of them with avocado slice and kale mixture.
7. Place the remaining muffin halves on top.
8. Serve fresh.

NUTRITION: Calories: 162, Fat: 4g, Fiber: 7g, Carbs: 9g, Protein: 4g

86. Apple Cinnamon Pancakes

Preparation Time: 30 Minutes

Servings: 4

INGREDIENTS

- White flour-1¾ cups
- Sugar-2 tbsp.
- Baking powder-2 tsp.
- Vanilla extract -¼ tbsp.
- Cinnamon powder-2 tsp.
- Milk -1¼ cups
- Egg whisked -1
- Apple, peeled, cored and chopped-1 cup
- Cooking spray

DIRECTIONS

1. Mix everything in a bowl except cooking spray.
2. Grease the Air fryer's pan with cooking spray.
3. Pour ¼ of the batter in the Air fryer pan and place it in the Fryer.
4. Seal it and cook for 5 minutes at 360 o F.
5. Once cooked half way through then flip it.
6. Cook the remaining pancakes following the same steps.
7. Serve fresh.

NUTRITION: Calories: 172, Fat: 4g, Fiber: 4g, Carbs: 8g, Protein: 3g

87. Romanesco Tofu Quinoa

Preparation Time: 25 Minutes

Servings: 4

INGREDIENTS

- Firm tofu, cubed-12 ounces
- Maple syrup-3 tbsp.
- Soy sauce-¼ cup
- Olive oil -2 tbsp.
- Lime juice -2 tbsp.
- Fresh Romanesco, torn-1 pound
- Carrots, chopped-3
- Red bell pepper, chopped-1
- Baby spinach, torn-8 ounces
- Red quinoa, cooked-2 cups

DIRECTIONS

1. Toss tofu with maple syrup, oil, lime juice and soy sauce in a bowl.
2. Add this tofu to the Air fryer basket and seal it.
3. Cook for 15 minutes at 370 o F on Air fryer mode.
4. Shake it halfway through.
5. Once done, add the tofu to a bowl.
6. Add carrots, Romanesco, quinoa, bell pepper and spinach.
7. Mix well then serve.
8. Enjoy.

NUTRITION: Calories: 209, Fat: 7g, Fiber: 6g, Carbs: 8g, Protein: 4g

88. Black Bean Cheese Burritos

Preparation Time: 19 Minutes

Servings: 2

INGREDIENTS

- Canned black beans, drained-2 cups
- Olive oil- a drizzle
- Red bell pepper, sliced -½
- Small avocado, peeled, pitted and sliced-1
- Mild salsa -2 tbsp.
- Salt and black pepper- to taste
- Mozzarella cheese, shredded-⅛ cup
- Tortillas -2

DIRECTIONS

1. Grease your Air fryer pan with oil.
2. Add beans, salsa, salt, pepper, and bell peppers.
3. Seal the fryer and cook for 6 minutes at 400 o F on Air fryer mode.
4. Spread the tortillas on the working surface then divide the beans mixture on top.
5. Add avocado and cheese, then roll the burritos.
6. Place the burritos in the Air fryer basket and seal the fryer.
7. Cook for 3 minutes at 300 o F on Air fryer mode.
8. Serve.

NUTRITION: Calories: 189, Fat: 3g, Fiber: 7g, Carbs: 12g, Protein: 5g

89. Mushroom Tofu Casserole

Preparation Time: 35 Minutes

Servings: 2

INGREDIENTS

- Yellow onion, chopped -1
- Garlic, minced-1 tbsp.
- Olive oil-1 tbsp.
- Carrot, chopped -1
- Celery stalks, chopped-2
- White mushrooms, chopped-½ cup

- Red bell pepper, chopped -½ cup
- Salt and black pepper- to taste
- Oregano, a dried-1 tbsp.
- Cumin, a ground-½ tbsp.
- Firm tofu, cubed-7 ounces
- Lemon juice -1 tbsp.
- Water -2 tbsp.
- Quinoa, already cooked-½ cup
- Cheddar cheese, grated-2 tbsp.

DIRECTIONS

1. Choose a pan and grease it with oil. Place it over medium heat.
2. Add onion and garlic. Sauté for 3 minutes.
3. Stir in celery, carrots, bell peppers, salt, mushrooms, pepper, cumin, and oregano.
4. Sauté for 6 minutes then take it off the heat.
5. Add tofu to the food processor along with cheese, quinoa, water, and lemon juice.
6. Blend until it is smooth then add this mixture to the sautéed veggies.
7. Mix well then add these veggies to the Air fryer pan.
8. Seal the Air fryer and cook for 15 minutes at 350 o F on Air fryer mode.
9. Serve warm.

NUTRITION: Calories: 230, Fat: 11g, Fiber: 7g, Carbs: 14g, Protein: 5g

90. Cinnamon Yam Pudding

Preparation Time: 13 Minutes

Servings: 4

INGREDIENTS

- Canned candied yams, drained-16 ounces
- Cinnamon powder-½ tbsp.
- Allspice, a ground-¼ tbsp.
- Coconut sugar -½ cup
- Eggs, whisked-2
- Heavy cream -2 tbsp.
- Maple syrup-½ cup
- Cooking spray

DIRECTIONS

1. Toss yams with allspice and cinnamon in a bowl.
2. Mash them with a fork and keep it aside.
3. Grease the Air fryer pan with pan and preheat it at 400 o F.
4. Spread the yams mixture at the bottom of the pan.
5. Whisk eggs with maple syrup, and cream in a separate bowl.
6. Pour this mixture over the yams layer.
7. Seal the fryer and cook for 8 minutes at 400 o F on Air fryer mode.
8. Serve fresh.

NUTRITION: Calories: 251, Fat: 11g, Fiber: 7g, Carbs: 9g, Protein: 5g

91. Tangy Cauliflower Hash

Preparation Time: 25 Minutes

Servings: 4

INGREDIENTS

- Cauliflower head stems discarded, florets separated and steamed -1
- Olive oil -2 tbsp.
- Salt and black pepper -to taste
- Hot paprika -1 tbsp.
- Sour cream -4 ounces

DIRECTIONS

1. Add everything to a pan, suitable to fit the Air Fryer.
2. Place this pan in the Air fryer basket then seal it.
3. Cook at 360 o F for 20 minutes on Air fryer mode.
4. Serve warm.

NUTRITION: Calories: 150, Fat: 3g, Fiber: 2g, Carbs: 10g, Protein: 3g

92. Nutmeg Mushroom Fritters

Preparation Time: 2hrs. 11 Minutes

Servings: 8

INGREDIENTS

- Mushrooms, chopped -4 ounces
- Red onion, chopped-1
- Salt and black pepper -to taste
- Nutmeg, a ground-¼ tbsp.
- Olive oil- 2 tbsp
- Panko breadcrumbs -1 tbsp.
- Milk -10 ounces

DIRECTIONS

1. Add 1 tbsp oil to a suitable pan and place it over medium-high heat.
2. Stir in mushrooms and onions, sauté for 3 minutes.
3. Add nutmeg, pepper, salt, and milk.
4. Take it off the heat and keep it aside for 2 hours.
5. Mix remaining oil with breadcrumbs in a separate plate.
6. Take a tbsp of the mushroom mixture and roll it.
7. Coat this ball with breadcrumbs mixture then flatten it.
8. Place it in the Air fryer basket.
9. Repeat the same steps and place the fritters in the basket.
10. Seal it and cook for 8 minutes at 400 o F on Air fryer mode.
11. Serve warm.

NUTRITION: Calories: 202, Fat: 8g, Fiber: 1g, Carbs: 11g, Protein: 6g

93. Tofu & Bell Peppers Medley

Preparation Time: 15 Minutes

Servings: 8

INGREDIENTS

- Yellow bell pepper, cut into strips-1
- Orange bell pepper, cut into strips -1
- Green bell pepper, cut into strips -1
- Salt and black pepper -to taste
- Firm tofu, crumbled-3 ounces
- Green onion, chopped-1
- Parsley, chopped-2 tbsp.

DIRECTIONS

1. Take a pan, suitable to fit your Air fryer.
2. Add bell pepper strips along with remaining things.
3. Toss well then place the pan in the Air fryer basket.
4. Seal it and cook for 10 minutes at 400 o F on Air fryer mode.
5. Serve warm.

NUTRITION: Calories: 135, Fat: 2g, Fiber: 2g, Carbs: 8g, Protein: 3g

94. Stuffed Feta Cheese Peppers

Preparation Time: 13 Minutes

Servings: 8

INGREDIENTS

- Small bell peppers, tops cut off and seeds removed-8
- Avocado oil -1 tbsp.
- Salt and black pepper -to taste
- Feta cheese, cubed-3½ ounces

DIRECTIONS

1. Toss cheese with oil, salt, and pepper in a bowl.
2. Stuff the peppers with cheese mixture then place these peppers in the Air fryer basket.
3. Seal the fryer and cook for 8 minutes at 400 o F on Air fryer mode.
4. Serve warm.

NUTRITION: Calories: 210, Fat: 2g, Fiber: 1g, Carbs: 6g, Protein: 5g

95. Citrus Pepper Salad

Preparation Time: 15 Minutes

Servings: 4

INGREDIENTS

- Lime juice -1 tbsp.
- Red bell peppers-4
- Lettuce head, torn-1
- Salt and black pepper- to taste
- Heavy cream-3 tbsp.
- Olive oil -2 tbsp.
- Rocket leaves -2 ounces

DIRECTIONS

1. Add bell peppers to the Air fryer's basket and seal it.
2. Cook at 400 o F on Air fryer mode for 10 minutes.
3. Remove the peppers from the Fryer.
4. Peel them and slice them into strips.
5. Toss the peppers with remaining things in a bowl.
6. Enjoy fresh.

NUTRITION: Calories: 200, Fat: 5g, Fiber: 3g, Carbs: 7g, Protein: 6g

96. Spinach Egg Pie

Preparation Time: 34 Minutes

Servings: 4

INGREDIENTS

- White flour-7 ounces
- Spinach, torn-7 ounces
- Olive oil-2 tbsp.
- Eggs whisked -2
- Milk-2 tbsp.
- Mozzarella cheese, crumbled-3 ounces
- Salt and black pepper -to taste
- Red onion, chopped -1

DIRECTIONS

1. Add flour, eggs, milk, pepper, salt and 1 tbsp oil to a food processor.
2. Blend well to form a dough then knead it.
3. Place the dough in a bowl and cover it. Refrigerate for 10 minutes.
4. Add 1 tbsp oil to a suitable pan and place it over medium heat.
5. Stir in remaining things and sauté for 4 minutes then take it off the heat.
6. Divide the dough into 4 pieces and spread each into a circle.
7. Place one dough circle in a ramekin.
8. Divide the prepared spinach mixture in the ramekin.
9. Place the ramekins in the Air fryer's basket and seal it.
10. Cook for 15 minutes on Air fryer mode at 350 o F.

NUTRITION: Calories: 200, Fat: 12g, Fiber: 2g, Carbs: 13g, Protein: 5g

97. Eggplant & Zucchini Mix

Preparation Time: 55 Minutes

Servings: 4

INGREDIENTS

- Eggplant, sliced-8 ounces
- Zucchini, sliced-8 ounces
- Bell peppers, chopped -8 ounces
- Garlic cloves, minced-2
- Olive oil-5 tbsp.
- Yellow onions, chopped-2
- Tomatoes, cut into quarters -8 ounces
- Salt and black pepper -to taste

DIRECTIONS

1. Add 1 tbsp oil to a pan, suitable to fit the Air fryer and place it over medium heat.

2. Stir in eggplant, pepper and salt. Sauté for 5 minutes.
3. Keep it aside in a bowl.
4. Add 1 tbsp oil more to the pan then add bell peppers and zucchini.
5. Stir cook for 4 minutes then add them to the sautéed eggplant.
6. Now add the remaining of the oil to the same pan and stir in onions.
7. Sauté for 3 minutes then add garlic, tomatoes, salt, and pepper.
8. Place this mixture along with all the sautéed veggie to the Air fryer pan.
9. Seal it and cook for 30 minutes at 300 o F on Air fryer mode.
10. Serve warm.

NUTRITION: Calories: 210, Fat: 1g, Fiber: 3g, Carbs: 14g, Protein: 6g

MAINS

98. Indian Chickpeas

Preparation time: 10 minutes

Cooking time: 25 minutes

Servings: 14

INGREDIENTS

- 6 cups canned chickpeas, drained
- 1cup veggie stock
- 1yellow onion, chopped
- 1tablespoon ginger, grated
- 20 garlic cloves, minced
- 8 Thai peppers, chopped
- 2tablespoons cumin, ground
- 2tablespoons coriander, ground
- 1tablespoons red chili powder
- 2tablespoons garam masala
- 2tablespoons vegan tamarind paste
- Juice of ½ lemon

DIRECTIONS

1. In your air fryer, mix chickpeas with stock, onion ginger, garlic, Thai peppers, cumin, coriander, chili powder, garam masala, tamarind paste and lemon juice, toss, cover and cook at 365 degrees F for 25 minutes.
2. Divide between plates and serve hot.
3. Enjoy!

NUTRITION: Calories 255, Fat 5, Fiber 14, Carbs 16, Protein 17

99. White Beans with Rosemary

Preparation time: 10 minutes

Cooking time: 20 minutes

Servings: 10

INGREDIENTS

- 2pounds white beans, cooked
- 3celery stalks, chopped
- 2carrots, chopped
- 1bay leaf
- 1yellow onion, chopped
- 3garlic cloves, minced
- 1teaspoon rosemary, dried
- 1teaspoon oregano, dried
- 1teaspoon thyme, dried
- A drizzle of olive oil
- Salt and black pepper to the taste
- 28ounces canned tomatoes, chopped
- 6cups chard, chopped

DIRECTIONS

1. In your air fryer's pan, mix white beans with celery, carrots, bay leaf, onion, garlic, rosemary, oregano, thyme, oil, salt, pepper, tomatoes and chard, toss, cover and cook at 365 degrees F for 20 minutes.
2. Divide into bowls and serve.
3. Enjoy!

NUTRITION: Calories 341, Fat 8, Fiber 12, Carbs 20, Protein 6

100. Squash Bowls

Preparation time: 10 minutes

Cooking time: 20 minutes

Servings: 5

INGREDIENTS

- 1big butternut squash, peeled and roughly cubed
- 2cups broccoli florets
- 1tablespoon sesame seeds
- For the salad dressing:

- 1 and ½ tablespoon stevia
- 3 tablespoons wine vinegar
- 3 tablespoons olive oil
- 1 tablespoon coconut aminos
- 1 tablespoon ginger, grated
- 2 garlic cloves, minced
- 1 teaspoon sesame oil

DIRECTIONS

1. In your blender, mix stevia with vinegar, oil, aminos, ginger, garlic and sesame oil, pulse really well and leave aside for now.
2. In your air fryer, mix squash with the dressing you've made, broccoli and sesame seeds, toss, cover and cook at 370 degrees F for 20 minutes.
3. Divide salad into bowls and serve.
4. Enjoy!

NUTRITION: Calories 250, Fat 4, Fiber 6, Carbs 26, Protein 6

101. Cauliflower Stew with Tomatoes and Green Chilies

Preparation time: 10 minutes

Cooking time: 15 minutes

Servings: 4

INGREDIENTS

- 30 ounces canned cannellini beans, drained
- 4 cups cauliflower florets
- 1 yellow onion, chopped
- 28 ounces canned tomatoes and juice
- 4 ounces canned roasted green chilies, chopped
- ½ cup hot sauce
- 1 tablespoon stevia
- 2 teaspoons cumin, ground
- 1 tablespoon chili powder
- A pinch of salt and cayenne pepper

DIRECTIONS

1. In your air fryer's pan, mix cannellini beans with cauliflower, onion, tomatoes and juice, roasted green chilies, hot sauce, stevia, cumin, chili powder, salt and cayenne pepper, stir, cover and cook at 360 degrees F for 15 minutes.
2. Divide into bowls and serve hot.
3. Enjoy!

NUTRITION: Calories 314, Fat 6, Fiber 6, Carbs 29, Protein 5

102. Simple Quinoa Stew

Preparation time: 10 minutes

Cooking time: 15 minutes

Servings: 6

INGREDIENTS

- ½ cup quinoa
- 30 ounces canned black beans, drained
- 28 ounces canned tomatoes, chopped
- 1 green bell pepper, chopped
- 1 yellow onion, chopped
- 2 sweet potatoes, cubed
- 1 tablespoon chili powder
- 2 tablespoons cocoa powder
- 2 teaspoons cumin, ground
- Salt and black pepper to the taste
- ¼ teaspoon smoked paprika

DIRECTIONS

1. In your air fryer, mix quinoa, black beans, tomatoes, bell pepper, onion, sweet potatoes, chili powder, cocoa, cumin, paprika, salt and pepper, stir, cover and cook on High for 6 hours.
2. Divide into bowls and serve hot.
3. Enjoy!

NUTRITION: Calories 342, Fat 6, Fiber 7, Carbs 18, Protein 4

103. Green Beans with Carrot

Preparation time: 10 minutes

Cooking time: 12 minutes

Servings: 4

INGREDIENTS

- 1pound green beans
- 1yellow onion, chopped
- 4carrots, chopped
- 4garlic cloves, minced
- 1tablespoon thyme, chopped
- 3tablespoons tomato paste
- Salt and black pepper to the taste

DIRECTIONS

1. In your air fryer's pan, mix green beans with onion, carrots, garlic, tomato paste,, salt and pepper, stir, cover and cook at 365 degrees F for 12 minutes.
2. Add thyme, stir, divide between plates and serve.
3. Enjoy!

NUTRITION: Calories 231, Fat 4, Fiber 6, Carbs 7, Protein 5

104. Chickpeas and Lentils Mix

Preparation time: 10 minutes

Cooking time: 15 minutes

Servings: 6

INGREDIENTS

- 1yellow onion, chopped
- 1tablespoon olive oil
- 1tablespoon garlic, minced
- 1teaspoons sweet paprika
- 1teaspoon smoked paprika
- Salt and black pepper to the taste
- 1cup red lentils, boiled
- 15ounces canned chickpeas, drained
- 29ounces canned tomatoes and juice

DIRECTIONS

1. In your air fryer, mix onion with oil, garlic, sweet and smoked paprika, salt, pepper, lentils, chickpeas and tomatoes, stir, cover and cook at 360 degrees F for 15 minutes.
2. Ladle into bowls and serve hot.
3. Enjoy!

NUTRITION: Calories 341, Fat 5, Fiber 8, Carbs 19, Protein 7

105. Creamy Corn with Potatoes

Preparation time: 10 minutes

Cooking time: 15 minutes

Servings: 6

INGREDIENTS

- 1yellow onion, chopped
- A drizzle of olive oil
- 1red bell pepper, chopped
- 3cups gold potatoes, chopped
- 4cups corn
- 2tablespoons tomato paste
- ½ teaspoon smoked paprika
- 1teaspoon cumin, ground
- Salt and black pepper to the taste
- ½ cup almond milk
- 2scallions, chopped

DIRECTIONS

1. In your air fryer, mix onion with the oil, bell pepper, potatoes, corn, tomato paste, paprika, cumin, salt, pepper, scallions and almond milk, stir, cover and cook at 365 degrees F for 15 minutes.
2. Divide between plates and serve
3. Enjoy!

NUTRITION: Calories 312, Fat 4, Fiber 6, Carbs 12, Protein 4

106. Spinach and Lentils Mix

Preparation time: 10 minutes

Cooking time: 15 minutes

Servings: 8

INGREDIENTS

- 10 ounces spinach
- 2 cups canned lentils, drained
- 1 tablespoon garlic, minced
- 15 ounces canned tomatoes, chopped
- 2 cups cauliflower florets
- 1 teaspoon ginger, grated
- 1 yellow onion, chopped
- 2 tablespoons curry paste
- ½ teaspoon cumin, ground
- ½ teaspoon coriander, ground
- 2 teaspoons stevia
- A pinch of salt and black pepper
- ¼ cup cilantro, chopped
- 1 tablespoon lime juice

DIRECTIONS

1. In a pan that fits your air fryer, mix spinach with lentils, garlic, tomatoes, cauliflower, ginger, onion, curry paste, cumin, coriander, stevia, salt, pepper and lime juice, stir, introduce in the fryer and cook at 370 degrees F for 15 minutes.
2. Add cilantro, stir, divide into bowls and serve.
3. Enjoy!

NUTRITION: Calories 265, Fat 1, Fiber 7, Carbs 12, Protein 7

107. Cajun Mushrooms with Veggies and Beans

Preparation time: 10 minutes

Cooking time: 15 minutes

Servings: 4

INGREDIENTS

- 3 garlic cloves, minced 2 tablespoons olive oil
- 1 green bell pepper, chopped
- 1 yellow onion, chopped
- 2 celery stalks, chopped
- 15 ounces canned tomatoes, chopped
- 8 ounces white mushrooms, sliced
- 15 ounces canned kidney beans, drained
- 1 zucchini, chopped
- 1 tablespoon Cajun seasoning
- Salt and black pepper to the taste

DIRECTIONS

1. In your air fryer's pan, mix oil with bell pepper, onion, celery, garlic, tomatoes, mushrooms, beans, zucchini, Cajun seasoning, salt and pepper, stir, cover and cook on at 370 degrees F for 15 minutes.
2. Divide veggie mix between plates and serve.
3. Enjoy!

NUTRITION: Calories 312, Fat 4, Fiber 7, Carbs 19, Protein 4

108. Eggplant Stew

Preparation time: 10 minutes

Cooking time: 15 minutes

Servings: 4

INGREDIENTS

- 24 ounces canned tomatoes, chopped
- 1 red onion, chopped
- 2 red bell peppers, chopped
- 2 big eggplants, roughly chopped
- 1 tablespoon smoked paprika

- 2 teaspoons cumin, ground
- Salt and black pepper to the taste
- Juice of 1 lemon
- 1 tablespoons parsley, chopped

DIRECTIONS

1. In your air fryer's pan, mix tomatoes with onion, bell peppers, eggplant, smoked paprika, cumin, salt, pepper and lemon juice, stir, cover and cook at 365 degrees F for 15 minutes
2. Add parsley, stir, divide between plates and serve cold.
3. Corn, Mushrooms and Cabbage Salad Enjoy!

NUTRITION: Calories 251, Fat 4, Fiber 6, Carbs 14, Protein 3

109. **Okra and Corn Mix**

Preparation time: 10 minutes

Cooking time: 15 minutes

Servings: 6

INGREDIENTS

- 1 green bell pepper, chopped
- 1 small yellow onion, chopped
- 3 garlic cloves, minced
- 16 ounces okra, sliced
- 2 cup corn
- 12 ounces canned tomatoes, crushed
- 1 and ½ teaspoon smoked paprika
- 1 teaspoon marjoram, dried
- 1 teaspoon thyme, dried
- 1 teaspoon oregano, dried
- Salt and black pepper to the taste

DIRECTIONS

1. In your air fryer, mix bell pepper with onion, garlic, okra, corn, tomatoes, smoked paprika, marjoram, thyme, oregano, salt and pepper, stir, cover and cook at 360 degrees F for 15 minutes.
2. Stir, divide between plates and serve.
3. Enjoy!

NUTRITION: Calories 243, Fat 4, Fiber 6, Carbs 10, Protein 3

110. **Potato and Carrot with Vegan Cheese**

Preparation time: 10 minutes

Cooking time: 16 minutes

Servings: 6

INGREDIENTS

- 2 potatoes, cubed
- 3 pounds carrots, cubed
- 1 yellow onion, chopped
- Salt and black pepper to the taste
- 1 teaspoon thyme, dried
- 3 tablespoons coconut milk
- 2 teaspoons curry powder
- 3 tablespoons vegan cheese, crumbled
- 1 tablespoon parsley, chopped

DIRECTIONS

1. In your air fryer's pan, mix onion with potatoes, carrots, salt, pepper, thyme and curry powder, stir, cover and cook at 365 degrees F for 16 minutes.
2. Add coconut milk, sprinkle vegan cheese, divide between plates and serve.
3. Enjoy!

NUTRITION: Calories 241, Fat 4, Fiber 7, Carbs 8, Protein 4

111. **Winter Green Beans**

Preparation time: 10 minutes

Cooking time: 16 minutes

Servings: 4

INGREDIENTS

- 1 and ½ cups yellow onion, chopped
- 1 pound green beans, halved
- 4 ounces canned tomatoes, chopped
- 4 garlic cloves, chopped
- 2 teaspoons oregano, dried
- 1 jalapeno, chopped
- Salt and black pepper to the taste
- 1 and ½ teaspoons cumin, ground
- 1 tablespoons olive oil

DIRECTIONS

1. Preheat your air fryer to 365 degrees F, add oil to the pan, also add onion, green beans, tomatoes, garlic, oregano, jalapeno, salt, pepper and cumin, cover and cook for 16 minutes.
2. Divide between plates and serve.
3. Enjoy!

NUTRITION: Calories 261, Fat 5, Fiber 8, Carbs 10, Protein 12

112. Spiced Green Beans with Veggies

Preparation time: 10 minutes

Cooking time: 20 minutes

Servings: 4

INGREDIENTS

- 1 teaspoon olive oil
- 2 red chilies, dried
- ¼ teaspoon fenugreek seeds
- ½ teaspoon black mustard seeds
- 10 curry leaves, chopped
- ½ cup red onion, chopped
- 3 garlic cloves, minced
- 2 teaspoons coriander powder
- 2 tomatoes, chopped
- 2 cups eggplant, chopped
- ½ teaspoon turmeric powder
- ½ cup green bell pepper, chopped
- A pinch of salt and black pepper
- 1 cup green beans, trimmed and halved
- 2 teaspoons tamarind paste
- 1 tablespoons cilantro, chopped

DIRECTIONS

1. In a baking dish that fits your air fryer, combine oil with chilies, fenugreek seeds, black mustard seeds, curry leaves, onion, coriander, tomatoes, eggplant, turmeric, green bell pepper, salt, pepper, green beans, tamarind paste and cilantro, toss, put in your air fryer and cook at 365 degrees F for 20 minutes.
2. Divide between plates and serve.

NUTRITION: Calories 251, Fat 5, Fiber 4, Carbs 8, Protein 12

113. Chipotle Green Beans

Preparation time: 10 minutes

Cooking time: 16 minutes

Servings: 6

INGREDIENTS

- 1 yellow onion, chopped
- 1 pound green beans, halved
- 2 teaspoons cumin, ground
- A drizzle of olive oil
- 12 ounces corn
- ¼ teaspoon chipotle powder
- 1 cup salsa

DIRECTIONS

1. In a pan that fits your air fryer, combine oil with onion, green beans, cumin, corn, chipotle powder and salsa, toss, introduce in your air fryer and cook at 365 degrees F for 16 minutes.
2. Divide between plates and serve.
3. Enjoy!

NUTRITION: Calories 224, Fat 2, Fiber 12, Carbs 14, Protein 10

114. Tomato and Cranberry Beans Pasta

Preparation time: 10 minutes

Cooking time: 15 minutes

Servings: 8

INGREDIENTS

- 2cups canned cranberry beans, drained
- 2celery ribs, chopped
- 1yellow onion, chopped
- 7garlic cloves, minced
- 1teaspoon rosemary, chopped
- 26ounces canned tomatoes, chopped
- ¼ teaspoon red pepper flakes
- 2teaspoons oregano, dried
- 3teaspoons basil, dried
- ½ teaspoon smoked paprika
- A pinch of salt and black pepper
- 10ounces kale, roughly chopped
- 2cups whole wheat vegan pasta, cooked

DIRECTIONS

1. In a pan that fits your air fryer, combine beans with celery, onion, garlic, rosemary, tomatoes, pepper flakes, oregano, basil, paprika, salt, pepper and kale, introduce in your air fryer and cook at 365 degrees F for 15 minutes.
2. Divide vegan pasta between plates, add cranberry mix on top and serve.
3. Enjoy!

NUTRITION: Calories 251, Fat 2, Fiber 12, Carbs 12, Protein 6

115. Mexican Casserole

Preparation time: 10 minutes

Cooking time: 15 minutes

Servings: 4

INGREDIENTS

- 1tablespoon olive oil
- 4garlic cloves, minced
- 1yellow onion, chopped
- 2tablespoons cilantro, chopped
- 1small red chili, chopped
- 2teaspoons cumin, ground
- Salt and black pepper to the taste
- 1teaspoon sweet paprika
- 1teaspoon coriander seeds
- 1pound sweet potatoes, cubed
- Juice of ½ lime
- 10ounces green beans
- 2cups tomatoes, chopped
- 1tablespoon parsley, chopped

DIRECTIONS

1. Grease a pan that fits your air fryer with the oil, add garlic, onion, cilantro, red chili, cumin, salt, pepper, paprika, coriander, potatoes, lime juice, green beans and tomatoes, toss, place in your air fryer and cook at 365 degrees F for 15 minutes.
2. Add parsley, divide between plates and serve.
3. Enjoy!

NUTRITION: Calories 223, Fat 5, Fiber 4, Carbs 7, Protein 8

116. Scallions and Endives with Rice

Preparation time: 10 minutes

Cooking time: 20 minutes

Servings: 4

INGREDIENTS

- 1tablespoon olive oil
- 2scallions, chopped

- 3 garlic cloves chopped
- 1 tablespoon ginger, grated
- 1 teaspoon chili sauce
- A pinch of salt and black pepper
- ½ cup white rice
- 1 cup veggie stock
- 3 endives, trimmed and chopped

DIRECTIONS

1. Grease a pan that fits your air fryer with the oil, add scallions, garlic, ginger, chili sauce, salt, pepper, rice, stock and endives, place in your air fryer, cover and cook at 365 degrees F for 20 minutes.
2. Divide casserole between plates and serve.
3. Enjoy!

NUTRITION: Calories 220, Fat 5, Fiber 8, Carbs 12, Protein 6

117. Cabbage and Tomatoes

Preparation time: 10 minutes

Cooking time: 12 minutes

Servings: 4

INGREDIENTS

- 1 tablespoon olive oil
- 1 green cabbage head, chopped
- Salt and black pepper to the taste
- 15 ounces canned tomatoes, chopped
- ½ cup yellow onion, chopped
- 2 teaspoons turmeric powder

DIRECTIONS

1. In a pan that fits your air fryer, combine oil with green cabbage, salt, pepper, tomatoes, onion and turmeric, place in your air fryer and cook at 365 degrees F for 12 minutes.
2. Divide between plates and serve.
3. Enjoy!

NUTRITION: Calories 202, Fat 5, Fiber 8, Carbs 9, Protein 10

118. Lemony Endive Mix

Preparation time: 10 minutes

Cooking time: 10 minutes

Servings: 4

INGREDIENTS

- 8 endives, trimmed
- Salt and black pepper to the taste
- 3 tablespoons olive oil
- Juice of ½ lemon
- 1 tablespoon tomato paste
- 2 tablespoons parsley, chopped
- 1 teaspoon stevia

DIRECTIONS

1. In a bowl, combine endives with salt, pepper, oil, lemon juice, tomato paste, parsley and stevia, toss, place endives in your air fryer's basket and cook at 365 degrees F for 10 minutes.
2. Divide between plates and serve.
3. Enjoy!

NUTRITION: Calories 160, Fat 4, Fiber 7, Carbs 9, Protein 4

119. Eggplant and Tomato Sauce

Preparation time: 10 minutes

Cooking time: 12 minutes

Servings: 2

INGREDIENTS

- 4 cups eggplant, cubed
- 1 tablespoon olive oil
- 1 tablespoon garlic powder
- A pinch of salt and black pepper

- 3 garlic cloves, minced
- 1 cup tomato sauce

DIRECTIONS

1. In a pan that fits your air fryer, combine eggplant cubes with oil, garlic, salt, pepper, garlic powder and tomato sauce, toss, place in your air fryer and cook at 370 degrees F for 12 minutes.
2. Divide between plates and serve.
3. Enjoy!

NUTRITION: Calories 250, Fat 7, Fiber 5, Carbs 10, Protein 4

120. Spiced Brown Rice with Mung Beans

Preparation time: 10 minutes

Cooking time: 16 minutes

Servings: 2

INGREDIENTS

- ½ teaspoon olive oil
- ½ cup brown rice, cooked
- ½ cup mung beans
- ½ teaspoon cumin seeds
- ½ cup red onion, chopped
- 2 tomatoes, chopped
- 1 small ginger piece, grated
- 4 garlic cloves, minced
- 1 teaspoon coriander, ground
- ½ teaspoon turmeric powder
- A pinch of cayenne pepper
- ½ teaspoon garam masala
- 1 cup veggie stock
- Salt and black pepper to the taste
- 1 teaspoon lemon juice

DIRECTIONS

1. In your blender, mix tomato with garlic, onions, ginger, salt, pepper, garam masala, cayenne, coriander and turmeric and pulse really well.
2. In a pan that fits your air fryer, combine oil with blended tomato mix, mung beans, rice, stock, cumin and lemon juice, place in your air fryer and cook at 365 degrees F for 16 minutes.
3. Divide everything between plates and serve.
4. Enjoy!

NUTRITION: Calories 200, Fat 6, Fiber 7, Carbs 10, Protein 8

121. Lentils and Spinach Casserole

Preparation time: 10 minutes

Cooking time: 16 minutes

Servings: 3

INGREDIENTS

- 1 teaspoon olive oil
- 1/3 cup canned brown lentils, drained
- 1 small ginger piece, grated
- 4 garlic cloves, minced
- 1 green chili pepper, chopped
- 2 tomatoes, chopped
- ½ teaspoon garam masala
- ½ teaspoon turmeric powder
- 2 potatoes, cubed
- Salt and black pepper to the taste
- ¼ teaspoon cardamom, ground
- ¼ teaspoon cinnamon powder
- 6 ounces spinach leaves

DIRECTIONS

1. In a pan that fits your air fryer combine oil with canned lentils, ginger, garlic, chili pepper, tomatoes, garam masala, turmeric, potatoes, salt, pepper, cardamom, cinnamon and spinach, toss, place in your air fryer and cook at 356 degrees F for 16 minutes.

2. Divide casserole between plates and serve.
3. Enjoy!

NUTRITION: Calories 250, Fat 3, Fiber 11, Carbs 16, Protein 10

122. Red Potatoes with Green Beans and Chutney

Preparation time: 10 minutes

Cooking time: 14 minutes

Servings: 4

INGREDIENTS

- 2pounds red potatoes, cubed
- 1cup green beans
- 1cup carrots, shredded
- 16ounces canned chickpeas, drained
- 2tablespoons olive oil
- 1teaspoon coriander seeds
- 1and ½ teaspoons cumin seeds
- 1and ½ teaspoons garam masala
- ½ teaspoon mustard seeds
- 1teaspoon garlic, minced

For the chutney:

- ¼ cup water
- ½ cup mint
- ½ cup cilantro
- 1small ginger piece, grated
- 2teaspoons lime juice
- A pinch of salt

DIRECTIONS

1. In a baking dish that fits your air fryer, combine oil with potatoes, green beans, carrots, chickpeas, coriander, cumin, garam masala, mustard seeds and garlic, place in your air fryer and cook at 365 degrees F for 20 minutes.
2. In your blender, mix water with mint, cilantro, ginger, lime juice and salt and pulse really well.
3. Divide potato mix between plates, add mint chutney on top and serve.
4. Enjoy!

NUTRITION: Calories 241, Fat 4, Fiber 7, Carbs 11, Protein 6

123. Simple Italian Veggie Salad

Preparation time: 10 minutes

Cooking time: 10 minutes

Servings: 8

INGREDIENTS

- 1and ½ cups tomatoes, chopped
- 3cups eggplant, chopped
- 2teaspoons capers
- Cooking spray
- 3garlic cloves, minced
- 2teaspoons balsamic vinegar
- 1tablespoon basil, chopped
- A pinch of salt and black pepper

DIRECTIONS

1. Grease a pan that fits your air fryer with cooking spray, add tomatoes, eggplant, capers, garlic, salt and pepper, place in your air fryer and cook at 365 degrees F for 10 minutes.
2. Divide between plates, drizzle balsamic vinegar all over, sprinkle basil and serve cold.
3. Enjoy!

NUTRITION: Calories 171, Fat 3, Fiber 1, Carbs 8, Protein 12

124. Roasted Cauliflower with Nuts & Raisins

Cooking Time: 15 minutes

Servings: 4

INGREDIENTS

- 1 small cauliflower head, cut into florets
- 2 tablespoons pine nuts, toasted
- 2 tablespoons raisins, soak in boiling water and drain
- 1 teaspoon curry powder
- ½ teaspoon sea salt
- 3 tablespoons olive oil

DIRECTIONS

1. Preheat your air fryer to 320°Fahrenheit for 2-minutes. Add ingredients into a bowl and toss to combine. Add the cauliflower mixture to air fryer basket and cook for 15-minutes.

NUTRITION: Calories: 264, Total Fat: 26g, Carbs: 8g, Protein: 2g

125. Spicy Herb Chicken Wings

Cooking Time: 15 minutes

Servings: 6

INGREDIENTS

- 4 lbs. chicken wings
- ½ tablespoon ginger
- 2 tablespoons vinegar
- 1 fresh lime juice
- 1 tablespoon olive oil
- 2 tablespoons soy sauce
- 6 garlic cloves, minced
- 1 habanero, chopped
- ¼ teaspoon cinnamon
- ½ teaspoon sea salt

DIRECTIONS

1. Preheat your air fryer to 390°Fahrenheit.
2. Add ingredients to a large bowl and combine well.
3. Place chicken wings into the marinade mix and store in the fridge for 2 hours.
4. Add chicken wings to the air fryer and cook for 15-minutes.
5. Serve hot!

NUTRITION: Calories: 673, Total Fat: 29g, Carbs: 9g, Protein: 39g

126. Lamb Meatballs

Cooking Time: 15 minutes

Servings: 4

INGREDIENTS

- 1 lb. ground lamb
- 1 egg white
- ½ teaspoon sea salt
- 2 tablespoons parsley, fresh, chopped
- 1 tablespoon coriander, chopped
- 2 garlic cloves, minced
- 1 tablespoon olive oil
- 1 tablespoon mint, chopped

DIRECTIONS

1. Preheat your air fryer to 320°Fahrenheit.
2. Add all the ingredients in a mixing bowl and combine well.
3. Shape small meatballs from the mixture and place them in air fryer basket and cook for 15-minutes.
4. Serve hot!

127. Sweet & Sour Chicken Skewer

Cooking Time: 18 minutes

Servings: 4

INGREDIENTS

- 1 lb. of chicken tenders
- ¼ teaspoon of pepper
- 4 garlic cloves, minced
- 1½ tablespoons soy sauce

- 2 tablespoons pineapple juice
- 1 tablespoon sesame oil
- ½ teaspoon ginger, minced

DIRECTIONS

1. Preheat your air fryer to 390°Fahrenheit. Combine ingredients in a bowl, except for the chicken.
2. Skewer the chicken tenders then place in a bowl and marinate for 2-hours.
3. Add tenders to the air fryer and cook for 18-minutes.
4. Serve hot!

128. Green Stuffed Peppers

Cooking Time: 25 minutes

Servings: 3

INGREDIENTS

- 3 green bell peppers, tops, and seeds removed
- 1 medium-sized onion, diced
- 1 carrot, thinly diced
- 1 small cauliflower, shredded
- 1 teaspoon garlic powder
- 1 teaspoon coriander
- 1 teaspoon mixed spices
- 1 teaspoon Chinese five spice
- 1 tablespoon olive oil
- 3 tablespoons any soft cheese
- 1 zucchini, thinly diced
- ¼ yellow pepper, thinly diced

DIRECTIONS

1. With the olive oil, sauté the onion in a wok over medium heat.
2. Add the cauliflower and seasonings. Cook for 5-minutes, stir to combine.
3. Add the vegetables (carrot, zucchini, yellow pepper and cook for an additional 5-minutes more.
4. Fill each of the green peppers with 1-tablespoon of soft cheese.
5. Then stuff them with cauliflower mixture.
6. Cap stuffed peppers with the tops and cook in air fryer for 15-minutes at 390°Fahrenheit.

NUTRITION: Calories: 272, Total Fat: 12.7g, Carbs: 26g, Protein: 17g

129. Beef Meatballs in Tomato Sauce

Cooking Time: 12 minutes

Servings: 3

INGREDIENTS

- 11-ounces of minced beef
- 1 onion, chopped finely
- 1 tablespoon fresh parsley, chopped
- 1 cup tomato sauce
- 1 egg
- Salt and pepper to taste
- 1 tablespoon fresh thyme, chopped

DIRECTIONS

1. Mix all ingredients in a mixing bowl, except the tomato sauce.
2. With the mixture form 11 balls. Preheat your air fryer to 390°Fahrenheit.
3. Add the meatballs to the air fryer basket and cook for 7-minutes.
4. Transfer the meatballs to an oven-safe dish and pour the tomato sauce over them.
5. Put the dish in the air fryer basket and return to air fryer and cook for an additional 5-minutes at 320°Fahrenheit.

NUTRITION: Calories: 275, Total Fat: 16g, Carbs: 2g, Protein: 20g

130. Mustard Pork Balls

Cooking Time: 15 minutes

Servings: 4

INGREDIENTS

- 7-ounces of minced pork
- 1 teaspoon of organic honey
- 1 teaspoon Dijon mustard
- 1 tablespoon cheddar cheese, grated
- 1/3 cup onion, diced
- Salt and pepper to taste
- A handful of fresh basil, chopped
- 1 teaspoon garlic puree

DIRECTIONS

1. In a bowl, mix the meat with all of the seasonings and form balls.
2. Place the pork balls into air fryer and cook for 15-minutes at 392°Fahrenheit.

NUTRITION: Calories: 121, Total Fat: 6.8g, Carbs: 2.7g, Protein: 11.3g

131. Garlic Pork Chops

Cooking Time: 16 minutes

Servings: 4

INGREDIENTS

- 4 pork chops
- 1 tablespoon coconut butter
- 2 teaspoons minced garlic cloves
- 1 tablespoon coconut butter
- 2 teaspoons parsley, chopped
- salt and pepper to taste

DIRECTIONS

1. Preheat your air fryer to 350°Fahrenheit. In a bowl, mix the coconut oil, seasonings, and butter.
2. Coat the pork chops with this mixture.
3. Place the chops on the grill pan of your air fryer and cook them for 8-minutes per side.

NUTRITION: Calories: 356, Total Fat: 30g, Carbs: 2.3g, Protein: 19g

132. Honey Ginger Salmon Steaks

Cooking Time: 10 minutes

Servings: 2

INGREDIENTS

- 2 salmon steaks
- 2 tablespoons fresh ginger, minced
- 2 garlic cloves, minced
- ¼ cup honey
- 1/3 cup orange juice
- 1/3 cup soy sauce
- 1 lemon, sliced

DIRECTIONS

1. Mix all the ingredients in a bowl. Marinate the salmon in the sauce for 2-hours in the fridge.
2. Add the marinated salmon to air fryer at 395°Fahrenheit for 10-minutes.
3. Garnish with fresh ginger and lemon slices.

NUTRITION: Calories: 514, Total Fat: 22g, Carbs: 39.5g, Protein: 41g

133. Rosemary & Lemon Salmon

Cooking Time: 10 minutes

Servings: 2

INGREDIENTS

- 2 salmon fillets
- Dash of pepper
- Fresh rosemary, chopped
- 2 slices of lemon

DIRECTIONS:

1. Rub the rosemary over your salmon fillets, then season them with salt and pepper, and place lemon slices on top of fillets.
2. Place in the fridge for 2-hours. Preheat your air fryer to 320°Fahrenheit.
3. Cook for 10-minutes.

NUTRITION: Calories: 363, Total Fat: 22g, Carbs: 8g, Protein: 40g

134. Fish with Capers & Herb Sauce

Cooking Time: 15 minutes

Servings: 4

INGREDIENTS

- 2 cod fillets
- ¼ cup almond flour
- 1 teaspoon Dijon Mustard
- 1 egg
- Sauce:
- 2 tablespoons of light sour cream
- 2 teaspoons capers
- 1 tablespoon tarragon, chopped
- 1 tablespoon fresh dill, chopped
- 2 tablespoons red onion, chopped
- 2 tablespoons dill pickle, chopped

DIRECTIONS

1. Add all of the sauce ingredients into a small mixing bowl and mix until well blended then place in the fridge.
2. In a bowl mix Dijon mustard and egg and sprinkle the flour over a plate.
3. Dip the cod fillets first into the egg and coat, then dip them into the flour, coating them on both sides.
4. Preheat your air fryer to 300°Fahrenheit, place fillets into air fryer and cook for 10-minutes.
5. Place fillets on serving dishes and drizzle with sauce and serve.

NUTRITION: Calories: 198, Total Fat: 9.4g, Carbs: 17.6g, Protein: 11g

135. Lemon Halibut

Cooking Time: 20 minutes

Servings: 4

INGREDIENTS

- 4 halibut fillets
- 1 egg, beaten
- 1 lemon, sliced
- Salt and pepper to taste
- 1 tablespoon parsley, chopped

DIRECTIONS

1. Sprinkle the lemon juice over the halibut fillets. In a food processor mix the lemon slices, salt, pepper, and parsley.
2. Take fillets and coat them with this mixture; then dip fillets into beaten egg.
3. Cook fillets in your air fryer at 350°Fahrenheit for 15-minutes.

NUTRITION: Calories: 48, Total Fat: 1g, Carbs: 2.5g, Protein: 9g

136. Fried Cod & Spring Onion

Cooking Time: 20 minutes

Servings: 4

INGREDIENTS

- 7-ounce cod fillet, washed and dried
- Spring onion, white and green parts, chopped
- A dash of sesame oil
- 5 tablespoons light soy sauce
- 1 teaspoon dark soy sauce
- 3 tablespoons olive oil
- 5 slices of ginger
- 1 cup of water

- Salt and pepper to taste

DIRECTIONS

1. Season the cod fillet with a dash of sesame oil, salt, and pepper. Preheat your air fryer to 356°Fahrenheit. Cook the cod fillet in air fryer for 12-minutes. For the seasoning sauce, boil water in a pan on the stovetop, along with both light and dark soy sauce and stir. In another small saucepan, heat the oil and add the ginger and white part of the spring onion. Fry until the ginger browns, then remove the ginger and onions. Top the cod fillet with shredded green onion. Pour the oil over the fillet and add the seasoning sauce on top.

NUTRITION: Calories: 233, Total Fat: 16g, Carbs: 15.5g, Protein: 6.7g

137. Medium-Rare Beef Steak

Cooking Time: 6 minutes

Servings: 1

INGREDIENTS

- 1-3cm thick beef steak
- 1tablespoon olive oil
- Salt and pepper to taste

DIRECTIONS

1. Preheat your air fryer to 350°Fahrenheit. Coat the steak with olive oil on both sides and season both sides with salt and pepper. Place the steak into the baking tray of air fryer and cook for 3-minutes per side.

NUTRITION: Calories: 445, Total Fat: 21g, Carbs: 0g, Protein: 59.6g

138. Spicy Duck Legs

Cooking Time: 30 minutes

Servings: 2

INGREDIENTS

- 2duck legs, bone-in, skin on
- Salt and pepper to taste
- 1teaspoon five spice powder
- 1tablespoon herbs that you like such as thyme, parsley, etc., chopped

DIRECTIONS

1. Rub the spices over duck legs. Place duck legs in the air fryer and cook for 25-minutes at 325°Fahrenheit. Then air fries them at 400°Fahrenheit for 5-minutes.

NUTRITION: Calories: 207, Total Fat: 10.6g, Carbs: 1.9g, Protein: 25g

139. Stuffed Turkey

Cooking Time: 63 minutes

Servings: 6

INGREDIENTS

- 1whole turkey, bone-in, with skin
- 2celery stalks, chopped
- 1lemon, sliced
- Fresh oregano leaves, chopped
- 1cup fresh parsley, minced
- 1teaspoon sage leaves, dry
- 2cups turkey broth
- 4cloves garlic, minced
- 1onion, chopped
- 2eggs
- 1½ lbs sage sausage
- 4tablespoons butter

DIRECTIONS

1. Preheat your air fryer to 390°Fahrenheit. In a pan over medium-heat melt 2 ½ tablespoons of butter. Add the sausage (remove sausage meat from skin and mash. Cook sausage meat in the pan for 8-minutes and stir. Add in celery, onions, garlic, and sage and cook for an additional 10-minutes, stir to combine. Remove sausage mixture from heat and add the broth. In a bowl, whisk eggs and two tablespoons of parsley. Pour egg mixture into sausage mix and stir. This will be the stuffing for your turkey. Fill the turkey with the stuffing mix. In a separate bowl, combine the remaining butter with parsley, oregano, salt, and pepper and rub this mix onto turkey skin. Place the turkey inside the air fryer and cook for 45-minutes. Garnish with lemon slices.

NUTRITION: Calories: 1046, Total Fat: 69.7g, Carbs: 12.7g, Protein: 91.5g

140. Turkey Breast with Maple Mustard Glaze

Cooking Time: 42 minutes

Servings: 6

INGREDIENTS

- 5lbs. of boneless turkey breast
- ¼ Maple Syrup sugar-free
- 2tablespoons Dijon Mustard
- 1tablespoon butter
- 2olive oil
- Dried herbs: sage, thyme, smoked paprika
- Salt and pepper to taste

DIRECTIONS

1. Preheat air fryer to 350°Fahrenheit. Rub turkey breasts with olive oil. Combine the spices and season the turkey on the outside with this mix of spices. Place the turkey in air fryer and cook for 25-minutes. Turn over and cook for an additional 12-minutes more. In a small saucepan over medium heat mix the maple syrup, mustard, and butter. Brush the turkey with the glaze in an upright position. Air fry for 5-minutes or until turkey breasts is golden in color.

NUTRITION: Calories: 464, Total Fat: 10g, Carbs: 25g, Protein: 64.6g

141. Garlic Chicken Kebab

Cooking Time: 10 minutes

Servings: 2

INGREDIENTS

- 1lb. chicken fillet, cut into small pieces
- 1tablespoon garlic, minced
- ½ cup plain yogurt
- 1tablespoon olive oil
- Juice of one lime
- 1teaspoon turmeric powder
- 1teaspoon red chili powder
- 1teaspoon black pepper
- 1tablespoon chicken masala

DIRECTIONS

1. Mix the yogurt and spices in a bowl. Add the oil and squeeze half a lime into it and stir. Coat the chicken pieces with mixture one at a time. Marinate the chicken pieces in the fridge for 2 hours. Preheat your air fryer to 356°Fahrenheit. Place the grill pan into the air fryer and put the chicken pieces into it. Cook chicken for 10-minutes.

NUTRITION: Calories: 355, Total Fat: 12.7g, Carbs: 7.8g, Protein: 49.6g

142. Mozzarella & Parmesan Chicken Breasts

Cooking Time: 15 minutes

Servings: 2

INGREDIENTS

- 2 chicken breasts, fat trimmed, halved
- 6 tablespoons mozzarella cheese, grated
- 2 tablespoons parmesan cheese, grated
- ½ cup marinara sauce
- 1 tablespoon butter, melted

DIRECTIONS

1. Preheat your air fryer to 360°Fahrenheit. Carefully coat chicken breasts with the melted butter and place them into the air fryer basket. Cook chicken for 10-minutes. Top with 1 tablespoon of marinara sauce and both kinds of cheese. Cook for an additional 5-minutes or until the cheese has melted.

NUTRITION: Calories: 251, Total Fat: 9.5g, Carbs: 14g, Protein: 31.5g

143. Rotisserie Style Chicken

Cooking Time: 60 minutes

Servings: 4

INGREDIENTS

- 1 whole chicken (under 6 lbs.
- Olive oil
- Seasoned salt

DIRECTIONS

1. Coat the chicken with olive oil. Season the chicken with salt. Cook in air fryer at 350°Fahrenheit for 30-minutes, then flip the chicken over and cook for an additional 30-minutes.

NUTRITION: Calories: 326, Total Fat: 22g, Carbs: 5g, Protein: 48g

144. Zucchini Manicotti

Cooking Time: 15 minutes

Servings: 4

INGREDIENTS

- 2 tablespoons fresh basil, chopped
- 1½ cups mozzarella, shredded
- 1 cup marinara sauce
- 4 medium zucchinis, sliced ¼-inch thick
- Salt and pepper to taste
- ½ teaspoon Italian seasoning
- 1 clove garlic, minced
- 1 large egg, lightly beaten
- 1 cup parmesan cheese, grated
- 1½ cups ricotta

DIRECTIONS

1. In a mixing bowl, combine ½ cup parmesan, ricotta, egg, garlic and Italian seasoning. Season with salt and pepper and mix well. On a clean working surface place three slices of zucchini so they are slightly overlapping. Add a spoonful of ricotta mixture on top. Roll up and transfer to a greased air fryer baking dish. Repeat with remaining zucchini and ricotta mixture. Add the marinara sauce on top of the zucchini manicotti, then sprinkle all over with the remaining ½ cup parmesan and mozzarella. Bake in the air fryer at 350°Fahrenheit for 15-minutes. Use fresh basil as garnish and serve right away.

NUTRITION: Calories: 356, Total Fat: 12.4g, Carbs: 10.2g, Protein: 34.2g

145. Steamed Salmon with Dill Sauce

Cooking Time: 15 minutes

Servings: 2

INGREDIENTS

- Sea salt about 2 pinches
- 2teaspoons olive oil
- 2tablespoons of dill, chopped
- ½ cup plain Greek yogurt
- ½ cup light sour cream
- 12-ounce salmon fillet

DIRECTIONS

2. First, set your air fryer to 300°Fahrenheit. Add one cup of water to the bottom of air
3. fryer. Cut the salmon into pieces and sprinkle one tablespoon of olive oil in the bowl and
4. mix with a pinch of salt. Add the pieces of salmon to the air fryer and cook for 12
5. minutes. Combine the chopped dill, salt, yogurt, sour cream in a bowl. Save
6. a teaspoon of chopped dill to garnish the top of the salmon.

NUTRITION: Calories: 278, Total Fat: 12.2g, Carbs: 8.2g, Protein: 34.2g

146. Thai Roast Beef Salad with Nam Jim Dressing

Cooking Time: 30 minutes

Servings: 2

INGREDIENTS

- ½ lb. fresh beef without bone
- Sea salt and pepper to taste
- 1teaspoon olive oil
- For Beef Dressing:
- 2tablespoons of fresh lime juice
- 2tablespoons of fish sauce
- A piece of ginger about 1-inch long
- 2garlic cloves
- 2tablespoons sesame oil
- 2tablespoons Tamari sauce
- 4tablespoons pure water
- Pinch of salt
- To Prepare Salad:
- 1carrot, diced
- 1small white cabbage, chopped
- 1red pepper, sliced
- 2teaspoons toasted sesame seeds
- ½ cup coriander leaves, chopped
- 2teaspoons bean sprouts, chopped
- Half a dozen sugar snap peas, finely sliced

DIRECTIONS

2. Set the air fryer to 375°Fahrenheit and cook beef for 30-minutes. Mix oil, salt, and pepper with roast beef. Cook at 300°Fahrenheit for an additional 10-minutes. Mix all the ingredients for the salad and set aside. Add all the salad ingredients into food processor and blend for 2-minutes to thin dressing. Allow the roast beef to cool down for about 20-minutes. Cut the beef into wafer thin slices. Garnish with coriander, lime wedges, and toasted sesame seeds. Mound salad on a dish then top with meat slices.

NUTRITION: Calories: 312, Total Fat: 11.6g, Carbs: 9.2g, Protein: 38.2g

147. Air Fried Chicken Thighs

Cooking Time: 12 minutes

Servings: 2

INGREDIENTS

- 2boneless chicken thighs
- Salt and pepper to taste
- 1teaspoon rosemary, dried
- 1tablespoon Worcestershire sauce
- 1tablespoon oyster sauce
- 1teaspoon liquid stevia
- 2garlic cloves, minced

DIRECTIONS

1. Add ingredients to a bowl and combine well. Place the marinated chicken in the fridge for an hour. Preheat your air fryer to 180°Fahrenheit for 3-minutes. Add marinated chicken to air fryer grill pan and cook for 12-minutes. Serve hot!

NUTRITION: Calories: 270, Total Fat: 17g, Carbs: 7g, Protein: 20g

148. Chicken Cheese Fillet

Cooking Time: 15 minutes

Servings: 4

INGREDIENTS

- 2large chicken fillets
- 4Gouda cheese slices
- 4ham slices
- Salt and Pepper to taste
- 1tablespoon of chives, chopped

DIRECTIONS

1. Preheat your air fryer to 180°Fahrenheit. Cut chicken fillet into four pieces. Make a slit horizontally to the edge. Open the fillet and season with salt and pepper. Cover each piece with chives and cheese slice. Close fillet and wrap in a ham slice. Place wrap chicken fillet into air fryer basket and cook for 15-minutes. Serve hot!

NUTRITION: Calories: 386, Total Fat: 21g, Carbs: 14.3g, Protein: 30g

149. Roasted Pepper Salad

Cooking Time: 10 minutes

Servings: 4

INGREDIENTS

- 1lettuce cut into broad strips
- 1red bell pepper
- 1tablespoon lemon juice
- 3tablespoons of rocket leaves
- Black pepper to taste
- 2tablespoons olive oil
- 3tablespoons plain yogurt

DIRECTIONS

1. Preheat your air fryer to 200°Fahrenheit. Place the bell pepper in air fryer basket and roast for 10-minutes. Add pepper to a bowl, cover with a lid and set aside for 10-minutes. Cut bell pepper into four parts and remove the seeds and skin. Chop the bell pepper into strips. Add lemon juice, yogurt, and oil in a bowl. Season with black pepper. Add lettuce and rocket leaves and toss. Garnish the salad with red bell pepper strips. Serve and enjoy!

NUTRITION: Calories: 91, Total Fat: 7g, Carbs: 3g, Protein: 2g

150. Pineapple Pizza

Cooking Time: 10 minutes

Servings: 3

INGREDIENTS

- 1large whole wheat tortilla
- ¼ cup tomato pizza sauce
- ¼ cup pineapple tidbits
- ¼ cup mozzarella cheese, grated
- ¼ cup ham slice

DIRECTIONS

1. Preheat your air fryer to 300°Fahrenehit. Place the tortilla on a baking sheet then spread pizza sauce over tortilla. Arrange ham slice, cheese,

pineapple over the tortilla. Place the pizza in the air fryer basket and cook for 10-minutes. Serve hot.

NUTRITION: Calories: 80, Total Fat: 2g, Carbs: 12g, Protein: 4g

151. Air Fryer Tortilla Pizza

Cooking Time: 7 minutes

Servings: 6

INGREDIENTS

- 1 large whole wheat tortilla
- 1 tablespoon black olives
- Salt and pepper to taste
- 4 tablespoons tomato sauce
- 8 pepperoni slices
- 3 tablespoons of sweet corn
- 1 medium, tomato, chopped
- ½ cup mozzarella cheese, grated

DIRECTIONS

1. Preheat your air fryer to 325°Fahrenheit. Spread tomato sauce over tortilla. Add pepperoni slices, olives, corn, tomato, and cheese on top of the tortilla. Season with salt and pepper. Place pizza in air fryer basket and cook for 7-minutes. Serve and enjoy!

NUTRITION: Calories: 110, Total Fat: 5g, Carbs: 10g, Protein: 4g

152. Air Fried Pork Apple Balls

Cooking Time: 15 minutes

Servings: 8

INGREDIENTS

- 2 cups pork, minced
- 6 basil leaves, chopped
- 2 tablespoons cheddar cheese, grated
- 4 garlic cloves, minced
- ½ cup apple, peeled, cored, chopped
- 1 large white onion, diced
- Salt and pepper to taste
- 2 teaspoons Dijon Mustard
- 1 teaspoon liquid Stevia

DIRECTIONS

1. Add pork minced in a bowl then add diced onion and apple into a bowl and mix well. Add the stevia, mustard, garlic, cheese, basil, salt and pepper and combine well. Make small round balls from the mixture and place them into air fryer basket. Cook at 350°Fahrenheit for 15-minutes. Serve and enjoy!

153. Stuffed Garlic Chicken

Cooking Time: 15 minutes

Servings: 2

INGREDIENTS

- ¼ cup of tomatoes, sliced
- ½ tablespoon garlic, minced
- 2 basil leaves
- Salsa for serving
- 1 prosciutto slice
- 2 teaspoons parmesan cheese, freshly grated
- 2 boneless chicken breasts
- Pepper and salt to taste

DIRECTIONS

1. Cut the side of the chicken breast to make a pocket. Stuff each pocket with tomato slices, garlic, grated cheese and basil leaves. Cut a slice of prosciutto in half to form 2 equal size pieces. Season chicken with salt and pepper and wrap each with a slice of prosciutto. Preheat your air fryer to 325°Fahrenheit. Place the stuffed chicken breasts into air fryer

basket and cook for 15-minutes. Serve chicken breasts with salsa.

154. Rosemary Citrus Chicken

Cooking Time: 15 minutes

Servings: 2

INGREDIENTS

- 1lb. chicken thighs
- 1/2 teaspoon rosemary, fresh, chopped
- 1/8 teaspoon thyme, dried
- ½ cup tangerine juice
- 2tablespoons white wine
- 1teaspoon garlic, minced
- Salt and pepper to taste
- 2tablespoons lemon juice

DIRECTIONS

1. Place the chicken thighs in a mixing bowl. In another bowl, mix tangerine juice, garlic, white wine, lemon juice, rosemary, pepper, salt, and thyme. Pour the mixture over chicken thighs and place in the fridge for 20-minutes. Preheat your air fryer to 350°Fahrenheit and place your marinated chicken in air fryer basket and cook for 15-minutes. Serve hot and enjoy!

NUTRITION: Calories: 473, Total Fat: 17g, Carbs: 7g, Protein: 66g

155. Air Fried Garlic Popcorn Chicken

Cooking Time: 15 minutes

Servings: 6

INGREDIENTS

- 1lb. chicken breasts, skinless, boneless, cut into bite-size chunks
- ¼ teaspoon garlic powder
- Salt and pepper to taste
- ¼ teaspoon paprika
- ¼ cup of buttermilk
- 1tablespoon olive oil
- ½ cup gluten-free flour
- 2cups corn flakes
- 2tablespoons parmesan cheese, grated

DIRECTIONS

1. Preheat your air fryer to 350°Fahrenheit. In a bowl, mix garlic, chicken, pepper, and salt. Add cornflakes, parmesan cheese, pepper, paprika, and salt into food processor and process mix until it forms a crumble. In a shallow dish add flour. In another bowl add the crumbled cornflake mixture. Add chicken pieces to the flour and coat well. Drizzle buttermilk over the coated chicken pieces and mix well. Coat chicken pieces with cornflakes mixture. Add coated chicken pieces onto a baking sheet and place in the air fryer basket. Drizzle the olive oil over popcorn chicken. Bake in preheated air fryer for 15-minutes. Serve warm!

NUTRITION: Calories: 235, Total Fat: 8g, Carbs: 14g, Protein: 23g

156. Macaroni Cheese Toast

Cooking Time: 5 minutes

Servings: 2

INGREDIENTS

- 1egg, beaten
- 4tablespoons cheddar cheese, grated
- Salt and pepper to taste
- ½ cup macaroni and cheese
- 4bread slices

DIRECTIONS

1. Spread the cheese and macaroni and cheese over the two bread slices. Place

the other bread slices on top of cheese and cut diagonally. In a bowl, beat egg and season with salt and pepper. Brush the egg mixture onto the bread. Place the bread into air fryer and cook at 300°Fahrenehit for 5-minutes.

NUTRITION: Calories: 250, Total Fat: 16g, Carbs: 9g, Protein: 14g

157. Cheese Burger Patties

Cooking Time: 15 minutes

Servings: 6

INGREDIENTS

- 1lb. ground beef
- 6cheddar cheese slices
- Pepper and salt to taste

DIRECTIONS

1. Preheat your air fryer to 390°Fahrenheit. Season beef with salt and pepper. Make six round shaped patties from the mixture and place them into air fryer basket. Air fry the patties for 10-minutes. Open the air fryer basket and place cheese slices on top of patties and place into air fryer with an additional cook time of 1-minute.

NUTRITION: Calories: 253, Total Fat: 14g, Carbs: 0.4g, Protein: 29g

158. Grilled Cheese Corn

Cooking Time: 15 minutes

Servings: 2

INGREDIENTS

- 2whole corn on the cob, peel husks and discard silk
- 1teaspoon olive oil
- 2teaspoons paprika
- ½ cup feta cheese, grated

DIRECTIONS

1. Rub the olive oil over corn then sprinkle with paprika and rub all over the corn. Preheat your air fryer to 300°Fahrenheit. Place the seasoned corn on the grill for 15-minutes. Place corn on a serving dish then sprinkle with grated cheese over corn. Serve and enjoy!

NUTRITION: Calories: 150, Total Fat: 10g, Carbs: 7g, Protein: 7g

159. Eggplant Fries

Cooking Time: 20 minutes

Servings: 4

INGREDIENTS

- 1eggplant, cut into 3-inch pieces
- ¼ cup of water
- 1tablespoon of olive oil
- 4tablespoons cornstarch
- sea salt to taste

DIRECTIONS

1. Preheat your air fryer to 390°Fahrenheit. In a bowl, combine eggplant, water, oil, and cornstarch. Place the eggplant fries in air fryer basket, and air fry them for 20-minutes. Serve warm and enjoy!

160. Air Fried Pita Bread Pizza

Cooking Time: 6 minutes

Servings: 3

INGREDIENTS

- 1large pita bread

- 1 teaspoon olive oil
- 7 pepperoni slices
- ¼ cup of sausage
- ½ teaspoon garlic, minced
- 1 tablespoon pizza sauce
- ¼ cup mozzarella cheese, shredded
- 1 small onion, finely diced

DIRECTIONS

1. Spread the pizza sauce over the pita bread evenly. Arrange pepperoni, onion, and sausage over pita bread. Sprinkle the top with garlic and cheese. Drizzle the pizza with olive oil then place in air basket. Place on top of trivet and air fry at 350°Fahrenheit for 6-minutes. Serve and enjoy!

161. Light & Crispy Okra

Cooking Time: 10 minutes

Servings: 4

INGREDIENTS

- 3 cups okra, wash and dry
- 1 teaspoon fresh lemon juice
- 1 teaspoon coriander
- 3 tablespoons gram flour
- 2 teaspoons red chili powder
- 1 teaspoon dry mango powder
- 1 teaspoon cumin powder
- Sea salt to taste

DIRECTIONS

1. Cut the top of okra then cut a deep horizontal cut in each okra and set aside. In a bowl, combine gram flour, salt, lemon juice, and all the spices. Add a little water in gram flour mixture and make a thick batter. Fill batter in each okra and place in the air fryer basket. Spray okra with cooking spray. Preheat your air fryer to 350°Fahrenheit for 5-minutes. Air fry the stuffed okra for 10-minutes or until lightly golden brown. Serve and enjoy!

NUTRITION: Calories: 56, Total Fat: 0.8g, Carbs: 9g, Protein: 2g

162. Chili Rellenos

Cooking Time: 35 minutes

Servings: 5

INGREDIENTS

- 2 cans of green chili peppers
- 1 cup of Monterey Jack cheese
- ½ cup milk
- 1 can tomato sauce
- 2 tablespoons almond flour
- 1 can evaporated milk
- 1 cup of cheddar cheese, shredded
- 2 large beaten eggs

DIRECTIONS

1. Preheat the air fryer to 350°Fahrenheit. Spray a baking dish with cooking spray. Take half of the chilies and arrange them in the baking dish. Sprinkle the chilies with half of the cheese and cover with the rest of chilies. In a medium bowl, combine milk, eggs, flour and pour the mixture over the chilies. Air fry for 25-minutes. Remove the chilies from the Air fryer pour tomato sauce over them and cook them for an additional 10-minutes. Remove them from air fryer and top with remaining cheese.

NUTRITION: Calories: 282, Total Fat: 6.2g, Carbs: 7.4g, Protein: 5g

163. Persian Mushrooms

Cooking Time: 20 minutes

Servings: 3

INGREDIENTS

- 6 Portobello large mushrooms
- 3-ounces of softened butter
- 1 cup parmesan cheese, grated
- A pinch of black pepper
- A pinch of sea salt
- 1 tablespoon parsley, fresh, chopped
- 2 cloves of garlic
- 2 large shallots

DIRECTIONS

1. Preheat your air fryer to 390°Fahrenheit. Clean the mushrooms and remove the stems. Slice the shallots and garlic cloves. Now, place the mushroom stems, garlic, shallots, parsley and softened butter into a blender. Arrange the caps of the mushrooms in the air fryer basket. Stuff the caps with the mixture and sprinkle tops with parmesan cheese. Cook for 20-minutes. Serve warm and enjoy!

NUTRITION: Calories: 278, Total Fat: 9.8g, Carbs: 7.2g, Protein: 4.3g

164. Air Fried Chicken Cordon Bleu

Cooking Time: 45 minutes

Servings: 4

INGREDIENTS

- 4 skinless and boneless chicken breasts
- 4 slices of ham
- 4 slices of Swiss cheese
- 3 tablespoons almond flour
- 1 cup of heavy whipping cream
- 1 teaspoon of chicken bouillon granules
- ½ cup dry white wine
- 5 tablespoons butter
- 1 teaspoon paprika

DIRECTIONS

1. Preheat your air fryer to 390°Fahrenheit. Pound the chicken breasts and put a slice of ham and Swiss cheese on each breast. Fold over edges of the chicken; cover the filling and secure the edges with toothpicks. In a bowl, combine flour, and paprika. Coat chicken with this mixture. Set the air fryer to cook the chicken for 15-minutes. In a large skillet, heat the butter, bouillon, and wine then reduce heat to low. Remove the chicken from air fryer and add it to the skillet. Allow the components to simmer for around 30-minutes. Serve warm and enjoy!

NUTRITION: Calories: 389, Total Fat: 12.7g, Carbs: 9.2g, Protein: 32.4g

165. Chicken Noodles

Cooking Time: 25 minutes

Servings: 4

INGREDIENTS

- 4 chicken breasts
- 1 teaspoon rosemary
- 1 teaspoon allspices
- 1 teaspoon red pepper
- 1 teaspoon tomato paste
- 1 tablespoon butter
- 5 cups chicken broth
- Sesame seeds for garnish
- For Noodles:
- 2 beaten eggs
- ½ teaspoon salt
- 2 cups almond flour

DIRECTIONS

1. Preheat your air fryer to 350°Fahrenheit. Coat the chicken with 1 tablespoon of butter, salt, and

pepper. Arrange the chicken breasts in the air fryer basket and cook for 20-minutes. For the noodles, combine egg, salt, and flour to make a dough. Put the dough on a floured surface knead it for a few minutes then cover it and set it aside for 30-minutes. Roll the dough on a floured surface. When the dough is thin, cut it into thin strips and allow them to dry for an hour. Meanwhile, take the chicken out of the air fryer and place aside. Boil the chicken broth and add the noodles, tomato paste and red pepper, cook for 5-minutes. Add the spices and stir noodles. Add salt and pepper to taste. Serve noodles with air fried chicken and garnish with sesame seeds. Serve hot and enjoy!

NUTRITION: Calories: 387, Total Fat: 12.7g, Carbs: 6.8g, Protein: 38.2g

166. Mushroom & Herb Stuffed Pork Chops

Cooking Time: 52 minutes

Servings: 5

INGREDIENTS

- 5thick pork chops
- 7mushrooms, chopped
- 1pinch of herbs
- 1tablespoon almond flour
- 1tablespoon lemon juice
- Salt and black pepper to taste

DIRECTIONS

1. Preheat your air fryer to 325°Fahrenheit. Season both sides of meat with salt and pepper. Arrange the chops in the air fryer and cook for 15-minutes at 350°Fahrenheit. Cook the mushrooms for 3-minutes in a pan over medium heat and stir in lemon juice. Add the flour and herbs to pan and stir. Cook the mixture for 4-minutes, then set aside. Cut five pieces of foil for each chop. O every piece of foil put a chop in the middle and cover it with mushroom mixture. Now, carefully fold the foil and seal around the chop. Place chops back into air fryer and cook for an additional 30-minutes. Serve with salad.

NUTRITION: Calories: 389, Total Fat: 14.2g, Carbs: 9.2g, Protein: 38.5g

167. Roasted Lamb with Pumpkin

Cooking Time: 33 minutes

Servings: 2

INGREDIENTS

- 1lamb rack
- 1tablespoon Dijon mustard
- 2-ounces of almond breadcrumbs
- 2tablespoons herbs, chopped
- Salt and pepper to taste
- 1tablespoon olive oil
- 1-ounce parmesan cheese, grated
- 1-medium pumpkin
- 1-lemon zest

DIRECTIONS

1. Preheat your air fryer to 390°Fahrenheit for 3-minutes. Pat the lamb dry using a towel. Remove the fat and rub the meat with mustard. Blitz the breadcrumbs with herbs, parmesan cheese, lemon zest, and seasonings. Season the joint. Place the meat into air fryer and roast for 15-minutes. For the pumpkin wedges, start by peeling and coring the pumpkin; then coat it with oil. Season the pumpkin then coat it with oil and place it aside. Take the lamb meat out of the air fryer and place it in serving the dish. Add pumpkin wedges to air fryer and roast them for 15-minutes. Once the pumpkin wedges are done, serve with meat!

NUTRITION: Calories: 386, Total Fat: 13.2g, Carbs: 9.3g, Protein: 37.3g

168. Liver Curry

Cooking Time: 35 minutes

Servings: 3

INGREDIENTS

- Coriander leaves
- 4 drops of liquid stevia
- ½ teaspoon ground coriander
- ½ teaspoon turmeric
- 1 teaspoon ginger
- 1 clove of garlic, minced
- 1 large tomato, chopped
- 1 onion, sliced
- ½ lb. of beef liver
- ½ teaspoon of Garam Masala
- 1 teaspoon cumin powder

DIRECTIONS

1. In a pan, fry the onion over medium heat for 5-minutes. Add the garlic and grated ginger and stir. Add the powdered spices, and fry for additional 3-minutes. Meanwhile, season the liver with salt and pepper. Place the liver in the air fryer and cook it for 15-minutes at 350°Fahrenheit. Remove the liver from the air fryer and transfer it to the skillet. Add the chopped tomato, and stevia and a little bit of water, and cook for a few more minutes. Serve and garnish with coriander.

NUTRITION: Calories: 292, Total Fat: 11.2g, Carbs: 8.2g, Protein: 42g

169. Minced Beef Kebab Skewers

Cooking Time: 25 minutes

Servings: 2

INGREDIENTS

- ½ lb. of minced beef
- ½ large onion, chopped
- 1 medium green chili
- ½ teaspoon chili powder
- 1 clove of garlic, minced
- 1 pinch of ginger
- 1 teaspoon Garam Masala
- 3 tablespoons of pork rinds

DIRECTIONS

Grate the ginger and garlic. Chop and deseed the chili. Chop the onion. Mix the ginger, chili, and onion with the minced beef. Add the powdered spices. Add a few pork rinds and salt. Shape the beef into fat sausages around short wooden skewers. Set the skewers aside for an hour, then cook them in your preheated air fryer for 25-minutes at 350°Fahrenheit.

170. Pomfret Fish Fry

Cooking Time: 15-minutes

Servings: 5

INGREDIENTS

- 4 onions
- 3 lbs. of silver Pomfret
- Salt and black pepper to taste
- 2 tablespoons olive oil
- 2 teaspoons lemon juice
- 3 pinches of cumin powder
- ¾ teaspoons of ginger
- 3 pinches of red chili powder
- 1 tablespoon turmeric powder
- 1 teaspoon garlic paste

DIRECTIONS

1. Wash the fish with clean water and soak it in lemon juice to remove any unpleasant smell. After 30-minutes, take the fish out and wash it with clean

water. Draw diagonal shaped slits on the fish. Combine the black pepper, salt, lemon juice, garlic paste, and turmeric powder. Rub the mixture inside and outside of fish and leave it in the fridge for 30-minutes to absorb the seasoning. Add the fish to air fryer basket with 2 tablespoons olive oil and cook for 12-minutes at 340°Fahrenheit.

NUTRITION: Calories: 278, Total Fat: 8.6g, Carbs: 7.4g, Protein: 32g

171. Cedar Planked Salmon

Cooking Time: 15 minutes

Servings: 6

INGREDIENTS

- 4 untreated cedar planks
- ½ cup olive oil
- 1½ tablespoons of rice vinegar
- 1 teaspoon sesame oil
- 2 lbs. of salmon fillets, skin removed
- 1 teaspoon garlic, minced
- 1 tablespoon ginger root, fresh, grated
- ¼ cup green onions, chopped
- ½ cup soy sauce

DIRECTIONS

1. Start by soaking the cedar planks for 2-hours. Take a shallow baking dish and stir in the olive oil, the rice vinegar, the sesame oil, soy sauce, ginger, and green onions. Place the salmon fillets in the prepared marinade for at least 20-minutes. Place the planks in the basket of your air fryer. Cook the salmon fillets for 15-minutes at 360°Fahrenheit.

NUTRITION: Calories: 273, Total Fat: 7.5g, Carbs: 5.2g, Protein: 34.2g

172. Crested Halibut

Cooking Time: 30 minutes

Servings: 4

INGREDIENTS

- 4 halibut fillets
- ¾ cup of pork rinds
- ½ cup of parsley, fresh, chopped
- ¼ cup dill, fresh, chopped
- ¼ cup chives, fresh, chopped
- 1 tablespoon olive oil
- 1 teaspoon lemon zest, finely grated
- Sea salt and black pepper to taste

DIRECTIONS

1. Preheat your air fryer to 390°Fahrenheit. In a mixing bowl, combine the pork rinds, parsley, dill, chives, olive oil, lemon zest, sea salt and black pepper. Rinse the halibut fillets and dry them on a paper towel. Arrange the halibut fillets and dry them on a paper towel. Arrange the halibut fillets onto a baking sheet. Spoon the pork rind crumb mixture onto fish fillets. Lightly press the mixture on the fillets. Bake the fillets in your preheated air fryer basket for 30-minutes. Serve warm.

NUTRITION: Calories: 272, Total Fat: 10.3g, Carbs: 9.4g, Protein: 32.2g

173. Creamy Halibut

Cooking Time: 20 minutes

Servings: 6

INGREDIENTS

- 2 lbs. of halibut fillets, cut into 6 pieces
- 1 teaspoon dill weed, dried
- ½ cup light sour cream
- ½ cup light mayonnaise

- 4 chopped green onions

DIRECTIONS

1. Preheat the air fryer to 390°Fahrenheit. Season the halibut with salt and pepper. In a bowl, mix the onions, sour cream, mayonnaise, and dill. Spread the onion mixture evenly over the halibut fillets. Cook in air fryer for 20-minutes. Serve warm.

NUTRITION: Calories: 286, Total Fat: 11.3g, Carbs: 6.9, Protein: 29.8g

174. Air Fried Catfish

Cooking Time: 20 minutes

Servings: 2

INGREDIENTS

- 5 catfish filets
- 1 pinch of salt
- 1 teaspoon garlic powder
- 1 teaspoon crab seasoning
- 1 cup almond flour
- 2 tablespoons olive oil for spraying
- 2 tablespoons hot sauce
- 1 cup buttermilk
- Black pepper as needed

DIRECTIONS

1. Season catfish fillets on both sides with salt and pepper. In a dish, combine the buttermilk with hot sauce. Add the catfish fillets and cover them with liquid. Let the ingredients soak while you prepare the rest of the ingredients. Whisk the flour, crab seasoning, and garlic powder in a casserole dish. Remove the catfish from the buttermilk and allow excess liquid to drip off. Dredge the catfish on both sides in the flour mixture. Place fillets into air fryer and drizzle with oil. Cook at 390°Fahrenheit for 15-minutes. When cooking is completed remove basket and gently turn the fillets over, spray some oil on them, and cook for an additional 5-minutes.

NUTRITION: Calories: 283, Total Fat: 8.6g, Carbs: 6.5g, Protein: 34.3g

175. Air Fried Spinach Fish

Cooking Time: 12 minutes

Servings: 2

INGREDIENTS

- 4 ounces of spinach leaves
- 1 large egg, beaten
- 2 tablespoons olive oil
- 2 cups almond flour
- 2 white fish fillets
- Pinch of sea salt
- Black pepper to taste

DIRECTIONS

1. In a deep bowl, place the beaten egg, almond flour, sea salt, black pepper, and spinach leaves. Marinate the fish for 2-hours in the fridge. Transfer the fish to air fryer and cook for 12-minutes at 370°Fahrenheit. Serve with lemon slices.

NUTRITION: Calories: 286, Total Fat: 11.2g, Carbs: 5.2g, Protein: 29.7g

176. Roly Poly Air Fried White Fish

Cooking Time: 10 minutes

Servings: 4

INGREDIENTS

- 4 lbs. of white fish fillets
- 2½ teaspoons of sea salt
- 4 mushrooms, sliced

- 1 teaspoon liquid stevia
- 2 tablespoons of Chinese winter pickle
- 2 tablespoons of vinegar
- 2 teaspoons chili powder
- 2 onions, thinly sliced
- 1 cup vegetable stock
- 2 tablespoons soy sauce

DIRECTIONS

1. Fill the fish fillets with mushrooms and pickle. Cut the onions into thinly sliced pieces. Spread the onions over the fish fillets. Combine the stock, soy sauce, vinegar, sea salt, and stevia. Sprinkle the mixture over the fish fillets. Place the fish fillets into your air fryer and cook at 350°Fahrenheit for 10-minutes. Serve warm.

NUTRITION: Calories: 278, Total Fat: 9.2g, Carbs: 7.4g, Protein: 33.2g

177. Air Fried Dragon Shrimp

Cooking Time: 15 minutes

Servings: 2

INGREDIENTS

- ½ lb. shrimp
- ¼ cup almond flour
- Pinch of ginger
- 1 cup chopped green onions
- 2 tablespoons olive oil
- 2 eggs, beaten
- ½ cup soy sauce

DIRECTIONS

1. Boil the shrimps for 5-minutes. Prepare a paste made of ginger and onion. Now, beat the eggs, add the ginger paste, soya sauce and almond flour and combine well. Add the shrimps to the mixture then place them in a baking dish and spray with oil. Cook shrimps at 390°Fahrenheit for 10-minutes.

NUTRITION: Calories: 278, Total Fat: 8.6g, Carbs: 6.2g, Protein: 28.6g

178. Lasagna Zucchini Cups

Cooking Time: 25 minutes

Servings: 6

INGREDIENTS

Chopped parsley, for garnish

- ¼ cup parmesan, freshly grated
- ½ cup mozzarella, shredded
- ½ cup ricotta
- 1-14.5-ounce can of crushed tomatoes
- Black pepper and salt to taste
- ½ teaspoon oregano, dried
- ½ lb. ground beef
- 2 garlic cloves, minced
- ½ onion, chopped
- 1 tablespoon olive oil
- 3 zucchinis

DIRECTIONS

1. In a large pan over medium heat, add the oil. Add onion and garlic and cook for 5-minutes. Add in the ground beef and cook for 10-minutes stirring often. Season with oregano, salt, pepper, cook until meat is no longer pink. Add crushed tomatoes and simmer mixture for 5-minutes. Stir in the ricotta and remove from heat. Cut zucchini in half crosswise in two. Using a spoon scoop out zucchini flesh to create wells. Fill wells with meat mixture. Top with mozzarella and parmesan cheese. Place directly in air fryer and cook at 350°Fahrenheit for 15-minutes. Garnish with parsley and parmesan.

179. Spinach Artichoke Stuffed Peppers

Cooking Time: 15 minutes

Servings: 4

INGREDIENTS

- 4 assorted bell peppers,
- halved and seeded
- Salt and black pepper to taste
- Olive oil for drizzling
- 2 cups shredded rotisserie chicken
- Fresh parsley, chopped for garnish
- 2 cloves garlic, minced
- ¼ cup mayonnaise
- ¼ cup sour cream
- ½ cup mozzarella, shredded, divided
- 6-ounces cream cheese, softened
- 1 (10-ounce package frozen spinach, thawed, well-drained, and chopped
- 1 (14-ounce can artichoke hearts, drained and chopped

DIRECTIONS

1. On a large, rimmed baking sheet, place bell peppers cut side-up and drizzle with olive oil, then season with salt and pepper. In a large bowl, combine chicken, artichoke hearts, spinach, cream cheese, ½ cup mozzarella, parmesan, sour cream, mayo and garlic. Season with more salt and pepper and mix until well blended. Divide the chicken mixture between pepper halves, top with remaining mozzarella, and bake in air fryer at 400°Fahrenheit for 15-minutes. Garnish with parsley and serve.

NUTRITION: Calories: 284, Total Fat: 13.4g, Carbs: 9.2g, Protein: 34.3g

180. Cauliflower Shepherd's Pie

Cooking Time: 43 minutes

Servings: 4

INGREDIENTS

- 1 medium head of cauliflower, cut into florets
- ¼ cup whole milk
- 3-ounces cream cheese, softened
- 1 tablespoon parsley, chopped for garnish
- 2/3 cup chicken broth
- 2 tablespoons almond flour
- 1 cup frozen peas
- 1 lb. ground beef
- 2 cloves garlic, minced
- 2 carrots, peeled, and chopped
- 1 large onion, chopped
- 1 tablespoon olive oil
- Salt and black pepper to taste

DIRECTIONS:

1. Make mashed cauliflower. Bring a pot of water to boil, add the florets and cook for 10-minutes. Drain pot and then use paper towel to absorb excess water. Return florets to pot and mash with potato masher until smooth. Stir in cream cheese, milk and season with salt and pepper. Set aside. Make the beef mixture: in large pan over medium heat, heat oil. Add onion, garlic and cook for 5-minutes.
2. Add ground beef for 5-minutes or until meat is no longer pink. Stir in frozen peas and corn and cook another 3-minutes. Sprinkle meat mixture with almond flour and stir to even distribute. Cook for another minute then add chicken broth. Bring to a simmer and let mixture thicken slightly, for 5-minutes. Place beef mixture in air fryer baking dish. Top beef mixture with an even layer of cauliflower and bake in air fryer at 400°Fahrenheit for 15-minutes. Garnish with parsley and serve.

NUTRITION: Calories: 279, Total Fat: 13.2g, Carbs: 10.2g, Protein: 34.2g

181. Coconut Lime Skirt Steak

Cooking Time: 5 minutes

Servings: 2

INGREDIENTS

- ½ cup coconut oil, melted
- Zest of one lime
- 2-1lb. grass fed skirt steaks
- ¾ teaspoon sea salt
- 1 teaspoon red pepper flakes
- 1 teaspoon ginger, fresh, grated
- 1 tablespoon garlic, minced
- 2 tablespoons freshly squeezed lime juice

DIRECTIONS

1. In a mixing bowl, combine lime juice, coconut oil, garlic, ginger, red pepper, salt, and zest. Add the steaks and toss and rub with marinade. Allow the meat to marinate for about 20-minutes at room temperature. Transfer steaks to your air fryer directly on the rack. Cook steaks in air fryer at 400°Fahrenhet for 5-minutes.

NUTRITION: Calories: 312, Total Fat: 12.3g, Carbs: 6.4g, Protein: 42.1g

182. Spicy Chicken Enchilada Casserole

Cooking Time: 40 minutes

Servings: 2

INGREDIENTS

- 1lb. of chicken breasts, skinless and boneless
- Salt and pepper to taste
- ½ cup cilantro, fresh, minced
- Olive oil spray
- 2 cups cheddar cheese, shredded
- Lime wedges (optional
- Sour cream (optional
- 1(4-ouncecan of green chilies, chopped
- 1 cup feta cheese, finely crumbled
- 1½ cup enchilada sauce

DIRECTIONS

1. Pat the chicken breasts dry and season with salt and pepper. Combine the chicken and enchilada sauce in a pan and simmer for 15-minutes over medium-low heat. Flip chicken over and cover and cook for an additional 15-minutes. Remove the chicken from pan and shred into bite-size pieces. Combine shredded chicken, feta cheese, enchilada sauce, chiles, and cilantro in a bowl. Add salt and pepper. Spray the air fryer basking dish with olive oil. Coat the entire bottom and sides. Evenly spread a cup of shredded cheese on the bottom of baking dish. Add the chicken mixture, then add another cup of cheese on top. Bake in your air fryer at 350°Fahrenheit for 10-minutes. Serve with optional lime wedges and sour cream.

NUTRITION: Calories: 338, Total Fat: 12.3g, Carbs: 8.3g, Protein: 32.2g

183. Kale & Ground Beef Casserole

Cooking Time: 16 minutes

Servings: 4

INGREDIENTS

- 4-ounces mozzarella, shredded
- 2 cups marinara sauce
- 10-ounces kale, fresh
- 1 teaspoon oregano
- 1 teaspoon onion powder
- ½ teaspoon sea salt
- 1lb. lean ground beef

- 2 tablespoons olive oil

DIRECTIONS

1. in a deep skillet, heat the olive oil for 2-minutes, add in the ground beef and cook for an additional 8-minutes or until meat is browned. stir in salt, pepper, garlic powder, onion powder and oregano. in batches, stir the kale into beef mixture, cooking for another 2-minutes. stir in the marinara sauce and cook for 2-minutes more. mix in half the cheese into mixture. transfer mixture into the air fryer baking dish. sprinkle the remaining cheese on top. broil in air fryer at 400°fahrenheit for 2-minutes. allow to rest for 5-minutes before serving.

NUTRITION: Calories: 312, Total Fat: 13.2, Carbs: 9.2g, Protein: 43.2g

184. Cauliflower-Cottage Pie

Cooking Time: 40 minutes

Servings: 4

INGREDIENTS

- Half a cup of bacon bits
- 2 cups cauliflower rice
- ¼ cup tomato puree
- 1 tablespoon coconut oil
- ½ white onion, chopped
- 2 lbs. lean ground beef
- 1 tablespoon mixed spice blend

DIRECTIONS

1. In the frying pan add coconut oil and onions cook for 2-minutes. Add the ground beef into pan and cook for an additional 5-minutes or until meat is browned. Add spices and stir to combine. Add the tomato puree and mix well and cook for another 10-minutes. Transfer to air fryer baking dish. Top with cauliflower rice and bacon bits. Bake in air fryer at 350°Fahrenheit for 20-minutes. Serve warm.

NUTRITION: Calories: 367, Total Fat: 13.4g, Carbs: 11.2g, Protein: 43.1g

185. Roasted Asian Shrimp & Brussels Sprouts

Cooking Time: 19 minutes

Servings: 4

INGREDIENTS

- 1 lb. jumbo frozen shrimp, thawed and drained
- 1 lb. brussels sprouts
- 2 tablespoons olive oil
- Salt and pepper to taste
- Asian Marinade Sauce:
- 2 tablespoons rice vinegar
- 2 tablespoons Splenda
- 2 teaspoons liquid stevia
- 1 tablespoon Asian sesame oil
- ½ teaspoon garlic powder
- 1/3 cup soy sauce

DIRECTIONS

1. About 20-minutes before you start cooking, place the shrimp into a colander and place it in the sink and let shrimp drain. Mix the soy sauce, stevia, rice vinegar, sesame oil, and garlic powder to make marinade mixture. After the shrimp have drained well, layer them on a paper towel an blot dry, so they are as dry as you can get them. Place dried shrimp into Ziploc bag with half of the marinade and allow the shrimp to marinate while you cook the brussels sprouts. Trim the stem ends off each brussels sprout and cut in half. Place brussels sprouts into a bowl and toss with

desired amount of olive oil, salt and pepper.
2. Spread brussels sprouts out in a single layer in your air fryer and roast at 400°Fahrenheit for 15-minutes. Keep brussels sprouts in air fryer and move to one side. Add shrimp beside them in air fryer. Roast for an additional 4-minutes. Remove from air fryer and place into serving bowl, add remaining marinade into bowl and give dish a stir. Serve immediately.

NUTRITION: Calories: 267, Total Fat: 11.2g, Carbs: 8.3g, Protein: 9.2g

186. Grilled Chicken with Garlic Sauce

Cooking Time: 15-minutes

Servings: 4

INGREDIENTS

- 1lb. chicken breast, cut into large cubes
- 2bell peppers, chopped
- 1zucchini
- 1onion, chopped
- For Garlic Sauce:
- 1head garlic, peeled
- ¼ cup lemon juice
- 1cup olive oil
- 1teaspoon salt
- Additional ingredients for the marinade:
- 1teaspoon salt
- ½ cup olive oil

DIRECTIONS

1. Soak 4 wooden skewers in water. For your garlic sauce, place garlic cloves and salt into blender. Then, add in about 1/8 of a cup of lemon juice and ½ a cup of olive oil. Blend for about 10-seconds. Keep half of the garlic sauce to serve with. Take the other half of garlic sauce and add an additional ½ cup of olive oil and a teaspoon of salt and mix well—this will make your marinade. Chop up the chicken, onion, bell peppers, and zucchini into 1-inch cubes or squares. Mix them in a bowl with the marinade. Place the cubes onto the skewers and cook them directly on the air fryer rack at 400°Fahrenheit for 15-minutes. Serve warm.

NUTRITION: Calories: 321, Total Fat: 12.5g, Carbs: 9.2g, Protein: 32.1g

187. Bacon-Wrapped Stuffed Zucchini Boats

Cooking Time: 15 minutes

Servings: 4

INGREDIENTS

- ½ a teaspoon of fresh ground black pepper
- 1teaspoon sea salt
- 5-ounces cream cheese
- 8-mushrooms, finely chopped
- 1tablespoon Italian parsley, chopped
- 1tablespoon finely chopped dill
- 3garlic cloves, peeled, pressed
- 1sweet red pepper, finely chopped
- 2large zucchinis
- 12bacon strips
- 1medium onion, chopped

DIRECTIONS

1. Preheat your air fryer to 350°Fahrenheit. Trim the ends off zucchini. Cut zucchini in half lengthwise. Scoop out pulp, leaving ¼-inch thick shells. Stir pulp in mixing bowl. Add onion, garlic, herbs, pepper, cream cheese, salt, and pepper. Mix well to combine. Fill individual shells with the same amount of stuffing. Wrap three bacon strips around each zucchini boat

such that the ends end up underneath. Place them directly on the air fryer rack and bake turning the temperature up to 375°Fahrenheit for 15-minutes. Remove and serve immediately.

NUTRITION: Calories: 282, Total Fat: 9.1g, Carbs: 6.3g, Protein: 24.2g

188. Parmesan Chicken Wings

Cooking Time: 22 minutes

Servings: 4

INGREDIENTS

- 2lbs. chicken wings
- 2tablespoons olive oil
- 1teaspoon sea salt
- 1teaspoon black pepper
- 3tablespoons butter
- 3tablespoons olive oil
- 3garlic cloves, minced
- 4tablespoons parmesan cheese
- 1/8 teaspoon smoked paprika
- ¼ teaspoon red pepper flakes
- Salt and pepper to taste

DIRECTIONS

1. Add chicken to a bowl and pat the chicken dry. Drizzle with 2 tablespoons of olive oil, 1 teaspoon of sea salt, and 1 teaspoon black pepper. Gently toss to coat chicken. Place chicken wings into air fryer directly on the rack. Bake at 400°Fahrenheit for 20-minutes, flipping wings half-way through cook time. In a pan over medium heat add butter and 3 tablespoons olive oil and melt the butter down, for about 3-minutes. Add 2 tablespoons of parmesan cheese, smoked paprika, red pepper flakes, salt and pepper to taste. Cook sauce for about 2-minutes. Remove the wings from air fryer and place in large bowl. Pour the garlic parmesan sauce over the wings toss to coat. Serve wings topped with additional a2 tablespoons of parmesan cheese.

NUTRITION: Calories: 324, Total Fat: 12.3g, Carbs: 9.3g, Protein: 39.3g

189. Beef Burgers

Cooking Time: 10 minutes

Servings: 4

INGREDIENTS

- 1lb. ground beef
- 1teaspoon parsley, dried
- ½ teaspoon oregano, dried
- ½ teaspoon ground black pepper
- ½ teaspoon salt
- ½ teaspoon onion powder
- ½ teaspoon garlic powder
- 1tablespoon Worcestershire sauce
- Olive oil cooking spray

DIRECTIONS

1. In a mixing bowl, mix the seasonings. Add the seasoning to beef in a bowl. Mix well to combine. Divide the beef into four patties, put an indent in the middle of patties with your thumb to prevent patties from bunching up in the middle. Place burgers into air fryer and spray the tops of them with olive oil. Cook for 10-minutes at 400°Fahrenheit, no need to flip patties. Serve on a bun with a side dish of your choice.

NUTRITION: Calories: 312, Total Fat: 11.3g, Carbs: 7.2g, Protein: 39.2g

190. Bacon Wrapped Avocado

Cooking Time: 10 minutes

Servings: 2

INGREDIENTS

- 2 avocados, fresh and firm
- Chili powder
- Ground cumin
- 4 thick slices of hickory smoked bacon

DIRECTIONS

1. Slice the avocados into wedges and peel off the skin. Stretch the bacon strips this will help to elongate them. Slice avocados in half. Next, take half a bacon strip and wrap one around each avocado wedge and tuck the ends under the bottom. Sprinkle wedges with chili powder and cumin. Bake the bacon wrapped avocado wedges in air fryer at 400°Fahrenheit for 10-minutes. Serve with your favorite salad!

NUTRITION: Calories: 276, Total Fat: 7.3g, Carbs: 6.3g, Protein: 21g

191. Buffalo Chicken Meatballs

Cooking Time: 20 minutes

Servings: 4

INGREDIENTS

- 1 lb. ground chicken
- 1 egg, beaten
- 1 celery stalk, trimmed and finely diced
- 1 cup buffalo wing sauce
- 1 teaspoon black pepper
- 1 teaspoon pink sea salt
- 1 teaspoon garlic powder
- 1 teaspoon onion powder
- 1 tablespoon mayonnaise
- 1 tablespoon almond flour
- 2 sprigs of green onion, finely chopped

DIRECTIONS

1. Place the baking pan in air fryer and spray with olive oil. In a bowl, combine all ingredients, except buffalo sauce. Mix well. Use your hands to form 2-inch balls. Place the meatballs in air fryer and bake at 350°Fahrenheit for 15-minutes. Remove the meatballs from the air fryer. Add them to a pan over medium-low heat. Coat meatballs with buffalo sauce and stir cooking in pan for 5-minutes. Serve.

NUTRITION: Calories: 302, Total Fat: 12.4g, Carbs: 7.6g, Protein: 32.1g

192. Caprese Grilled Chicken with Balsamic Vinegar

Cooking Time: 20 minutes

Servings: 6

INGREDIENTS

- 6 grilled chicken breasts, boneless, skinless
- 6 large basil leaves
- 6 slices of tomato
- 6 slices of mozzarella cheese
- 1 tablespoon butter
- ¼ cup balsamic vinegar

DIRECTIONS

1. Prepare chicken in air fryer at 400°Fahrenheit for 15-minutes or until chicken is cooked. As chicken is cooking, pour balsamic vinegar into the pan and cook until reduced by half, for about 5-minutes. Add in the butter and stir with a flat whisk until well combined. Set aside. Top chicken with mozzarella cheese slices, basil leaves, and tomato slice each. Drizzle with balsamic reduction and serve warm.

NUTRITION: Calories: 289, Total Fat: 11.3g, Carbs: 7.2g, Protein: 28g

193. Philly Cheese Steak Stuffed Peppers

Cooking Time: 40 minutes

Servings: 2

INGREDIENTS

- 8-ounces of roast beef, thinly sliced
- 8-slices of provolone cheese
- 2 large green bell peppers
- 1 medium sweet onion, diced
- 1 (6-ounce) package of baby Bella mushrooms
- 1 tablespoon garlic, minced
- 2 tablespoons olive oil
- 2 tablespoons butter

DIRECTIONS

1. Cut your peppers in half lengthwise, removing ribs and seeds. Slice onions and mushrooms. Sauté over medium heat with butter, olive oil, a dash of salt, pepper, and minced garlic. Cook for 20-minutes or until the mushrooms and onions are sweet and caramelized. Slice the roast beef into thin strips and add to the onion/mushroom mixture. Allow cooking for 10-minutes. In the inside of each pepper line it with a slice of provolone cheese. Fill each pepper with meat mixture. Garnish top of each pepper with another slice of provolone cheese. Bake in the air fryer at 375°Fahrenhiet for 10-minutes.

NUTRITION: Calories: 298, Total Fat: 11.5g, Carbs: 8.2g, Protein: 39.2g

194. Parmesan, Garlic, Lemon Roasted Zucchini

Cooking Time: 10 minutes

Servings: 4

INGREDIENTS

- 1½ lbs. zucchini (about 4 small zucchini)
- Salt and pepper to taste
- ¾ cup parmesan cheese, finely shredded
- 2 cloves garlic, minced
- Zest of 1 lemon
- 2 tablespoons olive oil

DIRECTIONS

1. Cut zucchini into thick wedges or halves (cut each zucchini in half then that half in half, so you have 4 wedges from each zucchini. In a bowl, stir olive oil, garlic, and lemon zest. Align zucchini in air fryer space them evenly apart. Brush olive oil mixture over tops of zucchini. Sprinkle tops with parmesan cheese and season lightly with salt and pepper. Bake in air fryer at 375°Fahrenheit for 10-minutes. Serve warm.

195. Chicken Filet Stuffed with Sausage

Cooking Time: 15 minutes

Servings: 4

INGREDIENTS

- 4 chicken fillets
- 4 sausages, casings removed

DIRECTIONS

1. Place the sausage inside the chicken filets and roll the fillets. Seal with 2 toothpicks each. Air fry the chicken filets at 375°Fahrenheit for 15-minutes. Serve warm.

NUTRITION: Calories: 276, Total Fat: 12.2g, Carbs: 8.2g, Protein: 28g

196. Bourbon Chicken

Cooking Time: 22 minutes

Servings: 4

INGREDIENTS

- 3lbs. of chicken wings
- ¾ cups ketchup
- ¼ teaspoon cayenne
- ¼ cup Bourbon
- 2 teaspoons smoked paprika
- ½ cup water
- 2 garlic cloves, crushed
- ¼ cup onion, minced
- 2 teaspoons stevia
- 1 tablespoon liquid smoke
- 1 teaspoon salt
- ½ teaspoon black pepper

DIRECTIONS

1. In a bowl, mix liquid smoke, onion, garlic, ketchup, stevia and cook for 5-minutes in an electric pressure cooker on Sauté function. Combine the rest of your ingredients and cook on high pressure for 5-minutes. Do a quick release of pressure and then transfer the chicken wings into the air fryer basket. Cook wings in air fryer for 6-minutes at 400°Fahrenheit. Dip wings into sauce and air fry for another 6-minutes. Serve hot!

NUTRITION: Calories: 302, Total Fat: 12.5g, Carbs: 8.4g, Protein: 32.4g

197. Roasted Chicken Legs

Cooking Time: 35 minutes

Servings: 2

INGREDIENTS

- 2 chicken legs
- 2 teaspoons sweet smoked paprika
- 1 teaspoon honey
- Salt and pepper to taste
- ½ teaspoon garlic powder
- Fresh parsley, chopped for garnish
- 1 lime sliced for garnish

DIRECTIONS

1. Combine all the ingredients except the chicken in a bowl. Rub the mixture over the chicken and preheat your air fryer for 3-minutes. Cook the chicken in air fryer at 390°Fahrenheit for 35-minutes. Serve with a favorite salad of your choice.

NUTRITION: Calories: 232, Total Fat: 9.3g, Carbs: 7.5g, Protein: 22.1g

198. Mongolian Chicken

Cooking Time: 17 minutes

Servings: 4

INGREDIENTS

- 4 chicken breasts, boneless, skinless, chopped small pieces
- 1 yellow onion, thinly sliced
- Olive oil for frying
- 1 Chili Padi, chopped
- 3 garlic cloves, minced
- 5 curry leaves
- 1 teaspoon ginger, grated
- ¾ cup evaporated milk
- Marinade:
- 1 egg
- 1 tablespoon light soy sauce
- Self-raising flour to coat
- ½ tablespoon cornstarch
- Seasonings:
- 1 teaspoon liquid stevia
- 1 tablespoon chili sauce
- ½ teaspoon sea salt
- Dash of black pepper

DIRECTIONS

1. Combine all of you marinade ingredients in a bowl and marinate the chicken with it for an hour. Dredge the chicken in the self-raising flour and spray some oil over. Cook in air fryer for 10-minutes at 390°Fahrenheit. Heat a wok and sauté the ginger, garlic, chili padi, curry leaves and onions for 2-minutes. Add the chicken and seasonings, stirring to combine well. Add your milk and cook until thickened. Serve hot!

NUTRITION: Calories: 286, Total Fat: 11.3g, Carbs: 6.4g, Protein: 28g

199. Chicken Drumsticks with Spinach Sauce

Preparation time: 15 minutes

Cooking time: 20 minutes

Servings: 4

INGREDIENTS

- 15oz chicken drumsticks
- 1up fresh spinach
- 1tablespoon olive oil
- ½ teaspoon minced garlic
- 1tablespoon walnuts
- 1teaspoon coconut oil
- ½ teaspoon thyme

DIRECTIONS

1. Pour the coconut oil into the air fryer basket.
2. Sprinkle the chicken drumsticks with the minced garlic and thyme and place them in the air fryer basket.
3. Cook the chicken for 5 minutes at 400 F. Stir it frequently.
4. Meanwhile, blend together the fresh spinach, olive oil, and walnuts.
5. Transfer the blended mixture over the drumsticks and cook them for 15 minutes at 370 F.
6. When the time is over and the chicken drumsticks are cooked – let them chill little.
7. Enjoy!

NUTRITION: Calories 234, Fat 11.9, Fiber 0.4, Carbs 0.7, Protein 30

200. Parsley Meatballs

Preparation time: 10 minutes

Cooking time: 10 minutes

Servings: 3

INGREDIENTS

- 1tablespoon fresh parsley, chopped
- 1teaspoon dried parsley
- 1cup ground pork
- ¼ teaspoon cayenne pepper
- ½ teaspoon salt
- 1tablespoon olive oil

DIRECTIONS

1. olive oil.
2. Add the meatballs and cook them for 10 minutes at 380 F. Stir the meatballs half-way.
3. Serve the cooked meatballs immediately!
4. Blend the chopped parsley and combine it together with the dried parsley, ground pork, cayenne pepper, and salt.
5. Mix the mixture up and make the medium meatballs.
6. Spray the air fryer with the

NUTRITION: calories 122, fat 6.7, fiber 0.1, carbs 0.2, protein 14.9

201. Paprika Beef Short Ribs

Preparation time: 20 minutes

Cooking time: 18 minutes

Servings: 8

INGREDIENTS

- 2-pound beef short ribs
- 1teaspoon salt
- 1tablespoon ground paprika
- 1teaspoon cilantro
- ½ teaspoon basil, dried
- 1tablespoon olive oil

DIRECTIONS

1. Sprinkle the ribs with the salt, ground paprika, cilantro, basil, and olive oil.
2. Stir the meat carefully and leave for 10 minutes to marinate.
3. After this, put the beef short ribs in the air fryer and cook at 400 F for 18 minutes. Stir the meat every 4 minutes.
4. Then transfer the cooked short ribs in the serving bowl and serve immediately!

NUTRITION: Calories 250, Fat 12.1, Fiber 0.3, Carbs 0.5, Protein 32.9

202. Lamb Burger

Preparation time: 15 minutes

Cooking time: 20 minutes

Servings: 6

INGREDIENTS

- 10oz lamb fillet
- 1teaspoon thyme
- ½ teaspoon minced garlic
- ½ teaspoon ground paprika
- ½ teaspoon salt
- 1teaspoon olive oil

DIRECTIONS

1. Chop the lamb fillet into the tiny pieces.
2. Sprinkle the meat with the thyme, minced garlic, ground paprika, and salt.
3. Stir it carefully until homogenous/
4. After this, make the medium burgers from the lamb meat mixture.
5. Pour the olive oil in the air fryer basket and add the lamb burgers.
6. Cook the lamb burgers for 20 minutes (10 minutes from each sideat 375 F.
7. Enjoy!

NUTRITION: Calories 271, Fat 11.2, Fiber 0.1, Carbs 0.3, Protein 39.8

203. Pesto Chicken

Preparation time: 10 minutes

Cooking time: 15 minutes

Servings: 6

INGREDIENTS

- 1tablespoon cashews
- 2cups fresh basil
- 1cup fresh spinach
- 2garlic cloves, chopped
- 4tablespoon olive oil
- ¼ teaspoon salt
- 2-pound chicken breast
- 1teaspoon ground black pepper
- 1teaspoon coconut oil
- ½ teaspoon cayenne pepper

DIRECTIONS

1. Place the cashews, fresh basil, fresh spinach, chopped garlic, olive oil, salt,

ground black pepper, and coconut oil in the blender.
2. Add cayenne pepper and blend the mixture until smooth.
3. Place the chicken breast in the air fryer basket.
4. Then pour the blended pesto mixture over the chicken breast and stir it gently.
5. Cook the chicken breast for 15 minutes at 380 F. Stir it time to time.
6. Check if the chicken is cooked and let it rest for 10 minutes.
7. Slice the chicken breast and serve it!

NUTRITION: Calories 273, Fat 14.7, Fiber 0.4, Carbs 1.5, Protein 32.8

204. Lemon Trout

Preparation time: 10 minutes

Cooking time: 12 minutes

Servings: 4

INGREDIENTS

- 1-pound trout
- ½ lemon
- ¼ teaspoon chili flakes
- ½ teaspoon salt
- ½ teaspoon ground coriander
- 1 tablespoon olive oil
- 1 tablespoon basil

DIRECTIONS

1. Slice the lemon.
2. Rub the fish with the chili flakes, salt, ground coriander, basil, and olive oil carefully.
3. Then fill the fish with the sliced lemon and transfer it to the air fryer basket.
4. Cook the trout for 12 minutes at 375 F.
5. When the trout is cooked – serve it hot!

NUTRITION: Calories 248, Fat 13.1, Fiber 0.2, Carbs 0.7, Protein 30.3

205. Stuffed Salmon Fillet with Tomatoes

Preparation time: 15 minutes

Cooking time: 15 minutes

Servings: 6

INGREDIENTS

- 2-pound salmon fillet
- 1 teaspoon minced garlic
- ¼ cup fresh basil
- ¼ cup cherry tomatoes
- 1 tablespoon olive oil
- ½ teaspoon dried dill

DIRECTIONS

1. Blend the fresh basil until smooth.
2. Then sprinkle the salmon fillet with the dried dill, olive oil, and minced garlic.
3. Make the cut in the salmon fillet and fill it with the blended basil and cherry tomatoes.
4. Secure the cut with the toothpicks if desired.
5. Place the salmon in the air fryer basket and cook it for 15 minutes at 385 F.
6. When the salmon is cooked – serve it only hot!

NUTRITION: Calories 222, Fat 11.7, Fiber 0.1, Carbs 0.5, Protein 29.5

206. Tomato Beef Brisket

Preparation time: 35 minutes

Cooking time: 30 minutes

Servings: 6

INGREDIENTS

- 17oz beef brisket
- ½ cup tomato
- 1cup fresh basil
- 1teaspoon cayenne pepper
- 1tablespoon olive oil
- 1teaspoon turmeric

DIRECTIONS

1. Put the tomatoes in the blender and blend them well.
2. Add fresh basil and blend the mixture until smooth.
3. After this, pour the tomato mixture over the beef brisket.
4. Sprinkle it with the cayenne pepper, olive oil, and turmeric and stir carefully.
5. Let it marinate for 20 minutes.
6. Then place the beef brisket in the air fryer basket and cook it at 370 F for 30 minutes. Stir the beef every 5 minutes.
7. When the meat is cooked – let it chill for 5 minutes and serve it!

NUTRITION: Calories 175, Fat 7.5, Fiber 0.4, Carbs 1.1, Protein 24.7

207. Seafood Bowl

Preparation time: 10 minutes

Cooking time: 11 minutes

Servings: 4

INGREDIENTS

- 10oz shrimps, peeled
- 8oz salmon fillet
- 7oz scallops
- 1teaspoon ground coriander
- 1teaspoon minced garlic
- 1tablespoon lemon juice
- 1tablespoon olive oil
- ¼ onion, diced

DIRECTIONS

1. Combine together the ground coriander, minced garlic, lemon juice, olive oil, and diced onion in the mixing bowl.
2. Stir the mixture well.
3. Then separate the mixture into 3 bowls.
4. Chop the salmon fillet and sprinkle with the 1 part of the spicy mixture.
5. Stir well and place in the air fryer basket.
6. Cook the salmon for 5 minutes at 400 F. Stir it after 3 minutes of cooking.
7. Then mix up together the shrimps and spice mixture.
8. After this, mix the scallops and spice mixture.
9. Add the shrimps and scallops in the air fryer basket and cook for 6 minutes. Stir the meal frequently.
10. Then let the cooked meal chill little and serve it!

NUTRITION: Calories 238, Fat 8.6, Fiber 0.2, Carbs 3.2, Protein 35.6

208. Spicy Meat Bowl

Preparation time: 15 minutes

Cooking time: 16 minutes

Servings: 6

INGREDIENTS

- 1cup ground pork
- 8oz bacon, chopped
- 1tablespoon chives
- 1teaspoon salt
- ½ teaspoon ground black pepper
- ½ teaspoon minced garlic

- ¼ teaspoon chili flakes
- 1 tablespoon olive oil
- ¼ cup almond milk

DIRECTIONS

1. Pour the olive oil into the air fryer basket.
2. Add ground pork, chopped bacon, chives, salt, ground black pepper, minced garlic, chili flakes, and almond milk.
3. Stir the mixture well and cook it at 380 F for 16 minutes. Stir the meat every 5 minutes.
4. When the meat is cooked – stir it one more time and serve!

NUTRITION: Calories 289, Fat 21.5, Fiber 0.3, Carbs 1.3, Protein 21.7

209. Stuffed Sweet Potato

Preparation time: 10 minutes

Cooking time: 10 minutes

Servings: 6

INGREDIENTS

- 3 sweet potatoes
- 6 teaspoon almond milk
- 1 teaspoon minced garlic
- 12oz ground chicken
- 1 teaspoon chives
- 1 tablespoon olive oil
- 1 tablespoon turmeric
- 1 teaspoon avocado oil

DIRECTIONS

1. Cut the sweet potatoes into the halves and remove the meat.
2. Then mix up together the almond milk, minced garlic, ground chicken, chives, olive oil, and turmeric.
3. Stir the mixture.
4. Sprinkle the sweet potato halves with the avocado oil.
5. Then fill the sweet potatoes with the meat mixture and wrap them in foil.
6. Place the sweet potatoes in the air fryer basket and cook at 380 F for 30 minutes.
7. When the time is over – discard the foil from the sweet potatoes and serve!

NUTRITION: Calories 145, Fat 7.9, Fiber 0.4, Carbs 1.3, Protein 16.7

210. Basil Beef Shank

Preparation time: 15 minutes

Cooking time: 30 minutes

Servings: 4

INGREDIENTS

- 1-pound beef shank
- 1 teaspoon paprika
- 1 teaspoon chili flakes
- 1 tablespoon olive oil
- ½ cup fresh basil
- 1 teaspoon minced garlic

DIRECTIONS

1. Sprinkle the beef shank with the paprika, chili flakes, and minced garlic.
2. Combine together the fresh basil and olive oil.
3. Blend it and rub the beef shank with the green mixture.
4. Transfer the beef shank in the air fryer and cook it for 30 minutes at 380 F.
5. Stir the meat time to time.
6. When the time is over – check if the meat is cooked and serve it immediately!

NUTRITION: Calories 244, Fat 10.7, Fiber 0.3, Carbs 0.6, Protein 34.6

211. Sesame Pork Cubes

Preparation time: 10 minutes

Cooking time: 15 minutes

Servings: 4

INGREDIENTS

- 1tablespoon avocado oil
- 16oz pork fillet
- 1tablespoon sesame seeds
- 1teaspoon ground black pepper
- 1teaspoon paleo mayo

DIRECTIONS

1. Chop the pork fillet into the cubes.
2. Sprinkle the pork cubes with the ground black pepper and Paleo mayo.
3. Stir the meat.
4. Then add avocado oil and stir it one more time.
5. After this, place the meat in the air fryer basket and cook it for 10 minutes at 370 F.
6. Then stir the meat and add sesame seeds.
7. Cook the meat for 5 minutes more at 365 F.
8. When the meat is cooked – let it chill little and serve!

NUTRITION: Calories 291, Fat 17, Fiber 0.6, Carbs 1.1, Protein 32.1

212. Thai Chicken

Preparation time: 10 minutes

Cooking time: 15 minutes

Servings: 4

INGREDIENTS

- 12oz chicken fillet
- 1tablespoon curry
- 1oz lemongrass
- ½ cup almond milk
- ¾ cup chicken stock
- ½ teaspoon salt
- 1teaspoon minced garlic

DIRECTIONS

1. Chop the chicken fillet roughly.
2. Then sprinkle the chicken with the curry, salt, and minced garlic.
3. Stir the meat and place it in the air fryer basket.
4. Add almond milk and lemongrass.
5. Cook the chicken for 15 minutes at 380 F.
6. When Thai chicken is cooked – let it chill little and serve!

NUTRITION: Calories 246, Fat 13.8, Fiber 1.2, Carbs 4.7, Protein 25.8

213. Vegetable and Chicken Bowl

Preparation time: 10 minutes

Cooking time: 10 minutes

Servings: 3

INGREDIENTS

- 6oz broccoli florets
- ½ red onion, chopped
- 1teaspoon ground cumin
- ½ teaspoon cilantro
- 1sweet pepper, roughly chopped
- 12oz chicken wings
- ½ cup chicken stock
- 1tablespoon coconut oil

DIRECTIONS

1. Place the broccoli florets in the air fryer basket.
2. Sprinkle them with the ground cumin, cilantro, and coconut oil.
3. Stir it carefully and add the chopped red onion.
4. After this, add chicken stock and cook the vegetables for 7 minutes at 400 F.
5. Then transfer the vegetables to the bowl.
6. Place the chicken wings in the air fryer basket and cook them for 10 minutes at 400 F.
7. Add the sweet pepper after 8 minutes of cooking/
8. When the time is over – transfer the chicken wings and sweet pepper in the vegetable bowl and serve.
9. Enjoy!

NUTRITION: Calories 298, Fat 13.5, Fiber 2.5, Carbs 8.9, Protein 35.2

214. Stuffed Cabbage

Preparation time: 20 minutes

Cooking time: 40 minutes

Servings: 6

INGREDIENTS

- 1zucchini, grated
- 1cup ground pork
- 1teaspoon ground nutmeg
- ½ teaspoon salt
- 1tomato, chopped
- 1tablespoon olive oil
- 1cup almond milk
- 1-pound cabbage

DIRECTIONS

1. Make the big hole in the cabbage.
2. Combine together the ground pork and grated zucchini.
3. Add ground nutmeg and salt.
4. After this, add chopped tomato and almond milk.
5. Stir the mixture well.
6. Spray the cabbage with the olive oil from all sides.
7. Then fill the cabbage hole with the ground pork mixture.
8. Wrap the cabbage in the foil and transfer it to the air fryer basket.
9. Cook the cabbage for 40 minutes at 380 F.
10. When the time is over – let it chill little and serve!

NUTRITION: Calories 180, Fat 13.2, Fiber 3.3, Carbs 8.3, Protein 9.8

215. Chili

Preparation time: 15 minutes

Cooking time: 25 minutes

Servings: 4

INGREDIENTS

- 1cup ground beef
- 1tablespoon avocado oil
- 1sweet pepper, chopped
- 1red onion, chopped
- 3garlic cloves, chopped
- ¼ teaspoon cumin
- 1teaspoon cayenne pepper
- ½ teaspoon chili pepper
- 2tomatoes, chopped
- 1cup beef broth
- 1teaspoon salt

DIRECTIONS

1. Place the ground beef in the air fryer basket and add avocado oil.
2. Cook the meat for 5 minutes at 400 F.

3. Then add the chopped sweet pepper, onion, garlic clove, cumin, cayenne pepper, chili pepper, chopped tomato, beef broth, and salt.
4. Stir the chili and cook for 25 minutes at 375 F.
5. When the chili is cooked – let it rest for 15 minutes.
6. Serve it!

NUTRITION: Calories 52, Fat 1.2, Fiber 2.1, Carbs 8.8, Protein 2.8

216. Lime Chicken with Pistachio

Preparation time: 10 minutes

Cooking time: 17 minutes

Servings: 4

INGREDIENTS

- 1-pound chicken breast, boneless
- ¼ cup pistachios, crushed
- 1 tablespoon avocado oil
- ¼ lime
- 2 tablespoons Paleo mayo
- ¼ cup chicken stock

DIRECTIONS

1. Squeeze the juice from the lime.
2. Sprinkle the chicken breast with the lime juice.
3. Then rub the chicken with Paleo mayo and crushed pistachios.
4. Place the chicken in the air fryer basket and sprinkle with the avocado oil.
5. Cook the chicken for 10 minutes at 365 F.
6. After this, add the chicken stock and cook the chicken for 7 minutes more at 375 F.
7. When the chicken is cooked – let it chill little and serve!

NUTRITION: Calories 206, Fat 11.1, Fiber 0.7, Carbs 1.7, Protein 24.9

217. Turkey Dill Meatballs

Preparation time: 10 minutes

Cooking time: 6 minutes

Servings: 6

INGREDIENTS:

- 2-pound ground turkey
- ¼ cup fresh dill
- 1 egg
- 1 tablespoon almond flour
- 1 teaspoon salt

DIRECTIONS

1. Blend the dill in the blender until smooth.
2. Then beat the egg in the blended dill and combine it with the almond flour, salt, and ground turkey.
3. Mix the mixture carefully with the help of the spoon.
4. After this, make the small meatballs.
5. Place the meatballs in the air fryer basket and cook them for 3 minutes from each side at 400 F.
6. Then chill the meatballs and serve!

NUTRITION: Calories 337, Fat 19.8, Fiber 0.8, Carbs 2.2, Protein 43.7

218. Mango Turkey

Preparation time: 8 minutes

Cooking time: 15 minutes

Servings: 3

INGREDIENTS

- 5oz mango, chopped

- 10oz ground turkey
- ¼ cup onion, grated
- ½ teaspoon salt
- 1teaspoon olive oil
- 1teaspoon paprika

DIRECTIONS

1. Place the chopped mango in the air fryer basket.
2. Add grated onion, salt, paprika, and olive oil.
3. Stir the mango mixture and cook it for 5 minutes at 375 F.
4. Then stir the mango mixture and add the ground turkey.
5. Stir the mixture well and cook it for 10 minutes at 375 F. Stir the meal frequently.
6. Transfer the cooked turkey to the serving bowl and serve!

NUTRITION: Calories 232, Fat 12.2, Fiber 1.2, Carbs 8.4, Protein 26.5

219. Turkey Burger with Jalapeno

Preparation time: 15 minutes

Cooking time: 15 minutes

Servings: 4

INGREDIENTS

- 13oz ground turkey
- 1jalapeno
- 1teaspoon olive oil
- 1tablespoon coconut flour
- ½ teaspoon paprika
- ¼ teaspoon nutmeg
- 1tablespoon chives

DIRECTIONS

1. Chop the jalapeno and blend it.
2. Combine together jalapeno and ground turkey.
3. Add coconut flour, paprika, nutmeg, and chives.
4. Stir the mixture well and make the medium burgers.
5. Place the burgers in the air fryer basket and spray them with the olive oil.
6. Cook the burgers for 15 minutes at 375 F.
7. When the burgers are cooked – chill them little and serve!

NUTRITION: Calories 208, Fat 11.9, Fiber 1.5, Carbs 2.5, Protein 25.8

220. Fennel Fish Fillet

Preparation time: 10 minutes

Cooking time: 15 minutes

Servings: 4

INGREDIENTS

- 1-pound white fish fillet
- 8oz fennel
- ½ teaspoon sea salt
- 1tablespoon vinegar
- 1teaspoon ground black pepper
- 1teaspoon olive oil

DIRECTIONS

1. Chop the fennel roughly.
2. Chop the white fish and place it in the air fryer.
3. Sprinkle the fish with the sea salt, vinegar, ground black pepper, and olive oil.
4. Stir the fish gently with the help of the spatula.
5. Cook the white fish for 5 minutes at 400F.
6. Then add the chopped fennel and stir the fish.
7. Cook the fish for 10 minutes more at 360 F.

8. When the meal is cooked – transfer it directly to the serving plate and serve!

NUTRITION: Calories 225, Fat 9.8, Fiber 1.9, Carbs 4.5, Protein 28.5

221. Shrimp Chowder

Preparation time: 10 minutes

Cooking time: 21 minutes

Servings: 4

INGREDIENTS:

- 10oz shrimps, peeled
- 3oz bacon, chopped, cooked
- 1tablespoon chives
- ½ carrot, chopped
- 1onion, diced
- 2potatoes, chopped
- 1teaspoon olive oil
- 4cups chicken stock
- ½ teaspoon ground coriander
- 1teaspoon salt

DIRECTIONS

1. Place the shrimps, bacon, chives, chopped carrot, and onion in the air fryer basket.
2. Add chopped potato and olive oil.
3. Sprinkle the mixture with the ground coriander and salt.
4. Stir it carefully and cook at 400 F for 5 minutes.
5. After this, stir the mixture and add the chicken stock.
6. Cook the chowder for 16 minutes more at 345 F.
7. When the chowder is cooked – let it rest for 10 minutes.
8. Enjoy!

NUTRITION: Calories 307, Fat 12, Fiber 3.4, Carbs 22.2, Protein 26.9

222. Ground Beef Bowl

Preparation time: 10 minutes

Cooking time: 15 minutes

Servings: 4

INGREDIENTS

- 2tablespoons chives
- 1onion, chopped
- 16oz ground beef
- 1teaspoon olive oil
- 1teaspoon paprika
- 1teaspoon cumin
- ½ teaspoon ground black pepper

DIRECTIONS

1. Put the ground beef in the air fryer basket.
2. Sprinkle the meat with the cumin, paprika, ground black pepper, and olive oil.
3. Stir it and cook for 7 minutes at 380 F. Stir the meat time to time.
4. After this, add chopped onion and chives.
5. Stir the meat mixture and cook it at 380 F for 8 minutes more or until all the ingredients are cooked.
6. Transfer the ground beef to the bowl and serve!

NUTRITION: Calories 236, Fat 8.5, Fiber 1, Carbs 3.3, Protein 35

223. Turmeric Chicken Liver

Preparation time: 10 minutes

Cooking time: 7 minutes

Servings: 5

INGREDIENTS

- 17oz chicken liver
- 2tablespoons almond flour
- 1tablespoon coconut oil
- ½ teaspoon salt
- ¼ teaspoon minced garlic
- ¾ cup chicken stock

DIRECTIONS

1. Place the coconut oil in the air fryer basket and preheat it for 20 seconds.
2. Then add chicken liver.
3. Stir it and cook for 2 minutes at 400 F.
4. Then sprinkle the chicken liver with the almond flour, salt, and minced garlic.
5. Add the chicken stock and stir liver and cook it for 5 minutes more or until cooked.
6. Serve the meal immediately!

NUTRITION: Calories 250, Fat 14.7, Fiber 1.2, Carbs 3.4, Protein 26.1

224. Chicken Burgers

Preparation time: 15 minutes

Cooking time: 12 minutes

Servings: 3

INGREDIENTS

- ¼ cup fresh parsley, chopped
- 1garlic clove, chopped
- 1tablespoon olive oil
- 1egg
- 10oz ground chicken
- 1teaspoon paprika
- 1teaspoon almond flour

DIRECTIONS

1. Place the ground chicken in the mixing bowl.
2. Beat the egg into the mixture and sprinkle it with the paprika, almond flour, chopped garlic clove, and chopped parsley.
3. Stir the meat mixture until homogenous.
4. Then make the medium burgers from the mixture.
5. Spray the air fryer basket with the olive oil inside and place the chicken burgers there.
6. Cook the meal for 12 minutes at 390 F. Turn the burgers into another side after 6 minutes of cooking.
7. Chill the cooked burgers little and serve!

NUTRITION: Calories 299, Fat 17.9, Fiber 1.5, Carbs 3.2, Protein 31.5

225. Zucchini Casserole

Preparation time: 10 minutes

Cooking time: 20 minutes

Servings: 5

INGREDIENTS

- 1carrot, sliced
- 1onion, sliced
- 1zucchini, sliced
- 1cup chicken stock
- 1cup kale, chopped
- 1teaspoon paprika
- 1teaspoon salt
- 3oz bacon, chopped, cooked
- 1tablespoon olive oil

DIRECTIONS

1. Combine together the carrot, onion, zucchini, and chopped kale in the mixing bowl.
2. Stir the mixture well.
3. Then add salt and paprika. Stir it.
4. Pour the olive oil into the air fryer basket.
5. Add the vegetable mixture and chopped bacon.
6. Stir it well.
7. Then add the chicken stock and cook the casserole for 20 minutes at 375 F. Stir it gently time to time.
8. When the time is over – check if all the ingredients are cooked.
9. Chill the casserole to the room temperature and serve!

NUTRITION: Calories 146, Fat 10.2, Fiber 1.6, Carbs 6.6, Protein 7.7

226. Cherry Tuscan Pork Loin

Preparation time: 15 minutes

Cooking time: 40 minutes

Servings: 5

INGREDIENTS

- -pound pork loin
- ½ lemon
- 1 cup cherry tomatoes
- 1 teaspoon chili pepper
- 1 tablespoon olive oil
- 1 onion, chopped
- 1 garlic clove, chopped

DIRECTIONS

1. Pour the olive oil into the air fryer basket.
2. Sprinkle the pork loin with the chili pepper and garlic clove.
3. Place the pork loin in the air fryer basket and cook it for 20 minutes from one side at 360 F.
4. After this, turn the pork loin into another side and cook it for 10 minutes more.
5. Add the cherry tomatoes.
6. Squeeze the lemon juice over the meat and tomatoes and cook the meal for 10 minutes more at 360 F.
7. When the meat is cooked – let it chill for 5 minutes.
8. Enjoy!

NUTRITION: Calories 262, Fat 15.6, Fiber 1.1, Carbs 4.3, Protein 25.5

227. Ground Chicken and Ground Pork Mix

Preparation time: 10 minutes

Cooking time: 20 minutes

Servings: 4

INGREDIENTS

- 7oz ground chicken
- 9oz ground pork
- 3oz cherry tomatoes
- 1 onion, chopped
- ¼ teaspoon minced garlic
- 1oz fresh cilantro, chopped
- 1 tablespoon olive oil
- ¼ teaspoon nutmeg

DIRECTIONS

1. Pour the olive oil into the air fryer basket.
2. Add ground pork and sprinkle the meat with the nutmeg and minced garlic.
3. Stir the mixture well and cook it for 5 minutes at 370 F.
4. After this, stir the ground pork and add the ground chicken.
5. Then add the chopped onion.

6. Chop the cherry tomatoes and add them too.
7. Add the chopped cilantro and stir the mix.
8. Cook the ground meat mix for 15 minutes more at 360 F.
9. Stir the mixture every 4 minutes.
10. When the time is over and all the ingredients are cooked – let it chill well.
11. Enjoy!

NUTRITION: Calories 233, Fat 9.6, Fiber 1.1, Carbs 3.8, Protein 31.7

228. Shrimp Salad with Greens and Avocado

Preparation time: 10 minutes

Cooking time: 5 minutes

Servings: 3

INGREDIENTS

- 8oz shrimps, peeled
- 1avocado, pitted
- 1cup fresh basil, chopped
- 1garlic clove, diced
- 1teaspoon olive oil
- 1teaspoon ground paprika
- 1teaspoon avocado oil
- 1cup fresh parsley, chopped

DIRECTIONS

1. Sprinkle the peeled shrimps with the olive oil and ground paprika.
2. Stir the mixture.
3. Place the shrimps in the air fryer basket and cook them for 5 minutes at 400 F. Stir them after 3 minutes of cooking.
4. Meanwhile, peel the avocado and chop it.
5. Place the chopped avocado in the mixing bowl.
6. Add diced garlic and chopped fresh basil.
7. After this, add the chopped parsley and avocado oil.
8. Stir salad well.
9. When the shrimps are cooked – place them over the salad and serve immediately!

NUTRITION: Calories 252, Fat 16.2, Fiber 5.6, Carbs 9.1, Protein 19.5

229. Cauliflower Fritters with Carrot

Preparation time: 10 minutes

Cooking time: 10 minutes

Servings: 6

INGREDIENTS

- 1-pound cauliflower head
- 1carrot, grated
- 1tablespoon almond flour
- 1egg, beaten
- 1tablespoon chopped dill
- 1tablespoon chopped parsley
- ½ teaspoon salt
- 1tablespoon olive oil
- ½ teaspoon chili flakes
- 1tablespoon coconut flakes

DIRECTIONS

1. Chop the cauliflower and place it in the blender.
2. Blend the cauliflower carefully.
3. Then place the blended cauliflower in the mixing bowl.
4. Add the grated carrot and almond flour.
5. After this, add the egg, chopped dill, chopped parsley, salt, coconut flakes, and chili flakes.
6. Stir the mixture carefully until smooth and homogenous.

7. Preheat the air fryer and pour the olive oil into the air fryer basket.
8. Then make the medium fritters from the cauliflower mixture with the help of the hands and place them in the air fryer basket.
9. Cook the fritters for 10 minutes at 400 F.
10. Turn the fritters into another side after 5 minutes of cooking.
11. When the fritters are cooked – chill them little.
12. Serve!

NUTRITION: Calories 85, Fat 5.8, Fiber 2.8, Carbs 6.5, Protein 3.7

230. Lamb Fillet with Tomato Gravy

Preparation time: 20 minutes

Cooking time: 10 minutes

Servings: 3

INGREDIENTS

- 9oz lamb fillet
- 2tomatoes, chopped
- 1orange
- 1teaspoon salt
- 1tablespoon vinegar
- 1tablespoon avocado oil
- 1teaspoon chili flakes
- 11tablespoon almond flour

DIRECTIONS

1. Place the chopped tomatoes in the blender.
2. Peel the orange and add it to the blender too.
3. After this, add the salt, avocado oil, vinegar, chili flakes, and almond flour.
4. Blend the mixture until smooth.
5. Then chop the lamb fillet roughly.
6. Pour the blended tomato mixture in the chopped lamb and stir it carefully.
7. Marinate the lamb fillet for 10 minutes.
8. After this, transfer the lamb fillet in the air fryer basket.
9. Sprinkle it with the remaining tomato mixture.
10. Cook the meat for 10 minutes at 400 F.
11. Stir the meat every 3 minutes.
12. When the meat is tender – transfer it in the serving bowls and sprinkle with the cooked gravy.
13. Serve it!

NUTRITION: Calories 262, Fat 11.7, Fiber 3.7, Carbs 12.7, Protein 27.3

231. Chicken Strips with Orange Zest

Preparation time: 10 minutes

Cooking time: 10 minutes

Servings: 4

INGREDIENTS

- 1-pound chicken fillet
- 1orange
- 1tablespoon dried oregano
- 1tablespoon olive oil
- ½ teaspoon salt

DIRECTIONS

1. Cut the chicken fillet into the strips.
2. Then sprinkle the chicken strips with the dried oregano and salt.
3. Squeeze the juice from the orange and pour it into the chicken strips.
4. Stir the mixture.
5. Pour the olive oil into the air fryer basket.
6. Add the chicken strips and cook the meal for 10 minutes at 390 F.

7. Stir the chicken strips after 5 minutes of cooking.
8. When the time is over – check if the meat is cooked and transfer it to the serving plate.
9. Serve it!

NUTRITION: Calories 271, Fat 12.1, Fiber 1.6, Carbs 6.1, Protein 33.4

232. Broccoli Casserole

Preparation time: 15 minutes

Cooking time: 15 minutes

Servings: 6

INGREDIENTS

- 12oz broccoli, chopped
- 1sweet potato, grated
- 1sweet pepper, chopped
- 1cup chicken stock
- ½ teaspoon dried basil
- ½ teaspoon salt
- 1tomato, chopped
- 8oz pork chop

DIRECTIONS

1. Chop the pork chops and place them in the air fryer basket.
2. Add salt, dried basil, and chicken stock.
3. Stir the mixture gently and cook it at 400 F for 8 minutes.
4. Meanwhile, combine together the chopped broccoli, grated sweet potato, and chopped sweet pepper.
5. Stir the vegetable mixture.
6. Add chopped tomato and shake it gently.
7. When the time is over – add the vegetable mixture in the air fryer basket and cook it for 7 minutes more.
8. Then check if all the ingredients are cooked and chill the casserole till the room temperature.
9. Serve it!

NUTRITION: Calories 167, Fat 9.8, Fiber 2.5, Carbs 9.7, Protein 10.9

233. Coconut Sour Shrimps with Greens

Preparation time: 20 minutes

Cooking time: 5 minutes

Servings: 4

INGREDIENTS

- 1tablespoon chives, chopped
- 1tablespoon fresh parsley, chopped
- 11oz shrimps, peeled
- 1/3 lemon
- 3tablespoons coconut milk
- 1tablespoon olive oil
- ¼ teaspoon salt

DIRECTIONS

1. Combine together the olive oil, salt, coconut milk, and chopped fresh parsley.
2. Add the chives and transfer the mixture to the blender.
3. Blend it well.
4. Then place the mixture in the mixing bowl and add the shrimps.
5. Stir the mixture with the help of the hands or spoon.
6. After this, squeeze the juice of the lemon.
7. Add the lemon juice to the shrimp mixture.
8. Marinate the shrimps for 10 minutes and transfer them to the air fryer basket.
9. Cook the shrimps for 5 minutes at 400 F.

10. Turn the shrimps into another side after 3 minutes of cooking.
11. Then let the cooked shrimps chill little and serve them!

NUTRITION: Calories 150, Fat 7.5, Fiber 0.4, Carbs 2.3, Protein 18.1

234. Seafood Casserole

Preparation time: 15 minutes

Cooking time: 12 minutes

Servings: 6

INGREDIENTS

- 1-pound salmon fillet
- 1teaspoon minced garlic
- ¼ cup almond milk
- 1onion, chopped
- 7oz broccoli, chopped
- 1sweet pepper, chopped
- 1teaspoon olive oil
- 1teaspoon salt
- 1teaspoon chili flakes

DIRECTIONS

1. Chop the salmon fillet into the medium cubes and sprinkle them with the minced garlic.
2. Then pour the olive oil into the air fryer basket.
3. Place the salmon in the air fryer.
4. Add the chopped onion and broccoli.
5. Then sprinkle the mixture with the salt, chili flakes, and add the sweet pepper.
6. Then pour the almond milk and cook the casserole for 12 minutes at 380 F.
7. You can stir the casserole during the cooking.
8. When the time is over and the meal is cooked – let it chill little and serve!

NUTRITION: Calories 155, Fat 8, Fiber 1.8, Carbs 6.1, Protein 16.3

235. Stuffed Chicken Breast with Avocado

Preparation time: 20 minutes

Cooking time: 13 minutes

Servings: 4

INGREDIENTS

- 1-pound chicken breast, boneless
- 1cup spinach, chopped
- 1tablespoon olive oil
- 3oz almonds, crushed
- ½ teaspoon salt
- ½ teaspoon ground black pepper
- 1onion, chopped

DIRECTIONS

1. Make a cut the chicken breast.
2. Place the fresh spinach in the blender and blend it well.
3. Add olive oil and crushed almond.
4. Blend the mixture for 10 seconds more.
5. Then transfer the mixture to the mixing bowl.
6. Add salt and ground black pepper.
7. Add onion and stir the mixture.
8. Fill the chicken breast with the spinach mixture and secure the cut with the help of the toothpicks.
9. Spread the chicken breast with the remaining spinach mixture and place in the air fryer basket.
10. Cook the chicken breast for at 380 F for 13 minutes.
11. Turn the chicken into another side after 7 minutes of cooking.
12. When the time is over – check if the chicken is cooked and transfer it to the serving plate.
13. Slice it and serve with the greens!

NUTRITION: Calories 296, Fat 17, Fiber 3.5, Carbs 7.6, Protein 29.1

236. Spiralized Casserole

Preparation time: 15 minutes

Cooking time: 15 minutes

Servings: 3

INGREDIENTS

- 1 carrot, spiralized
- 1 zucchini, spiralized
- 1 onion, sliced
- ½ teaspoon ground black pepper
- 1 teaspoon ground paprika
- 1 tablespoon coconut flakes
- 1 tablespoon almond flour
- 1 tablespoon olive oil
- ¼ cup chicken stock

DIRECTIONS

1. Spray the air fryer basket with the olive oil inside.
2. After this, combine together the spiralized carrot, zucchini, and sliced onion.
3. Stir the mixture gently and sprinkle it with the ground black pepper, ground paprika, and coconut flakes.
4. Then add almond flour.
5. Stir the vegetable mixture with the help of 2 forks and transfer it to the air fryer basket.
6. Pour the chicken stock and cook the casserole for 15 minutes at 380 F.
7. When the casserole is cooked – all the vegetables should be soft.
8. Serve it!

NUTRITION: Calories 136, Fat 10.2, Fiber 3.5, Carbs 10.5, Protein 3.6

237. Crunchy Chicken Fingers

Preparation time: 15 minutes

Cooking time: 12 minutes

Servings: 4

INGREDIENTS

- 12oz chicken fillet
- ½ cup coconut flakes
- 2 eggs
- ¼ cup almond milk
- 1 tablespoon almond flour
- ½ teaspoon chili flakes
- ½ teaspoon salt
- ½ teaspoon ground black pepper
- 1 tablespoon olive oil

DIRECTIONS

1. Cut the chicken fillet in the shape of the fingers.
2. Then take the bowl and beat the eggs in it.
3. Whisk the eggs and add almond milk and almond flour.
4. Then add the chili flakes and salt.
5. Sprinkle the mixture with the ground black pepper and whisk it well until homogenous.
6. Dip the chicken fingers in the egg batter and after this, coat them in the coconut flakes.
7. Pour the olive oil into the air fryer basket and place the chicken fingers there too.
8. Cook the meal for 12 minutes (6 minutes from each side at 380 F.
9. When the meal is cooked – let it chill little and serve!

NUTRITION: Calories 334, Fat 22.4, Fiber 2.1, Carbs 4.2, Protein 29.6

238. Egg Salad with Avocado

Preparation time: 12 minutes

Cooking time: 15 minutes

Servings: 6

INGREDIENTS

- 2 sweet peppers, chopped
- 1 red onion, sliced
- 1 avocado, chopped
- 3 eggs
- 1 tomato, chopped
- 1 tablespoon olive oil
- 1 teaspoon minced garlic

DIRECTIONS

1. Place the eggs on the air fryer rack and cook them at 250 F for 15 minutes.
2. After this, place them in the ice water to chill.
3. Then place the chopped sweet peppers in the bowl.
4. Add the sliced onion and chopped avocado.
5. After this, add the minced garlic.
6. Peel the eggs and chop them roughly.
7. Add the eggs to the vegetable bowl.
8. Sprinkle the salad with the olive oil and stir gently.
9. Serve it immediately!

NUTRITION: Calories 142, Fat 11.2, Fiber 3.3, Carbs 8.3, Protein 4.1

239. Juicy Scallops

Preparation time: 15 minutes

Cooking time: 6 minutes

Servings: 2

INGREDIENTS

- 11oz scallops
- 1 orange
- ¼ lime
- 1 tablespoon olive oil
- ½ teaspoon dried rosemary
- ¼ teaspoon salt
- ¼ teaspoon ground black pepper

DIRECTIONS

1. Grate the orange zest and squeeze the juice.
2. Mix up together the orange juice and orange zest.
3. Stir it carefully and add dried rosemary and salt.
4. Sprinkle the mixture with the ground black pepper.
5. Squeeze the juice from the lime and add it to the mixture.
6. Whisk it well.
7. Pour the liquid mixture over the scallops and leave them for at least 6 minutes to marinate.
8. After this, pour the olive oil in the air fryer basket and add the marinated scallops.
9. Cook the seafood for 6 minutes at 400 F. Flip the scallops into another side after 3 minutes of cooking.
10. Serve the cooked meal immediately.

NUTRITION: Calories 245, Fat 8.4, Fiber 2.6, Carbs 15.7, Protein 27.1

240. Stuffed Pepper Halves with Ground Meat

Preparation time: 15 minutes

Cooking time: 13 minutes

Servings: 6

INGREDIENTS

- 3 sweet peppers, halved
- 8oz ground pork
- 1 teaspoon chili flakes
- 1 tablespoon fresh parsley, chopped
- 1 tablespoon olive oil
- 1 teaspoon ground black pepper
- ½ onion, diced

DIRECTIONS

1. Remove the seeds from the pepper halves.
2. Then combine together the ground pork, chili flakes, chopped parsley, ground black pepper, and diced onion in the mixing bowl.
3. Stir it carefully.
4. Pour the olive oil into the air fryer basket and add the meat mixture.
5. Stir it carefully and cook the mixture for 7 minutes at 380F.
6. Stir the mixture twice during the cooking.
7. After this, transfer the cooked ground pork in the mixing bowl.
8. Fill the pepper halves with the pork mixture.
9. Transfer the pepper halves in the air fryer basket and cook them for 6 minutes at 400 F (depend on the size of the vegetables).
10. When the time is over – let the cooked meal chill little and serve it.

NUTRITION: Calories 98, Fat 3.8, Fiber 1.1, Carbs 5.6, Protein 10.7

241. Pear Bowl with Nuts and Flax Seeds

Preparation time: 10 minutes

Cooking time: 10 minutes

Servings: 6

INGREDIENTS

- 2 pears
- 4oz walnuts
- 2 tablespoons flax seeds
- ¼ teaspoon ground cinnamon
- 1 teaspoon vanilla extract
- 5oz bacon, chopped
- 1 tablespoon sesame seeds

DIRECTIONS

1. Cut the pears into the halves and remove the seeds.
2. Then chop the pears and place them in the air fryer basket.
3. Sprinkle the fruits with the vanilla extract and ground cinnamon.
4. Stir the fruits and cook them for 4 minutes at 400 F.
5. After this, transfer the fruits in the bowl.
6. Place the chopped bacon in the air fryer and cook it at 400 F for 6 minutes.
7. Stir it time to time.
8. Meanwhile, sprinkle the cooked pears with the sesame seeds and flax seeds.
9. Stir the mixture gently.
10. Crush the walnuts and add them to the pear bowl.
11. After this, add the cooked sesame seeds and stir the mixture.
12. Serve it immediately!

NUTRITION: Calories 308, Fat 22.6, Fiber 4.3, Carbs 14, Protein 14.3

242. Sweet Potato Toasts

Preparation time: 15 minutes

Cooking time: 11 minutes

Servings: 4

INGREDIENTS

- 1 avocado, pitted
- 6oz bacon, chopped
- 2 sweet potatoes, peeled
- 1 onion, sliced
- ¼ teaspoon salt
- 1 teaspoon ground paprika
- 1 tablespoon avocado oil

DIRECTIONS

1. Slice the sweet potatoes into the medium slices.
2. Then place the chopped bacon in the air fryer basket and cook it for 6 minutes at 400 F. Stir it after 3 minutes of cooking.
3. Then transfer the cooked bacon to the mixing bowl.
4. Place the sliced sweet potato in the air fryer basket and sprinkle it with the avocado oil.
5. Cook the sweet potato slices for 4 minutes from one side and for 4 minutes from another side at 400 F.
6. Meanwhile, mash the avocado well and combine it together with the chopped bacon, salt, ground paprika, and sliced onion.
7. Stir the mixture carefully until homogenous.
8. When the sliced sweet potato is cooked – let it chill for 4 minutes.
9. Then spread each slice of the sweet potato with the avocado mash and make the sandwiches.
10. Serve the meal warm!

NUTRITION: Calories 345, Fat 27.7, Fiber 4.2, Carbs 7.9, Protein 17.1

243. Bacon Red Potato Halves

Preparation time: 10 minutes

Cooking time: 14 minutes

Servings: 5

INGREDIENTS

- 1-pound red potato
- 8oz bacon
- 1 tablespoon dried dill
- 1 teaspoon dried basil
- 1 teaspoon salt
- 1 tablespoon olive oil

DIRECTIONS

1. Wash the red potatoes carefully and cut them into the halves.
2. Then sprinkle the red potatoes with the dried basil, dried dill, and salt.
3. Stir the potatoes carefully.
4. After this, chop the bacon and place it in the air fryer basket.
5. Cook the bacon for 4 minutes at 380 F. Stir it after 2 minutes of cooking.
6. After this, add the red potato halves and stir the mixture carefully.
7. Cook the meal at 400 F for 10 minutes.
8. Stir the potatoes every 3 minutes.
9. Then check if the meal is cooked and transfer it to the serving plates.
10. Serve it!

NUTRITION: Calories 335, Fat 21.9, Fiber 1.6, Carbs 15.4, Protein 18.6

244. Hash Brown

Preparation time: 10 minutes

Cooking time: 10 minutes

Servings: 3

INGREDIENTS:

- 3 potatoes, peeled
- 1 tablespoon olive oil
- ¼ teaspoon ground white pepper
- ¾ teaspoon salt

- 1 teaspoon ground paprika

DIRECTIONS

1. Grate the peeled carrot and combine it together with the ground white pepper, salt, and ground paprika.
2. Stir the mixture well.
3. Pour the olive oil into the air fryer basket and place the grated potato mixture there with the help of the spoon.
4. Cook the potato hash brown for 10 minutes at 400 F.
5. Stir the hashbrown after 6 minutes of cooking. The cooked meal should have light brown color.
6. Chill the hash brown to the room temperature and serve!

NUTRITION: Calories 189, Fat 5, Fiber 5.4, Carbs 34, Protein 3.7

245. Mixed Meat Sausages

Preparation time: 15 minutes

Cooking time: 13 minutes

Servings: 6

INGREDIENTS

- 11oz ground chicken
- 8oz ground pork
- 1 teaspoon minced garlic
- 1 onion, grated
- ½ teaspoon salt
- ½ teaspoon ground nutmeg
- ½ teaspoon turmeric
- 1 teaspoon olive oil
- 1 tablespoon almond flour

DIRECTIONS

1. Place the ground chicken and ground pork in the mixing bowl.
2. Add the minced garlic and grated onion.
3. After this, sprinkle the meat mixture with the salt, ground nutmeg, and turmeric.
4. Add almond flour and stir the mixture with the help of the spoon until homogenous.
5. Make the medium sausages from the meat mixture with the help of the hands.
6. Spray the air fryer basket with the olive oil inside.
7. Place the sausages in the air fryer basket and cook them at 380 F for 13 minutes.
8. Turn the sausages into another side after 6 minutes of cooking.
9. When the sausages are cooked – let them chill little and transfer in the serving plate.
10. Serve the meal with the fresh vegetables.

NUTRITION: Calories 196, Fat 8.4, Fiber 1, Carbs 3.1, Protein 26.2

246. Asparagus with Chicken

Preparation time: 10 minutes

Cooking time: 14 minutes

Servings: 5

INGREDIENTS

- 9oz asparagus
- 8oz chicken breast
- 1 tablespoon olive oil
- 1 sweet pepper, chopped
- ½ teaspoon salt
- 1 tablespoon chicken stock

DIRECTIONS

1. Wash the asparagus carefully and chop it roughly.

2. Then sprinkle the chicken breast with the salt and olive oil.
3. Place the chicken breast in the air fryer basket and cook it for 9 minutes at 380 F.
4. Flip the chicken to another side after 5 minutes of cooking.
5. After this, add the asparagus and chicken stock.
6. Stir the mixture and cook it at 400 F for 5 minutes more.
7. When the time is over – let the cooked meal chill little and serve it.

NUTRITION: Calories 94, Fat 4.1, Fiber 1.4, Carbs 3.8, Protein 11

SIDES

247. Grilled Pineapple with Cinnamon

Cooking Time: 20 minutes

Servings: 2

INGREDIENTS

- 4 pineapple slices
- 2 tablespoons Truvia
- 1 teaspoon cinnamon

DIRECTIONS

1. Add the cinnamon and Truvia into a Ziploc bag and shake well. Add the pineapple slices to it and shake and coat. Leave to marinate in the fridge for 20-minutes. Preheat your air fryer for 5-minutes at 360°Fahrenheit. Place the pineapple pieces on the air fryer rack and grill them for 10-minutes. Flip and grill them for an additional 10-minutes.

NUTRITION: Calories: 276, Total Fat: 5.3g, Carbs: 4.2g, Protein: 4.6g

248. Bell Peppers with Potato Stuffing

Cooking Time: 20 minutes

Servings: 4

INGREDIENTS

- 4 green bell peppers, top cut and deseeded
- 4 potatoes, boiled, peeled and mashed
- 2 onions, finely chopped
- 1 teaspoon lemon juice
- 2 tablespoons coriander leaves, chopped
- 2 green chilies, finely chopped
- Olive oil as needed
- Salt to taste
- ¼ teaspoon Garam Masala
- ½ teaspoon chili powder
- ¼ teaspoon turmeric powder
- 1 teaspoon cumin seeds

DIRECTIONS

1. Heat the oil in a pan and sauté the onion, chilies and cumin seeds. Add the rest of the ingredients except the bell peppers and mix well. Preheat your air fryer to 390°Fahrenheit for 10-minutes. Brush your bell peppers with olive oil, inside and out and stuff each pepper with potato mixture. Place in air fryer basket and grill for 10-minutes. Check and grill for an additional 5-minutes.

NUTRITION: Calories: 282, Total Fat: 9.2g, Carbs: 7.1g, Protein: 4.2g

249. Chickpea & Zucchini Burgers

Cooking Time: 10 minutes

Servings: 4

INGREDIENTS

- 1 can of chickpeas, strained
- 1 red onion, diced
- 2 eggs, beaten
- 1 ounce almond flour
- 3 tablespoons coriander
- 1 teaspoon garlic puree
- 1 ounce cheddar cheese, shredded
- 1 Courgette, spiralized
- 1 teaspoon chili powder
- Salt and pepper to taste
- 1 teaspoon mixed spice

DIRECTIONS

1. Add your ingredients to a bowl and mix well. Shape portions of the mixture into

burgers. Place in the air fryer for 15-minutes until cooked.

NUTRITION: Calories: 263, Total Fat: 11.2g, Carbs: 8.3g, Protein: 6.3g

250. 36Spanish Style Spiced Potatoes

Cooking Time: 23 minutes

Servings: 4

INGREDIENTS

- 3potatoes, peeled and chopped into chips
- 1onion, diced
- ½ cup tomato sauce
- 1tomato, thinly sliced
- 1tablespoon red wine vinegar
- 2tablespoons olive oil
- 1teaspoon paprika
- 1teaspoon chili powder
- Salt and pepper to taste
- 1teaspoon rosemary
- 1teaspoon oregano
- 1teaspoon mixed spice
- 2teaspoons coriander

DIRECTIONS

1. Toss the chips in the olive oil and cook in your air fryer for 15-minutes at 360°Fahrenheit. Mix remaining ingredients in a baking dish. Place the sauce in air fryer for 8-minutes. Toss the potatoes in the sauce and serve warm!

NUTRITION: Calories: 265, Total Fat: 7,3g, Carbs: 6.2g, Protein: 5.2g

251. Spicy Cheesy Breaded Mushrooms

Cooking Time: 7 minutes

Servings: 2

INGREDIENTS

- 8-ounces of Button mushrooms (pat dried)
- 1egg
- Almond flour as required
- 3ounces parmesan cheese, freshly grated
- Breadcrumbs as needed
- Salt and pepper to taste
- 1teaspoon paprika

DIRECTIONS

1. Mix the cheese and the breadcrumbs and paprika in a mixing bowl. Whisk the egg in another bowl. Dredge the Button mushrooms in the flour, dip in egg then coat them in breadcrumb mix. Cook for 7-minutes in your air fryer at 360° Fahrenheit, tossing once halfway through cook time.

NUTRITION: Calories: 203, Total Fat: 4.2g, Carbs: 3.2g, Protein: 3.6g

252. Broccoli with Cheese & Olives

Cooking Time: 15 minutes

Servings: 4

INGREDIENTS

- 2lbs. broccoli florets
- ¼ cup parmesan cheese, shaved
- 2teaspoons lemon zest, grated
- 1/3 cup Kalamata olives, halved, pitted
- ½ teaspoon ground black pepper
- 1teaspoon sea salt
- 2tablespoons olive oil

DIRECTIONS

1. Boil the water in a pan and cook the broccoli for 4-minutes. Drain broccoli. Toss the broccoli with oil, salt, and pepper. Place broccoli in your air fryer basket and cook for 15-minutes at

400°Fahrenheit. Toss twice during cook time. Move to a serving bowl and toss in lemon zest, olives, and cheese.

NUTRITION: Calories: 242, Total Fat: 7.2g, Carbs: 3.2g, Protein: 5.6g

253. French Beans with Walnuts & Almonds

Cooking Time: 27 minutes

Servings: 6

INGREDIENTS

- 1½ lbs. of French green beans
- (stems removed
- ¼ cup slivered almonds (lightly toasted
- ¼ cup walnuts, finely chopped
- ½ teaspoon ground white pepper
- ½ lb. shallots, peeled and quartered
- 1 teaspoon sea salt
- 2 tablespoons olive oil

DIRECTIONS:

1. Boil some water in a pan, adding the green beans to it. Cook beans for 2-minutes with salt. Drain the beans. Place the green beans into a bowl and toss with the rest of the ingredients except the walnuts and almonds. Mix nuts together in small bowl and set aside. Place into air fryer basket and cook for 25-minutes at 400°Fahrenheit. Toss twice during cook time. Serve garnished with mixed nuts.

NUTRITION: Calories: 213, Total Fat: 5.2g, Carbs: 3.4g, Protein: 4.3g

254. Fried Zucchini, Squash, & Carrot Mix

Cooking Time: 35 minutes

Servings: 4

INGREDIENTS

- ½ lb. carrots, peeled and cubed
- 6 teaspoons olive oil
- 1 lb. zucchini, chopped into half-moons
- 1 lb. yellow squash, chopped in half-moons
- 1 teaspoon sea salt
- ½ teaspoon white pepper
- 1 tablespoon Tarragon leaves, chopped

DIRECTIONS

1. Toss carrots in a bowl with 2 teaspoons of olive oil, then place them into air fryer basket. Cook for 5-minutes at 400°Fahrenheit. Toss the zucchini and squash in the rest of the oil, salt and pepper and place into air fryer. Cook for 30-minutes, tossing three times during cook time. Toss with tarragon and serve.

NUTRITION: Calories: 217, Total Fat: 4.2g, Carbs: 3.9g, Protein: 6.2g

255. Hot Spicy Thyme Cherry Tomatoes

Cooking Time: 25 minutes

Servings: 4

INGREDIENTS

- 1 dozen cherry tomatoes
- 1 tablespoon olive oil
- ½ teaspoon thyme, dried
- Salt and pepper to taste
- 1 garlic clove, minced
- 1 teaspoon paprika

DIRECTIONS

1. Chop the tomatoes in half and discard the seeds. Toss the tomatoes with the rest of the ingredients in a bowl. Place in the air fryer at 390°Fahrenheit for 15-minutes.

NUTRITION: Calories: 232, Total Fat: 5.2g, Carbs: 4.3g, Protein: 5.1g

256. Honey Roasted Carrots

Cooking Time: 25 minutes

Servings: 4

INGREDIENTS

- 3cups baby carrots
- 1tablespoon olive oil
- 1tablespoon honey
- Salt and pepper to taste

DIRECTIONS

1. Toss all the ingredients in a bowl. Cook for 12-minutes in an air fryer at 390°Fahrenheit.

NUTRITION: Calories: 82, Total Fat: 3.2g, Carbs: 2.1g, Protein: 1.0g

257. Spicy Mango Okra

Cooking Time: 25 minutes

Servings: 5

INGREDIENTS

- 35-ounces Okra, washed, drained and wiped dry
- 1teaspoon red chili powder
- 2tablespoons coriander powder
- 2tablespoons almond flour
- 1½ tablespoons olive oil
- Pinch of caraway seeds
- Pinch of Fenugreek seeds
- Pinch of Asafoetida
- ½ teaspoon turmeric
- 2green chilies
- 4teaspoons dry mango powder
- Salt to taste

DIRECTIONS

1. Slit the okra lengthwise into half. Brush some olive oil on okra then fry in the air fryer. Heat some oil in a pan and add the asafetida, heating it for 10-seconds. Add the fenugreek and caraway seeds, fry them for 10-seconds. Stir in the almond flour and cook for 10-minutes. Mix in the air fried okra and sprinkle the spices on top. Cook for 10-minutes, adding the green chilies cook for an additional 2-minutes.

NUTRITION: Calories: 35, Total Fat: 0.11g, Carbs: 7.7g, Protein: 2.27g

258. Parsley & Garlic Flavored Potatoes

Cooking Time: 40 minutes

Servings: 4

INGREDIENTS

- 3Idaho baking potatoes (pricked with a fork
- 2tablespoons olive oil
- 1teaspoon parsley
- 1tablespoon garlic, minced
- Salt to taste

DIRECTIONS

1. Stir ingredients together in a bowl. Rub the potatoes with the mix. Place them into air fryer basket and cook for 40-minutes at 390°Fahrenheit. Toss twice during cook time.

NUTRITION: Calories: 97, Total Fat: 0.64g, Carbs: 25.2g, Protein: 10.2g

259. Turmeric & Garlic Roasted Carrots

Cooking Time: 20 minutes

Servings: 4

INGREDIENTS

- 21-ounces of carrots, peeled
- 1 handful of fresh coriander
- 1 teaspoon turmeric
- 1 tablespoon olive oil
- 1 teaspoon garlic, minced

DIRECTIONS

1. Lightly drizzle the olive oil over the carrots and sprinkle the turmeric and garlic over them. Place in pan in air fryer and cook for 20-minutes at 290°Fahrenheit. Toss once during cook time. Serve carrots garnished with fresh coriander.

NUTRITION: Calories: 60, Total Fat: 0.35g, Carbs: 10.2g, Protein: 0.48g

260. Paprika Chips

Cooking Time: 40 minutes

Servings: 4

INGREDIENTS

- 31-ounces of sweet potatoes, peeled and cut into chips
- ½ teaspoon salt
- 2 tablespoons olive oil
- ½ tablespoon paprika

DIRECTIONS

1. Toss all the ingredients together in a bowl. Place in a pan inside your air fryer and cook for 40-minutes at 300°Fahrenheit.

NUTRITION: Calories: 62, Total Fat: 6.5g, Carbs: 41.5g, Protein: 5.3g

261. Bacon & Veggie Mash

Cooking Time: 1 hour and 15 minutes

Servings: 8

INGREDIENTS:

- 4 strips of bacon, chopped into pieces
- 1 tablespoon butter
- ¾ cup Yellow onion, diced
- ½ cup red bell pepper, diced
- ¼ cup celery, diced
- 2 teaspoons garlic, minced
- ¾ teaspoon fresh thyme leaves
- 1½ cups whole milk
- 3 eggs
- ½ cup heavy cream
- 1 teaspoon sea salt
- ¼ teaspoon cayenne pepper
- 3 cups day-old bread, cubed
- 3 tablespoons parmesan cheese, grated
- 1 cup Monterey Jack cheese grated
- Seasoning:
- 2½ teaspoons paprika
- 2 teaspoons salt
- 2 teaspoons garlic powder
- 1 teaspoon black pepper
- 1 teaspoon onion powder
- 1 teaspoon cayenne pepper
- 1 teaspoon oregano, dried
- 1 teaspoon thyme, dried

DIRECTIONS

1. Grease a casserole dish with the butter. Cook bacon in small frying pan until crisp, then place aside. Cook the corn in the pan until caramelized for about 10-minutes, then add in celery, onion, bell pepper and cook for an additional 5-minutes. Mix in the thyme and garlic and remove from heat. Stir in the eggs, milk, and cream, whisking well to combine. Add in salt, cayenne pepper, bread and Monterey Jack cheese. Transfer to casserole dish and place in air fryer basket. Cook for 30-minutes at 320°Fahrenheit. Sprinkle with parmesan cheese and cook for another 30-minutes.

NUTRITION: Calories: 42, Total Fat: 8.3g, Carbs: 9.5g, Protein: 16.2g

262. Garlic & Parsley Roasted Mushrooms

Cooking Time: 30 minutes

Servings: 4

INGREDIENTS

- 2lbs. mushrooms, washed, quartered, dried
- 1tablespoon duck fat
- ½ teaspoon garlic powder
- 2teaspoons Herbes de Provence
- 2tablespoons white vermouth
- 1teaspoon parsley, fresh, finely chopped

DIRECTIONS

1. Place the duck fat, garlic powder, Herbes de Provence in an air fryer pan and heat for 2-minutes. Stir in the mushrooms. Cook for 25-minutes at 300°Fahrenheit. Mix in the vermouth and cook for an additional 5-minutes. Sprinkle mushrooms with parsley for garnish.

NUTRITION: Calories: 92, Total Fat: 0.23g, Carbs: 0.52g, Protein: 1.2g

263. Ginger & Honey Cauliflower Bites

Cooking Time: 20 minutes

Servings: 4

INGREDIENTS

- 1head of cauliflower, cut into florets
- 1/3 cup oats
- 1/3 cup almond flour
- 1egg, beaten
- 1teaspoon mixed spice
- 2tablespoons soy sauce
- 2tablespoons honey
- Salt and pepper to taste
- ½ teaspoon mustard powder
- 1teaspoon mixed herbs
- 1/3 cup desiccated coconut
- 1teaspoon ginger powder

DIRECTIONS

1. Preheat your air fryer to 360°Fahrenheit. In a bowl, combine flour, oats, ginger powder and coconut. Season it with salt and pepper. Add egg into another bowl. Season the cauliflower florets with the mixed herbs, salt, and pepper. Dip florets into the egg and then dredge in coconut mix. Cook in your air fryer for 15-minutes at 315°Fahrenheit. Mix remaining ingredients in a bowl. Dip the cauliflower in the honey mixture and cook for an additional 5-minutes in air fryer.

NUTRITION: Calories: 42, Total Fat: 2.3g, Carbs: 3.1g, Protein: 3.2g

264. Vegetable Fries

Cooking Time: 18 minutes

Servings: 4

INGREDIENTS

- 5-ounces sweet potatoes, peeled and chopped as chips
- 5-ounces Courgette, peeled and chopped as chips
- 5-ounces carrots, peeled and chopped as chips
- 2tablespoons olive oil
- Salt and pepper to taste
- Pinch of basil
- Pinch of mixed spice

DIRECTIONS

1. Toss the veggies in olive oil and place in an air fryer preheated to 360°Fahrenehit

for 18-minutes. Toss twice during cook time. Season with salt, pepper, and other seasonings.

NUTRITION: Calories: 42, Total Fat: 1.3g, Carbs: 2.1g, Protein: 1.4g

265. Hot Pepper Pin Wheel

Cooking Time: 6 minutes

Servings: 3

INGREDIENTS

- 2lbs. dill pickles
- 3almond tortillas
- Salt and pepper to taste
- 3-ounces sliced ham
- 1lb. softened cream
- 1hot pepper, finely diced

DIRECTIONS

1. Mix diced hot pepper in with cheese. On one side of the tortilla spread cheese over it. Place the ham slice over it. Spread a layer of cheese on top of ham slice. Roll 1 pickle up in the tortilla. Preheat the air fryer to 340°Fahrenheit. Place the rolls in air fryer basket and cook for 6-minutes.

NUTRITION: Calories: 67, Total Fat: 2.1g, Carbs: 0.11g, Protein: 3.2g

266. Crab & Cheese Soufflé

Cooking Time: 18 minutes

Servings: 2

INGREDIENTS

- 1lb. cooked crab meat
- 1capsicum
- 1small onion, diced
- 1cup cream
- 1cup milk
- 4-ounces Brie
- Brandy to cover crab meat
- 3eggs
- 5drops liquid stevia
- 3-ounces cheddar cheese, grated
- 4cups bread, cubed

DIRECTIONS

1. Soak the cram meat in brandy and 4-parts water. Loosen the meat in brandy. Sauté onion and bread. Grate cheddar cheese and mix ingredients. In the same pan, add some of the butter and stir for a minute. Add the crab to pan. Add ½ of the milk and 1 tablespoon of brandy and cook for 2-minutes. Add the bread cubes to frying pan and mix well. Sprinkle with cheese and pepper. Put the stuffing in 5 ramekins, without brushing them with oil. Distribute the brie evenly. In a bowl, combine ½ cup of cream with stevia. Heat the cream in a pan and add remaining milk. Pour mixture into ramekins. Preheat your air fryer to 350°Fareneheit add dish and cook for 20-minutes.

NUTRITION: Calories: 202, Total Fat: 5.6g, Carbs: 6.2g, Protein: 14.3g

267. Lemon Courgette Caviar

Cooking Time: 20 minutes

Servings: 3

INGREDIENTS

- 2medium Courgettes
- 1tablespoon olive oil
- 1½ tablespoons balsamic vinegar
- ½ red onion
- Juice of one lemon

DIRECTIONS

1. Preheat your air fryer. Wash, then dry courgettes. Add lemon juice to over courgettes. Arrange courgettes in a baking dish, then bake them in the air fryer for 20-minutes. Remove the courgettes from the oven and allow them to cool. Blend the onion in a blender. Slice the courgettes in half, lengthwise, then remove their insides using a spoon. Place courgettes into mixer and process everything. Add the vinegar, the olive oil and a little bit of salt, then blend again. Serve cool with tomato sauce.

NUTRITION: Calories: 76, Total Fat: 0.3g, Carbs: 18g, Protein: 3g

268. Chopped Liver with Eggs

Cooking Time: 12 minutes

Servings: 2

INGREDIENTS

- 2large eggs
- 1lb. sliced liver
- Salt and pepper to taste
- 1tablespoon cream
- ½ tablespoon black truffle oil
- 1tablespoon butter

DIRECTIONS

1. Preheat your air fryer to 340°Fahrenheit. Cut liver into thin slices and place in the fridge. Separate the whites from the yolks of the eggs and put each yolk in a cup. In another bowl, add the cream, the black truffle oil, salt, pepper and beat to combine. Take the liver and arrange half of the mixture in a small ramekin. Pour the white of the egg and divide equally between two ramekins. Put the yolks on top. Surround the yolks with the liver and cook for 12-minutes. Serve cool.

NUTRITION: Calories: 374, Total Fat: 10g, Carbs: 8.5g, Protein: 59g

269. Baked Tomato & Egg

Cooking Time: 20 minutes

Servings: 2

INGREDIENTS

- 2tomatoes
- 4eggs
- 1cup mozzarella cheese, shredded
- Salt and pepper to taste
- 1tablespoon olive oil
- A few basil leaves

DIRECTIONS

1. Preheat your air fryer to 360°Fahrenheit. Cut each tomato into two halves and place them in a bowl. Season with salt and pepper. Place cheese around the bottom of the tomatoes and add the basil leaves. Break one egg into each tomato slice. Garnish with cheese and drizzle with olive oil. Set the temperature to 360°Fahrenheit and bake for 20-minutes.

NUTRITION: Calories: 28.9, Total Fat: 2.4g, Carbs: 2.0g, Protein: 0.4g

270. Parmesan Asparagus Fries

Cooking Time: 10 minutes

Servings: 5

INGREDIENTS

- 1lb. asparagus spears
- ¼ cup almond flour
- Salt and pepper to taste

- 2 eggs, beaten
- ½ cup Parmesan cheese, grated
- 1 cup pork rinds

DIRECTIONS

1. Preheat your air fryer to 380°Fahrenheit. Combine pork rinds and parmesan cheese in a small bowl. Season with salt and pepper. Line baking sheet with parchment paper. First, dip half the asparagus spears into flour, then into eggs, and finally into pork rind mixture. Place asparagus spears on the baking sheet and bake for 10-minutes. Repeat with remaining spears.

NUTRITION: Calories: 20, Total Fat: 0.1g, Carbs: 3.9g, Protein: 2.2g

271. Spicy Mozzarella Stick

Cooking Time: 5 minutes

Servings: 3

INGREDIENTS

- 8-ounces mozzarella cheese, cut into strips
- 2 tablespoons olive oil
- ½ teaspoon salt
- 1 cup pork rinds
- 1 egg
- 1 teaspoon garlic powder
- 1 teaspoon paprika

DIRECTIONS

1. Cut the mozzarella into 6 strips. Whisk the egg along with salt, paprika, and garlic powder. Dip the mozzarella strips into egg mixture first, then into pork rinds. Arrange them on a baking platter and place in the fridge for 30-minutes. Preheat your air fryer to 360°Fahrenheit. Drizzle olive oil into the air fryer. Arrange the mozzarella sticks in the air fryer and cook for about 5-minutes. Make sure to turn them at least twice, to ensure they will become golden on all sides.

NUTRITION: Calories: 156, Total Fat: 9.6g, Carbs: 1.89g, Protein: 16g

272. Cheese Croquettes with Prosciutto

Cooking Time: 7 minutes

Servings: 6

INGREDIENTS

- 1 lb. cheddar cheese
- 12 slices of prosciutto
- 1 cup pork rinds
- 4 tablespoons olive oil
- 2 eggs, beaten
- 1 cup almond flour

DIRECTIONS

1. Cut your cheese into 6 equal pieces. Wrap each piece of cheese with 2 prosciutto slices. Place them in the freezer for 5-minutes. Preheat your air fryer to 380°Fahrenheit. Dip the croquettes into the flour first, then the egg, and finally coat them with pork rinds. Place them in air fryer basket and drizzle them with olive oil and cook for 7-minutes.

NUTRITION: Calories: 107, Total Fat: 8.02g, Carbs: 10.3g, Protein: 9.4g

273. Fried Garlic Calamari

Total Time: 10 minutes

Servings: 4

INGREDIENTS

- 1 lb. calamari, cut into rings

- ¼ cup of almond flour
- 1 cup pork rinds
- 3 mashed garlic cloves
- 2 large beaten eggs

DIRECTIONS

1. Coat the calamari rings with flour. Dip the calamari in the mixture of the eggs and the mashed garlic. Dip them in the pork rinds. Cool the calamari rings in the fridge for 2-hours. Then, put them into your air fryer and apply oil generously. Cook for 10-minutes at 380°Fahrenheit. Serve with garlic mayonnaise or lemon wedges.

NUTRITION: Calories: 106, Total Fat: 1.84g, Carbs: 8.42g, Protein: 12.86g

274. Crispy Cheese & Garlic Sticks

Cooking Time: 4 minutes

Servings: 4

INGREDIENTS

- 1 cup almond flour
- 1 teaspoon garlic, minced
- ¼ teaspoon chili powder
- 1 teaspoon butter
- 3 cubes of cheddar cheese grated
- 1 teaspoon baking powder

DIRECTIONS

1. Mix the flour and baking powder. Add the chili powder, garlic, salt, butter and grated cheese, along with a few drops of water. Make sure to make a stiff dough. Knead the dough for a while. Now, sprinkle a small amount of flour on the counter. Take a rolling pin and roll the dough. Slice the dough into any shape you want. Preheat your air fryer to 370°Fahrenheit. Set the time to 4-minutes and add cheese sticks to the basket. Serve with hot sauce!

NUTRITION: Calories: 143, Total Fat: 8.4g, Carbs: 1.78g, Protein: 15.2g

275. Mushroom, Onion and Feta Frittata

Cooking Time: 30 minutes

Servings: 4

INGREDIENTS

- 4 cups button mushrooms
- 1 red onion
- 2 tablespoons olive oil
- 6 tablespoons feta cheese, crumbled
- Pinch of salt
- 6 eggs
- Cooking spray

DIRECTIONS

1. Peel and slice the red onion into ¼ inch thin slices. Clean the button mushrooms, then cut them into ¼ inch thin slices. Add olive oil to pan and sauté mushrooms over medium heat until tender. Remove from heat and pan so that they can cool. Preheat your air fryer to 330°Fahrenheit. Add cracked eggs into a bowl, and whisk them, adding a pinch of salt. Coat an 8-inch heat resistant baking dish with cooking spray. Add the eggs into the baking dish, then onion and mushroom mixture, and then add feta cheese. Place the baking dish into air fryer for 30-minutes and serve warm.

NUTRITION: Calories: 246, Total Fat: 12.3g, Carbs: 9.2g, Protein: 10.3g

276. Bacon, Lettuce, Tempeh & Tomato Sandwiches

Cooking Time: 5 minutes

Servings: 4

INGREDIENTS

- 8-ounce package tempeh
- 1cup warm vegetable broth
- Tomato slices and lettuce, to serve
- ¼ teaspoon chipotle chili powder
- ½ teaspoon garlic powder
- ½ teaspoon onion powder
- 1teaspoon Liquid smoke
- 3tablespoons soy sauce

DIRECTIONS

1. Begin by opening the packet of tempeh and slice into pieces about ¼ inch thick. Grab a medium bowl and add the remaining ingredients except for lettuce and tomato and stir well. Place the pieces of tempeh onto a baking tray that will fit into your air fryer and pour over the flavor mix. Put the tray in air fryer and cook for 5-minutes at 360°Fahrenheit. Remove from air fryer and place on sliced bread with the tomato and lettuce and any other extra toppings you desire.

NUTRITION: Carbs: 265, Total Fat: 11.3g, Carbs: 9.2g, Protein: 12.4g

277. Curried Cauliflower Florets

Cooking Time: 10 minutes

Servings: 4

INGREDIENTS:

- 1/4 cup sultanas or golden raisins
- ¼ teaspoon salt
- 1tablespoon curry powder
- 1head cauliflower, broken into small florets
- ¼ cup pine nuts
- ½ cup olive oil

DIRECTIONS

1. In a cup of boiling water, soak your sultanas to plump. Preheat your air fryer to 350°Fahrenheit. Add oil and pine nuts to air fryer and toast for a minute or so. In a bowl toss the cauliflower and curry powder as well as salt, then add the mix to air fryer mixing well. Cook for 10-minutes. Drain the sultanas, toss with cauliflower, and serve.

NUTRITION: Calories: 275, Total Fat: 11.3g, Carbs: 8.6g, Protein: 9.5g

278. Parsnip Fries

Cooking Time: 12 minutes

Servings: 2

INGREDIENTS

- 2tablespoons of olive oil
- A pinch of sea salt
- 1large bunch of parsnips

DIRECTIONS

1. Wash and peel the parsnips, then cut them into strips. Place the parsnips in a bowl with the olive oil and sea salt and coat well. Preheat your air fryer to 360°Fahrenheit. Place the parsnip and oil mixture into the air fryer basket. Cook for 12-minutes. Serve with sour cream or ketchup.

NUTRITION: Calories: 262g, Total Fat: 11.3g, Carbs: 10.4g, Protein: 7.2g

279. Coconut Chips

Cooking Time: 5 minutes

Servings: 2

INGREDIENTS

- 2 cups large pieces of shredded coconut
- 1/3 teaspoon liquid Stevia
- 1 tablespoon chili powder

DIRECTIONS

1. Preheat your air fryer to 390°Fahrenheit. Combine the shredded coconut pieces with spices. Cook for 5-minutes in air fryer and enjoy!

NUTRITION: Calories: 261, Total Fat: 9.2g, Carbs: 7.3g, Protein: 6.2g

280. Sweet Potato Chips

Cooking Time: 15 minutes

Servings: 2

INGREDIENTS

- 2 large sweet potatoes, thinly sliced with Mandoline
- 2 tablespoons olive oil
- Salt to taste

DIRECTIONS

1. Preheat your air fryer to 350°Fahrenheit. Stir the sweet potato slices, in a large bowl with the oil. Arrange slices in your air fryer and cook them until crispy, for about 15-minutes.

NUTRITION: Calories: 253, Total Fat: 11.2g, Carbs: 8.4g, Protein: 6.5g

281. Vegetable Spring Rolls

Cooking Time: 23 minutes

Servings: 10

INGREDIENTS

- 10 spring roll wrappers
- 2 tablespoons cornstarch
- Water
- 3 green onions, thinly sliced
- 1 tablespoon black pepper
- 1 teaspoon soy sauce
- Pinches of salt
- 2 tablespoons cooking oil, plus more for brushing
- 8-cloves of garlic, minced
- ½ bell pepper, cut into thin matchsticks
- 2 large onions, cut into thin matchsticks
- 1 large carrot, cut into thin matchsticks
- 2 cups cabbage, shredded
- 2-inch piece of ginger, grated

DIRECTIONS

1. To prepare the filling: add to a large bowl the carrot, bell pepper, onion, cabbage, ginger, and garlic. Gently add two tablespoons of olive oil in a pan over high heat. Add the filling mixture and stir in salt and a dash of stevia sweetener if you like. Cook for 3-minutes. Add soy sauce, black pepper and mix well.
2. Add green onions, stir and set aside. In a small bowl, combine enough water and cornstarch to make a creamy paste. Fill the rolls with a tablespoon of filling in center of each wrapper and roll tightly, dampening the edges with cornstarch paste to ensure a good seal. Repeat until all wrappers and filling are used. Preheat your air fryer to 350°Fahrenheit. Brush the rolls with oil, and arrange them in the air fryer, and cook them until crisp and golden for about 20-minutes. Halfway through the cook time flip them over.

NUTRITION: Calories: 263, Total Fat: 11.2g, Carbs: 8.6g, Protein: 8.2g

282. Onion Pakora

Cooking Time: 6 minutes

Servings: 6

INGREDIENTS:

- 1cup graham flour
- ¼ teaspoon turmeric powder
- Salt to taste
- 1/8 teaspoon chili powder
- ¼ teaspoon carom
- 1tablespoon fresh coriander, chopped
- 2green chili peppers, finely chopped
- 4onions, finely chopped
- 2teaspoons vegetable oil
- ¼ cup rice flour

DIRECTIONS

1. Combine the flours and oil in a mixing bowl. Add water as needed to create a dough-like consistency. Add peppers, onions, coriander, carom, chili powder, and turmeric. Preheat air fryer to 350°Fahrenheit. Roll vegetable mixture into small balls, add to the fryer and cook for about 6-minutes. Serve with hot sauce!

NUTRITION: Calories: 253, Total Fat: 12.2g, Carbs: 11.4g, Protein: 7.6g

283. Semolina Veggie Cutlets

Cooking Time: 23 minutes

Servings: 2

INGREDIENTS

- 1cup semolina
- Olive oil for frying
- Salt and pepper to taste

Sides

- 1½ cups of your favorite veggies(suggestion: carrot, peas, green beans, bell pepper and cauliflower
- 5cups milk

DIRECTIONS:

1. Stir and warm the milk in a saucepan over medium heat. Add vegetables when it becomes hot and cook until they are softened for about 3-minutes. Season with salt and pepper. Add the semolina to milk mixture and cook for another 10-minutes. Remove from heat and spread thin across a piece of parchment on a baking sheet, and chill for 4 hours in the fridge. Take out the baking sheet from the fridge, cut semolina mixture into cutlets. Preheat your air fryer to 350°Fahrenheit. Brush the cutlets with oil and bake for 10-minutes in your air fryer and serve with hot sauce!

NUTRITIONAL Value per serving: Calories: 252, Total Fat: 11.2g, Carbs: 10.3g, Protein: 7.3g

284. Charred Shishito Peppers

Cooking Time: 5 minutes

Servings: 4

INGREDIENTS

- 20Shishito peppers
- 1teaspoon vegetable oil
- Sea salt to taste
- 1lemon, juiced

DIRECTIONS

1. Preheat your air fryer to 390°Fahrenheit. Toss Shishito peppers with salt and oil adding to the air basket. Air fry for 5-minutes and transfer peppers to bowl. Squeeze lemon juice over peppers and season with coarse sea salt. Serve as finger food.

NUTRITION: Calories: 243, Total Fat: 8.4g, Carbs: 6.3g, Protein: 6.2g

285. Samosas

Cooking Time: 20 minutes

Servings: 4

INGREDIENTS

- 2cups all-purpose flour
- ½ teaspoon cumin seeds
- 2tablespoons olive oil
- 1teaspoon turmeric
- 1teaspoon chili powder
- 1teaspoon ginger-garlic paste
- 2teaspoons garam masala powder
- ½ cup green peas
- 2russet potatoes, peeled and cubed
- 1teaspoon carom seeds
- 2teaspoons ghee butter

DIRECTIONS

1. Prepare the crust in a bowl, combining the carom seeds, flour, water as needed to make a dough. Knead dough and chill in the fridge for 30-minutes. Prepare the filling: in a saucepan, cover the potatoes with water and bring to a boil. Add peas and continue to boil until vegetables are tender. Drain and mash well. Add the garam masala, ginger-garlic paste, chili powder, and turmeric to potato mixture. Season with salt and mix well.
2. In a small pan sauté oil over medium heat. Add the cumin seeds and toast they are sizzling and aromatic. Add the cumin to potato mixture, mix well, then set aside. Retrieve the dough out of the fridge, roll it out on the counter, and cut into several squares about 4-inches across. Place a spoonful of filling in each square and fold samosa to a triangle-like shape, carefully sealing edges. Preheat your air fryer to 350°Fahrenheit. Brush the samosas with oil, place them into air fryer, cook them until they are golden brown for about 20-minutes and serve warm or cold.

NUTRITION: Calories: 253, Total Fat: 11.3g, Carbs: 8.6g, Protein: 7.2g

286. Baked Tomatoes with Feta & Pesto

Cooking Time: 14 minutes

Servings: 4

INGREDIENTS

- Pesto:
- ½ cup fresh parsley and basil, chopped
- ½ cup Parmesan cheese, grated
- Pinch of salt
- 1tablespoon olive oil
- 1clove garlic, toasted
- 3tablespoons pine nuts, toasted
- Tomatoes & Feta:
- 2Heirloom tomatoes, cut into ½ inch slices
- 8-ounces feta cheese, cut into ½ inch slices
- 1tablespoon olive oil
- Pinch of salt
- ½ cup red onion, sliced paper-thin

DIRECTIONS

1. Prepare the pesto by combining all the pesto ingredients excluding olive oil and salt into a food processor. Run the food processor on slow until thick paste forms. Season with salt to taste. Toss tomatoes, feta, and red onion with the olive oil. Briefly, preheat your air fryer to 350°Fahrenheit. Arrange tomato mixture in food tray and cook for 14-minutes. Portion the tomato mixture onto individual serving plates and top with some pesto and serve!

NUTRITION: Calories: 246, Total Fat: 10.4g, Carbs: 8.6g, Protein: 8.4g

287. Cumin, Chili & Squash

Cooking Time: 20 minutes

Servings: 4

INGREDIENTS

- 1 medium butternut squash
- 1 bunch coriander
- 2/3 cup Greek yogurt
- ¼ cup pine nuts
- 1 tablespoon olive oil
- 1 pinch chili flakes
- 2 teaspoons cumin seeds
- Salt and pepper to taste

DIRECTIONS

1. Slice the squash into small chunks. Mix with the spices and oil in a baking pan. Roast the squash in your air fryer at 380°Fahrenheit for 20-minutes. Toast the pine nuts and serve with Greek yogurt and sprinkle coriander on top.

NUTRITION: Calories: 252, Total Fat: 10.3g, Carbs: 7.6g, Protein: 8.7g

288. Pineapple Sticks with Yogurt Dip

Cooking Time: 10 minutes

Servings: 2

INGREDIENTS

- ¼ cup dried coconut
- ½ pineapple
- Yogurt Dip:
- 1 cup vanilla yogurt
- 1 sprig of fresh mint

DIRECTIONS

1. Preheat your air fryer to 390°Fahrenheit. Cut the pineapple into sticks. Dip pineapple sticks into the dried coconut. Place the sticks covered with desiccated coconut into air fryer basket and cook for 10-minutes. Prepare the yogurt dip. Dice the mint leaves and combine with vanilla yogurt and stir. Serve pineapple sticks with yogurt dip and enjoy!

NUTRITION: Calories: 246, Total Fat: 8.4g, Carbs: 7.2g, Protein: 6.3g

289. Low-Carb Zucchini Roll-Ups

Cooking Time: 5 minutes

Servings: 4

INGREDIENTS

- 3 zucchinis, sliced thin, lengthwise
- Sea salt to taste
- 1 cup goat cheese
- ¼ teaspoon black pepper
- 1 tablespoon olive oil

DIRECTIONS

1. preheat air fryer to 390°fahrenheit. brush each zucchini strip with olive oil. mix sea salt and black pepper with goat cheese. spoon the goat cheese into the middle of each strip of zucchini and roll it up and fasten with a toothpick. place into air fryer and cook for 5-minutes.

NUTRITION: Calories: 243, Total Fat: 8.7g, Carbs: 6.4g, Protein: 6.5g

290. Zucchini Fries & Roasted Garlic Aioli

Cooking Time: 12 minutes

Servings: 4

INGREDIENTS

- Roasted Garlic Aioli:
- ½ cup mayonnaise
- Sea salt and pepper to taste
- 1 teaspoon roasted garlic, pureed
- 2 tablespoons olive oil
- ½ lemon, juiced
- Zucchini Fries:
- Sea salt and pepper to taste
- ½ cup almond flour
- 2 eggs, beaten
- 1 cup breadcrumbs
- 1 large zucchini, cut into ½-inch sticks
- 1 tablespoon olive oil
- Cooking spray

DIRECTIONS

1. Take three bowls and line them up on the counter. In the first, combine flour, salt, and pepper. Place eggs in the second bowl. Place breadcrumbs combined with salt and pepper in the third bowl. Take zucchini sticks and dip first into flour, then in the eggs, and then into crumbs. Preheat your air fryer to 400°Fahrenheit.
2. Cover sticks with cooking spray and layer in the basket. There should be two layers, pointing in opposite directions. Halfway through the 12-minute cook time rotate and turn the fries and spray with more cooking spray. Prepare the roasted garlic aioli in a medium bowl by mixing mayonnaise, pureed roasted garlic, olive oil and lemon juice. Stir in some pepper and salt. Serve the fries with the roasted garlic aioli and enjoy!

NUTRITION: Calories: 246, Total Fat: 9.3g, Carbs: 8.1g, Protein: 7.4g

291. <u>Zucchini, Carrots & Yellow Squash</u>

Cooking Time: 35 minutes

Servings: 4

INGREDIENTS

- ½ lb carrots, diced
- 1 lime, cut into wedges
- ½ teaspoon ground white pepper
- 1 lb. zucchini, trim stem and root ends, cut into ¾ inch semicircles
- 1 lb. yellow squash, with roots and stems, trimmed
- 6 teaspoons olive oil, divided
- 1 teaspoon sea salt
- 1 tablespoon tarragon leaves, chopped

DIRECTIONS

1. In a bowl add carrots and cover with 2 teaspoons of oil and stir. Put the carrots in fryer basket and set to 400°Fahrenheit and cook for 5-minutes. Place the zucchini and yellow squash into a bowl. Cover with the remaining 4 teaspoons of olive oil. Season with pepper and salt. When air fryer timer goes off, stir in zucchini and yellow squash with carrots. Cook for 30-minutes. Stir from time to time. Garnish with lime wedges and tarragon leaves.

NUTRITION: Calories: 256, Total Fat: 9.4g, Carbs: 8.6g, Protein: 7.4g

292. <u>Roast Butternut Pumpkin with Nuts & Balsamic Vinaigrette</u>

Cooking Time: 20 minutes

Servings: 4

INGREDIENTS

- 1 butternut pumpkin, cut into 1-inch slices
- Sprigs of thyme for garnishing
- 2½ tablespoons toasted pine nuts
- Sea salt and pepper to taste
- 1½ tablespoons olive oil

- Vinaigrette:
- 6 tablespoons olive oil
- 1 tablespoon Dijon mustard
- Sea salt and black pepper to taste
- 2 tablespoons balsamic vinegar

DIRECTIONS

1. Preheat air fryer to 390°Fahrenheit for 5-minutes. Cover the slices of pumpkin with olive oil and season with thyme, salt, and pepper. Set the air fryer to cook for 20-minutes, and place seasoned pumpkin slices into air fryer. Prepare the vinaigrette by combining all the vinaigrette ingredients in a bowl. Serve pumpkin covered with vinaigrette, sprinkle top with toasted pine nuts and sprigs of thyme.

NUTRITION: Calories: 257, Total Fat: 11.3g, Carbs: 10.6g, Protein: 8.3g

293. Crispy Black-Eyed Peas

Cooking Time: 10 minutes

Servings: 6

INGREDIENTS

- 15-ounces black-eyed peas
- 1/8 teaspoon chipotle chili powder
- ¼ teaspoon salt
- ½ teaspoon chili powder
- 1/8 teaspoon black pepper

DIRECTIONS

1. Rinse the beans well with running water then set aside. In a large bowl, mix the spices until well combined. Add the peas to spices and mix. Place the peas in the wire basket and cook for 10-minutes at 360°Fahrenheit. Serve and enjoy!

NUTRITION: Calories: 262, Total Fat: 9.4g, Carbs: 8.6g, Protein: 9.2g

294. Lemony Green Beans

Cooking Time: 12 minutes

Servings: 4

INGREDIENTS

- 1 lb. green beans washed and destemmed
- Sea salt and black pepper to taste
- 1 lemon
- ¼ teaspoon extra virgin olive oil

DIRECTIONS

1. Preheat your air fryer to 400°Fahrenheit. Place the green beans in the air fryer basket. Squeeze lemon over beans and season with salt and pepper. Cover ingredients with oil and toss well. Cook green beans for 12-minutes and serve!

NUTRITION: Calories: 263, Total Fat: 9.2g, Carbs: 8.6g, Protein: 8.7g

295. Roasted Orange Cauliflower

Cooking Time: 20 minutes

Servings: 2

INGREDIENTS

- 1 head cauliflower
- ½ lemon, juiced
- ½ tablespoon olive oil
- 1 teaspoon curry powder
- Sea salt and black pepper to taste

DIRECTIONS

1. Prepare your cauliflower by washing and removing the leaves and core. Slice it into florets of comparable size. Grease your air fryer with oil and preheat it for 2-minutes at 390°Fahrenheit. Combine fresh lemon juice and curry powder, add

296. Eggplant Parmesan Panini

Cooking Time: 25 minutes

Servings: 2

INGREDIENTS

- 1 medium eggplant, cut into ½ inch slices
- ½ cup mayonnaise
- 2 tablespoons milk
- Black pepper to taste
- ½ teaspoon garlic powder
- ½ teaspoon onion powder
- 1 tablespoon dried parsley
- ½ teaspoon Italian seasoning
- ½ cup breadcrumbs
- Sea salt to taste
- Fresh basil, chopped for garnishing
- ¾ cup tomato sauce
- 2 tablespoons parmesan, grated cheese
- 2 cups grated mozzarella cheese
- 2 tablespoons olive oil
- 4 slices artisan Italian bread
- Cooking spray

DIRECTIONS

1. Cover both sides of eggplant with salt. Place them between sheets of paper towels. Set aside for 30-minutes to get rid of excess moisture. In a mixing bowl, combine Italian seasoning, breadcrumbs, parsley, onion powder, garlic powder and season with salt and pepper. In another small bowl, whisk mayonnaise and milk until smooth.
2. Preheat your air fryer to 400°Fahrenheit. Remove the excess salt from eggplant slices. Cover both sides of eggplant with mayonnaise mixture. Press the eggplant slices into the breadcrumb mixture. Use cooking spray on both sides of eggplant slices. Air fry slices in batches for 15-minutes, turning over when halfway done. Each bread slice must be greased with olive oil. On a cutting board, place two slices of bread with oiled sides down. Layer mozzarella cheese and grated parmesan cheese. Place eggplant on cheese. Cover with tomato sauce and add remaining mozzarella and parmesan cheeses. Garnish with chopped fresh basil. Put the second slice of bread oiled side up on top. Take preheated Panini press and place sandwiches on it. Close the lid and cook for 10-minutes. Slice panini into halves and serve.

NUTRITION: Calories: 267, Total Fat: 11.3g, Carbs: 8.7g, Protein: 8.5g

297. Spinach Samosa

Cooking Time: 15 minutes

Servings: 2

INGREDIENTS

- 1½ cups of almond flour
- ½ teaspoon baking soda
- 1 teaspoon garam masala
- 1 teaspoon coriander, chopped
- ¼ cup green peas
- ½ teaspoon sesame seeds
- ¼ cup potatoes, boiled, small chunks
- 2 tablespoons olive oil
- ¾ cup boiled and blended spinach puree
- Salt and chili powder to taste

DIRECTIONS

1. In a bowl, mix baking soda, salt, and flour to make the dough. Add 1-tablespoon of oil. Add the spinach puree and mix until the dough is smooth. Place in fridge for twenty-minutes. In the pan add one tablespoon of oil, then add potatoes,

peas and cook for 5-minutes. Add the sesame seeds, garam masala, coriander, and stir. Knead the dough and make the small ball using a rolling pin. Form balls, make into cone shapes, which are then filled with stuffing that is not yet fully cooked. Make sure flour sheets are well sealed. Preheat air fryer to 390°Fahrenheit. Place samosa in air fryer basket and cook for 10-minutes.

NUTRITION: Calories: 254, Total Fat: 12.2g, Carbs: 9.3g, Protein: 10.2g

298. Avocado Fries

Cooking Time: 10 minutes

Servings: 4

INGREDIENTS

- 1-ounce aquafina
- 1 avocado, sliced
- ½ teaspoon salt
- ½ cup panko breadcrumbs

DIRECTIONS

1. Toss the panko breadcrumbs and salt together in a bowl. Pour Aquafina into another bowl. Dredge the avocado slices in Aquafina and then panko breadcrumbs. Arrange the slices in single layer in air fryer basket. Air fry at 390°Fahrenheit for 10-minutes.

NUTRITION: Calories: 263, Total Fat: 7.4g, Carbs: 6.5g, Protein: 8.2g

299. Honey Roasted Carrots

Cooking Time: 12 minutes

Servings: 2

INGREDIENTS

- 1 tablespoon honey
- Salt and pepper to taste
- 3 cups of baby carrots
- 1 tablespoon olive oil

DIRECTIONS

1. In a mixing bowl, combine carrots, honey, and olive oil. Season with salt and pepper. Cook in air fryer at 390°Fahrenheit for 12-minutes.

NUTRITION: Calories: 257, Total Fat: 11.6g, Carbs: 8.7g, Protein: 7.3g

300. Crispy & Crunchy Baby Corn

Cooking Time: 10 minutes

Servings: 4

INGREDIENTS

- 1 cup almond flour
- 1 teaspoon garlic powder
- ¼ teaspoon chili powder
- 4 baby corns, boiled
- Salt to taste
- ½ teaspoon carom seeds
- Pinch of baking soda

DIRECTIONS

1. In a bowl, add flour, chili powder, garlic powder, baking soda, carom seed, and salt. Mix well. Pour a little water into the batter to make a nice batter. Dip boiled baby corn into the batter to coat. Preheat your air fryer to 350°Fahrenheit. Line the air fryer basket with foil and place the baby corns on foil. Cook baby corns for 10-minutes.

NUTRITION: Calories: 243, Total Fat: 9.6g, Carbs: 8.2g, Protein: 10.3g

301. Tasty Tofu

Cooking Time: 12 minutes

Servings: 4

INGREDIENTS

- ¼ cup cornmeal
- 15-ounces extra firm tofu, drained, cubed
- Salt and pepper to taste
- 1 teaspoon chili flakes
- ¾ cup cornstarch

DIRECTIONS

1. Line the air fryer basket with aluminum foil and brush with oil. Preheat your air fryer to 370°Fahrenheit. Mix all ingredients in a bowl. Place in air fryer and cook for 12-minutes.

NUTRITION: Calories: 246, Total Fat: 11.2g, Carbs: 8.7g, Protein: 7.6g

302. Crispy Herb Cauliflower Florets

Cooking Time: 20 minutes

Servings: 2

INGREDIENTS

- 1 egg, beaten
- 2 tablespoons parmesan cheese, grated
- 2 cups cauliflower florets, boiled
- ¼ cup almond flour
- 1 tablespoon olive oil
- Salt to taste
- ½ tablespoon mixed herbs
- ½ teaspoon chili powder
- ½ teaspoon garlic powder
- ½ cup breadcrumbs

DIRECTIONS

1. In a bowl, combine garlic powder, breadcrumbs, chili powder, mixed herbs, salt, and cheese. Add olive oil to the breadcrumb mixture and mix well. Place flour in a bowl and place the egg in another bowl. Dip the cauliflower florets into the beaten egg, then in flour, and coat with breadcrumbs. Preheat your air fryer to 350°Fahrenheit. Place the coated cauliflower florets inside air fryer basket and cook for 20-minutes.

Nutrition: Calories: 253, Total Fat: 11.3g, Carbs: 9,5g, Protein: 8.5g

303. Roasted Corn

Cooking Time: 10 minutes

Servings: 8

INGREDIENTS

- 4 ears of corn
- Salt and pepper to taste
- 3 teaspoons vegetable oil

DIRECTIONS

1. Remove the husks from corn, wash and pat them dry. Cut if needed to fit into air fryer basket. Drizzle with vegetable oil and season with salt and pepper. Cook at 400°Fahrenheit for 10-minutes.

NUTRITION: Calories: 256, Total Fat: 9.4g, Carbs: 8.7g, Protein: 9.2g

304. Spicy Nuts

Cooking Time: 4 minutes

Servings: 8

INGREDIENTS

- 2cups mixed nuts
- 1teaspoon chipotle chili powder
- 1teaspoon salt
- 1teaspoon pepper
- 1tablespoon butter, melted
- 1easpoon ground cumin

DIRECTIONS

1. In a bowl, add all ingredients and toss to coat. Preheat your air fryer to 350°Fahrenheit for 5-minutes. Add mixed nuts into air fryer basket and roast for 4-minutes.

NUTRITION: Calories: 252, Total Fat: 8.6g, Carbs: 7.2g, Protein: 8.4g

305. Tawa Veggies

Cooking Time: 25 minutes
Servings: 4

INGREDIENTS

- ¼ cup okra
- 2teaspoons garam masala
- 1teaspoon red chili powder
- 1teaspoon amchur powder
- ¼ cup taro root
- ¼ cup potato
- ¼ cup eggplant
- Salt to taste
- Olive oil for brushing

DIRECTIONS

1. Cut potato and taro root into fries and soak in salt water for 10 minutes. Cut okra and eggplant into four pieces. Rinse potatoes and taro root and pat dry. Add the spices to potatoes, taro roots, okra, and eggplant. Brush pan with oil and preheat to 390°Fahrenheit and cook for 10-minutes. Lower the heat to 355°Fahrenheit and cook for an additional 15-minutes.

NUTRITION: Calories: 264, Total Fat: 11.3g, Carbs: 10.4g, Protein: 8.7g

306. Mediterranean Veggie Mix

Cooking Time: 20 minutes
Servings: 4

INGREDIENTS

- 1large zucchini, sliced
- 1green pepper, sliced
- 1large parsnip, peeled and cubed
- Salt and black pepper to taste
- 2tablespoons honey
- 2cloves garlic, crushed
- 1teaspoon mixed herbs
- 1teaspoon mustard
- 6tablespoons olive oil, divided
- 4cherry tomatoes
- 1medium carrot, peeled and cubed

DIRECTIONS

1. Add the zucchini, green pepper, parsnip, cherry tomatoes, carrot to bottom of air fryer.
2. Cover ingredients with 3 tablespoons of oil and adjust the time to 15-minutes.
3. Cook at 360°Fahrenheit. Prepare your marinade by combining remaining ingredients in air fryer safe baking dish.
4. Combine marinade and vegetables in baking dish and stir well.
5. Sprinkle with salt and pepper. Cook it at 390°Fahrenheit for 5-minutes.

NUTRITION: Calories: 262, Total Fat: 11.3g, Carbs: 9.5g, Protein: 7.4g

SEAFOOD

307. Ginger Salmon Mix

Preparation time: 4 minutes

Cooking time: 15 minutes

Servings: 4

INGREDIENTS

- 1pound salmon fillets, boneless
- 1tablespoon ginger, grated
- 1tablespoon olive oil
- 2teaspoons garlic powder
- 1tablespoon lemon juice
- 1tablespoon dill, chopped
- Salt and black pepper to the taste

DIRECTIONS

1. In the air fryer's pan, mix the salmon with the ginger and the other ingredients, toss, introduce the pan in the air fryer and cook at 380 degrees F for 15 minutes.
2. Divide between plates and serve..

NUTRITION: Calories 236, Fat 8, Fiber 12, Carbs 17, Protein 16

308. Salmon Fillets and Green Olives

Preparation time: 4 minutes

Cooking time: 20 minutes

Servings: 4

INGREDIENTS

- 1cup green olives, pitted
- 1pound salmon fillets, boneless
- Salt and black pepper to the taste
- 1tablespoon avocado oil
- Juice of 1 lime
- 1tablespoon dill, chopped

DIRECTIONS

1. In a baking dish that fits your air fryer, mix the salmon with the green olives and the other ingredients, toss gently, introduce in your air fryer and cook at 370 degrees F for 20 minutes.
2. Divide everything between plates and serve.

NUTRITION: Calories 281, Fat 8, Fiber 14, Carbs 17, Protein 16

309. Chervil Cod

Preparation time: 10 minutes

Cooking time: 20 minutes

Servings: 4

INGREDIENTS

- 4cod fillets, boneless
- 1tablespoon chervil, chopped
- Juice of 1 lime
- Salt and black pepper to the taste
- ½ cup coconut milk
- A drizzle of olive oil

DIRECTIONS

1. In a baking dish that fits your air fryer, mix the cod with the chervil and the other ingredients, toss gently, introduce in your air fryer and cook at 380 degrees F for 20 minutes.
2. Divide between plates and serve hot.

NUTRITION: Calories 250, Fat 5, Fiber 6, Carbs 15, Protein 18

310. Honey Salmon

Preparation time: 5 minutes

Cooking time: 15 minutes

Servings: 4

INGREDIENTS

- 4 salmon fillets, boneless
- 2 tablespoons lemon juice
- A pinch of salt and black pepper
- 1 tablespoon honey
- 2 tablespoons olive oil
- 2 tablespoons chives, chopped

DIRECTIONS

1. In the air fryer's pan, mix the salmon with the lemon juice, honey and the other ingredients and cook at 350 degrees F for 15 minutes.
2. Divide the mix between plates and serve.

NUTRITION: Calories 272, Fat 8, Fiber 12, Carbs 15, Protein 16

311. Scallops Mix

Preparation time: 10 minutes

Cooking time: 15 minutes

Servings: 4

INGREDIENTS

- 1 pound scallops
- 1 red bell pepper, chopped
- ½ cup white wine
- ½ teaspoon sweet paprika
- Salt and black pepper to the taste
- A drizzle of olive oil

DIRECTIONS

1. In the air fryer's pan, mix the scallops with the wine and the other ingredients and cook at 380 degrees F and cook for 15 minutes, stirring halfway.
2. Divide between plates and serve.

NUTRITION: Calories 290, Fat 12, Fiber 2, Carbs 16, Protein 19

312. Shrimp and Cucumber Mix

Preparation time: 5 minutes

Cooking time: 10 minutes

Servings: 4

INGREDIENTS

- 1 pound shrimp, deveined and peeled
- 1 cup cucumber, roughly cubed
- 1 tablespoon avocado oil
- 1 tablespoon balsamic vinegar
- ½ cup coconut cream
- 1 tablespoon parsley, chopped
- Salt and black pepper to the taste

DIRECTIONS

1. In a pan that fits your air fryer, mix the shrimp with the cucumber and the other ingredients, toss, introduce in the fryer and cook at 360 degrees F for 10 minutes.
2. Divide into bowls and serve.

NUTRITION: Calories 272, Fat 4, Fiber 3, Carbs 14, Protein 4

313. Shrimp and Potatoes

Preparation time: 5 minutes

Cooking time: 20 minutes

Servings: 4

INGREDIENTS

- 1pound, peeled and deveined
- ½ cup chicken stock
- ½ pound gold potatoes, peeled and cut into wedges
- Salt and black pepper to the taste
- ½ teaspoon Italian seasoning
- 1tablespoon avocado oil
- ¼ teaspoon sweet paprika
- ½ teaspoon coriander, ground

DIRECTIONS

1. In the air fryer's pan, mix the potatoes with the oil and the other ingredients except the shrimp and cook at 380 degrees F for 10 minutes.
2. Add the shrimp, cook for 10 minutes more, divide into bowls and serve,

NUTRITION: Calories 219, Fat 6, Fiber 4, Carbs 14, Protein 15

314. Shrimp and Red Pepper Sauce

Preparation time: 10 minutes

Cooking time: 10 minutes

Servings: 4

INGREDIENTS

- 1pound big shrimp, peeled and deveined
- 1teaspoon red pepper flakes, crushed
- 1cup heavy cream
- 2teaspoons olive oil
- ½ teaspoon coriander, ground
- 1teaspoon basil, dried
- Salt and black pepper to the taste
- 1tablespoon tarragon, chopped

DIRECTIONS

1. In the air fryer's pan, mix the shrimp with the pepper flakes and the other ingredients, cook at 370 degrees F for 10 minutes, divide into bowls, and serve.

NUTRITION: Calories 210, Fat 7, Fiber 6, Carbs 13, Protein 8

315. Sage Shrimp

Preparation time: 3 minutes

Cooking time: 10 minutes

Servings: 4

INGREDIENTS

- 2pounds shrimp, peeled and deveined
- 1tablespoon sage, chopped
- ½ cup chicken stock
- 4garlic cloves, minced
- Salt and black pepper to the taste
- 1tablespoon dill, chopped

DIRECTIONS

1. In the air fryer, mix the shrimp with the sage and the other ingredients, toss, cook at 360 degrees F for 10 minutes, divide into bowls and serve.

NUTRITION: Calories 210, Fat 11, Fiber 12, Carbs 16, Protein 9

316. Dill Sea Bass

Preparation time: 10 minutes

Cooking time: 14 minutes

Servings: 4

INGREDIENTS

- 1pound sea bass fillets, boneless
- 1tablespoon olive oil
- 1tablespoon dill, chopped
- Salt and black pepper to the taste
- ½ teaspoon cumin, ground

- ½ teaspoon rosemary, dried
- 1 tablespoon lemon juice

DIRECTIONS

1. In your air fryer, mix the sea bass with the oil, dill and the other ingredients, toss and cook at 360 degrees F for 14 minutes.
2. Divide the fish between plates and serve.

NUTRITION: Calories 280, Fat 11, Fiber 1, Carbs 12, Protein 18

317. Baked Snapper

Preparation time: 10 minutes

Cooking time: 15 minutes

Servings: 4

INGREDIENTS

- 1 pound snapper fillets, boneless
- 1 tablespoon lemon juice
- 1 tablespoon olive oil
- ½ teaspoon cumin, ground
- Salt and black pepper to the taste

DIRECTIONS

1. In the air fryer's basket, mix the snapper with the lemon juice and the other ingredients, cook at 380 degrees F for 15 minutes, divide everything between plates and serve with a side salad.

NUTRITION: Calories 191, Fat 2, Fiber 3, Carbs 18, Protein 12

318. Trout and Red Chili Mix

Preparation time: 10 minutes

Cooking time: 15 minutes

Servings: 4

INGREDIENTS

- 4 trout fillets, boneless
- Salt and black pepper to the taste
- 1 red chili pepper, chopped
- 1 green chili pepper, chopped
- 1 cup heavy cream
- 1 tablespoon lemon juice

DIRECTIONS

1. In the air fryer's pan, mix the fish with the chilies and the other ingredients, toss, cook at 360 degrees F for 15 minutes, divide between plates and serve.

NUTRITION: Calories 271, Fat 4, Fiber 2, Carbs 15, Protein 11

319. Cilantro Shrimp and Apples Mix

Preparation time: 10 minutes

Cooking time: 12 minutes

Servings: 4

INGREDIENTS

- 1 pound shrimp, peeled and deveined
- 1 cup green apples, cored and cubed
- Juice of 1 lime
- 1 tablespoon avocado oil
- 1 tablespoon cilantro, chopped
- 1 teaspoon chili powder

DIRECTIONS:

1. In your air fryer, mix the shrimp with the apples and the other ingredients, cook at 360 degrees F for 12 minutes, divide into bowls and serve.

NUTRITION: Calories 251, Fat 7, Fiber 3, Carbs 16, Protein 12

320. Saffron Salmon

Preparation time: 5 minutes

Cooking time: 20 minutes

Servings: 4

INGREDIENTS

- 1pound salmon fillets, boneless
- ½ teaspoon saffron powder
- Juice of 1 lime
- Salt and black pepper to the taste
- 1tablespoon butter, melted
- ¼ tablespoon chives, chopped

DIRECTIONS

1. In a pan that fits your air fryer, mix the salmon with the saffron and the other ingredients, and cook at 380 degrees F for 20 minutes.
2. Divide everything between plates and serve.

NUTRITION: Calories 271, Fat 8, Fiber 9, Carbs 15, Protein 8

321. Salmon and Parsnips

Preparation time: 10 minutes

Cooking time: 20 minutes

Servings: 4

INGREDIENTS

- 4salmon fillets, boneless
- 1cup parsnips, peeled and cubed
- Juice of 1 lime
- 1tablespoon olive oil
- ¼ cup veggie stock
- 1teaspoon sweet paprika
- Salt and black pepper to the taste

DIRECTIONS

1. In your air fryer, mix the salmon with the parsnips and the other ingredients, cook at 370 degrees F for 20 minutes, divide everything between plates and serve.

NUTRITION: Calories 200, Fat 6, Fiber 6, Carbs 18, Protein 11

322. Spiced Cod

Preparation time: 4 minutes

Cooking time: 20 minutes

Servings: 4

INGREDIENTS

- 4cod fillets, boneless
- 1teaspoon nutmeg, ground
- 1teaspoon allspice, ground
- 1teaspoon cinnamon powder
- 1teaspoon turmeric powder
- Juice of 1 lemon
- 1tablespoon avocado oil
- Salt and black pepper to the taste

DIRECTIONS

1. In your air fryer, mix the cod with the spices and the other ingredients, cook at 370 degrees F for 20 minutes, divide between plates and serve.

NUTRITION: Calories 200, Fat 4, Fiber 8, Carbs 16, Protein 7

323. Salmon and White Onions Mix

Preparation time: 10 minutes

Cooking time: 20 minutes

Servings: 4

INGREDIENTS

- 4 salmon fillets, boneless
- 2 white onions, sliced
- Juice of 1 lime
- ½ teaspoon sweet paprika
- 3 tablespoons olive oil
- Salt and black pepper to the taste

DIRECTIONS:

1. In your air fryer, mix the salmon with the white onions and the other ingredients, and cook at 380 degrees F for 20 minutes.
2. Divide everything between plates and serve.

NUTRITION: Calories 200, Fat 5, Fiber 5, Carbs 16, Protein 15

324. Sherry Salmon Mix

Preparation time: 10 minutes

Cooking time: 15 minutes

Servings: 4

INGREDIENTS

- 4 salmon fillets, boneless
- 1 tablespoon avocado oil
- 1 cup orange juice
- salt and white pepper to the taste
- 1 teaspoon sherry
- 1 tablespoon chives, chopped

DIRECTIONS

1. In a pan that fits your air fryer, mix the salmon with the oil and the other ingredients, introduce in the fryer and cook at 370 degrees F for 15 minutes.
2. Divide everything between plates and serve.

NUTRITION: Calories 261, Fat 8, Fiber 6, Carbs 15, Protein 14

325. Sake Shrimp Mix

Preparation time: 5 minutes

Cooking time: 12 minutes

Servings: 4

INGREDIENTS

- 1 pound shrimp, peeled and deveined
- ½ teaspoon cumin, ground
- 1/3 cup sake
- 1 tablespoon soy sauce
- A pinch of cayenne pepper
- 1 teaspoon mustard
- 1 teaspoon sugar

DIRECTIONS

1. In a pan that fist your air fryer, mix the shrimp with the sake and the other ingredients, introduce the pan in the fryer and cook at 370 degrees F for 12 minutes.
2. Divide into bowls and serve.

NUTRITION: Calories 271, Fat 11, Fiber 7, Carbs 16, Protein 6

326. Trout and Avocado Mix

Preparation time: 10 minutes

Cooking time: 20 minutes

Servings: 4

INGREDIENTS

- 4 trout fillets, boneless
- 1 cup avocado, peeled, pitted and cubed
- 1 tablespoon olive oil
- Juice of 1 lemon
- 1 tablespoon chives, chopped
- Salt and black pepper to the taste

DIRECTIONS

1. In the air fryer, mix the trout with the avocado and the other ingredients, cook at 370 degrees F for 20 minutes.
2. Divide the mix into bowls and serve.

NUTRITION: Calories 214, Fat 8, Fiber 8, Carbs 17, Protein 7

327. Shrimp and Sausage Mix

Preparation time: 5 minutes

Cooking time: 12 minutes

Servings: 4

INGREDIENTS

- 1pound shrimp, peeled and deveined
- 1cup sausages, sliced
- Juice of 1 lime
- 1tablespoon olive oil
- 1yellow onion, chopped
- 1tablespoon chives, chopped

DIRECTIONS

1. In a pan that fits your air fryer, mix the shrimp with the sausages and the other ingredients, introduce the pan in the air fryer and cook at 380 degrees F for 12 minutes.
2. Divide the mix into bowls and serve.

NUTRITION: Calories 201, Fat 6, Fiber 7, Carbs 17, Protein 7

328. Marjoram Shrimp

Preparation time: 10 minutes

Cooking time: 15 minutes

Servings: 4

INGREDIENTS

- 2pounds big shrimp, peeled and deveined
- 2tablespoons olive oil
- 1tablespoon marjoram
- 1cup caned tomatoes, chopped
- Salt and black pepper to the taste

DIRECTIONS

1. In a pan that fits your air fryer, mix the shrimp with the marjoram and the other ingredients, introduce in the fryer and cook at 380 degrees F for 15 minutes.
2. Divide into bowls and serve.

NUTRITION: Calories 261, Fat 7, Fiber 7, Carbs 16, Protein 8

329. Clams and Beer Sauce

Preparation time: 10 minutes

Cooking time: 15 minutes

Servings: 4

INGREDIENTS

- 1pound clams
- 1red onion, chopped
- A pinch of salt and black pepper
- ½ teaspoon sweet paprika
- 1cup beer
- 2tablespoons cilantro, chopped
- 1teaspoon olive oil

DIRECTIONS

1. In a pan that fits your air fryer, mix the clams with the onion and the other ingredients, introduce in the fryer and cook at 390 degrees F for 15 minutes.
2. Divide into bowls and serve.

NUTRITION: Calories 231, Fat 6, Fiber 8, Carbs 16, Protein 16

330. Oregano Clams

Preparation time: 5 minutes

Cooking time: 12 minutes

Servings: 4

INGREDIENTS

- 1pound clams
- 4tablespoons butter, soft
- ¼ cup oregano, chopped
- 1cup orange juice
- A pinch of salt and black pepper

DIRECTIONS

1. In the air fryer, mix the clams with the melted butter and the other ingredients, toss and cook at 380 degrees F for 12 minutes.
2. Divide into bowls and serve.

NUTRITION: Calories 100, Fat 7, Fiber 4, Carbs 15, Protein 6

331. Turmeric Trout and Beans

Preparation time: 5 minutes

Cooking time: 20 minutes

Servings: 4

INGREDIENTS

- 1pound trout fillets, boneless
- 1cup canned red kidney beans, drained
- 1tablespoon lemon juice
- 1teaspoon turmeric powder
- 2tablespoons butter, melted
- Salt and black pepper to the taste
- 1tablespoon parsley, chopped

DIRECTIONS

1. In a pan that fits your air fryer, mix the trout with the beans and the other ingredients, introduce in the fryer and cook at 380 degrees F for 8 minutes.
2. Divide between plates and serve hot.

NUTRITION: Calories 261, Fat 7, Fiber 9, Carbs 16, Protein 7

332. Shrimp and Black Beans

Preparation time: 5 minutes

Cooking time: 10 minutes

Servings: 4

INGREDIENTS

- 1pound shrimp, peeled and deveined
- 1red onion, sliced
- 1cup canned black beans, drained
- A drizzle of olive oil
- ¼ cup chicken stock
- 1tablespoon chives, chopped
- A pinch of salt and black pepper
- 3garlic cloves, crushed

DIRECTIONS

1. In the air fryer's pan, mix the shrimp with the onion, beans and the other ingredients, toss, introduce the pan in the fryer and cook at 390 degrees F for 10 minutes.
2. Divide everything into bowls and serve.

NUTRITION: Calories 261, Fat 7, Fiber 6, Carbs 17, Protein 11

333. Salmon, Cauliflower and Red Quinoa

Preparation time: 3 minutes

Cooking time: 20 minutes

Servings: 4

INGREDIENTS

- 1pound salmon fillets, boneless
- 1cup cauliflower florets
- 1cup red quinoa, cooked
- 1cup chicken stock
- 2tablespoons olive oil
- 1tablespoon chives, chopped
- 1teaspoon sweet paprika

DIRECTIONS

1. In a pan that fits your air fryer, mix the salmon with the cauliflower, quinoa and the other ingredients, introduce the pan in the fryer and cook at 380 degrees F for 20 minutes.
2. Divide into bowls and serve.

NUTRITION: Calories 261, Fat 6, Fiber 8, Carbs 16, Protein 6

334. Corn, Okra and Shrimp

Preparation time: 10 minutes

Cooking time: 15 minutes

Servings: 4

INGREDIENTS

- 2pounds shrimp, peeled and deveined
- 1cup corn
- 1cup okra
- ½ teaspoon chili powder
- ¼ cup veggie stock
- Salt and black pepper to the taste
- 2tablespoons olive oil
- 1teaspoon rosemary, dried

DIRECTIONS

1. In a pan that fits your air fryer, mix the shrimp with the corn, okra and the other ingredients, introduce the pan in the fryer and cook at 360 degrees F for 15 minutes.
2. Divide into bowls and serve.

NUTRITION: Calories 161, Fat 1, Fiber 6, Carbs 17, Protein 7

335. Tomato Clams

Preparation time: 5 minutes

Cooking time: 20 minutes

Servings: 4

INGREDIENTS

- 1pound clams
- 1cup canned tomatoes, crushed
- ½ tablespoon balsamic vinegar
- Salt and black pepper to the taste
- 1teaspoons chili powder
- 1tablespoon chives, chopped

DIRECTIONS

1. In a pan that fits your air fryer, mix the clams with the tomatoes and the other ingredients, toss, introduce in the fryer and cook at 370 degrees F for 20 minutes.
2. Divide into bowls and serve.

NUTRITION: Calories 251, Fat 7, Fiber 7, Carbs 18, Protein 11

336. Shrimp, Cod and Sauce

Preparation time: 4 minutes

Cooking time: 15 minutes

Servings: 4

INGREDIENTS

- 1pounds shrimp, peeled and deveined
- ½ pound cod fillets, boneless and cubed
- 1cup orange juice

- 1 teaspoon turmeric powder
- 2 tablespoons soy sauce
- 1 tablespoon chives, chopped

DIRECTIONS

1. In a pan that fits your air fryer, mix the shrimp with the cod and the other ingredients, toss, introduce in the fryer and cook at 380 degrees F for 15 minutes.
2. Divide into bowls and serve.

NUTRITION: Calories 251, Fat 4, Fiber 3, Carbs 14, Protein 5

337. Caraway Shrimp Mix

Preparation time: 10 minutes

Cooking time: 10 minutes

Servings: 4

INGREDIENTS

- 1 pound shrimp, peeled and deveined
- Salt and black pepper to the taste
- ½ teaspoon caraway seeds
- 1 tablespoon olive oil
- 2 spring onions, chopped
- ¼ cup chicken stock

DIRECTIONS

1. In a pan that fits your air fryer, mix the shrimp with the caraway and the other ingredients, toss, introduce in the fryer and cook at 380 degrees F for 10 minutes.
2. Divide into bowls and serve.

NUTRITION: Calories 251, Fat 3, Fiber 7, Carbs 15, Protein 8

338. Shrimp and Butternut Squash

Preparation time: 10 minutes

Cooking time: 10 minutes

Servings: 4

INGREDIENTS

- 1 pound shrimp, cooked, peeled and deveined
- 2 tablespoons avocado oil
- 1 cup butternut squash, peeled and cubed
- ½ cup canned tomatoes, crushed
- ¼ teaspoon oregano, dried
- 1 tablespoon chives, chopped

DIRECTIONS:

1. In a pan that fits your air fryer, mix the shrimp with the squash and the other ingredients, introduce in the fryer and cook at 380 degrees F for 10 minutes.
2. Divide the mix between plates and serve.

NUTRITION: Calories 271, Fat 12, Fiber 4, Carbs 14, Protein 5

339. Calamari and Sauce

Preparation time: 10 minutes

Cooking time: 20 minutes

Servings: 4

INGREDIENTS

- 2 cups calamari rings
- 1 cup canned tomatoes, crushed
- 1 tablespoon balsamic vinegar
- 1 tablespoon olive oil
- Salt and black pepper to the taste
- 1 teaspoon chili powder

DIRECTIONS

1. In the air fryer's pan, mix the calamari rings with the tomatoes and the other ingredients, cook at 390 degrees F for 20 minutes, divide into bowls and serve.

NUTRITION: Calories 191, Fat 6, Fiber 7, Carbs 15, Protein 7

340. Calamari Salsa Mix

Preparation time: 10 minutes

Cooking time: 20 minutes

Servings: 4

INGREDIENTS

- 2tablespoons olive oil
- 2cups calamari rings
- 1red onion, chopped
- 1cup mild salsa
- Salt and black pepper to the taste
- ¼ cup parsley, chopped

DIRECTIONS

1. In a pan that fits your air fryer, mix the calamari rings with the onion and the other ingredients, introduce in the air fryer and cook at 380 degrees F for 20 minutes.
2. Divide everything between plates and serve.

NUTRITION: Calories 271, Fat 8, Fiber 8, Carbs 17, Protein 11

341. Maple Walnut Salmon

Preparation time: 10 minutes

Cooking time: 15 minutes

Servings: 4

INGREDIENTS

- ½ cup chopped walnuts
- 1tsp smoked paprika
- ½ tsp onion powder
- ½ tsp garlic powder
- 3Tbsp keto maple syrup
- 1Tbsp apple cider vinegar
- 1tsp coconut aminos
- 2Tbsp butter
- 24oz salmon filets

DIRECTIONS:

1. Preheat your air fryer to 400 degrees F and line the air fryer tray with foil.
2. In a large bowl, combine the walnuts, paprika, onion powder, garlic powder, keto syrup, vinegar and coconut aminos.
3. Place the salmon on the prepared tray and spoon the walnut mix over the top of the fish.
4. Place the tray in the fridge and let cool for 2 hours.
5. Remove the tray from the fridge and dot the butter throughout the tray, dispersing it around the fish.
6. Place in the air fryer and bake for 15 minutes
7. Servings hot!

NUTRITION: Calories 449, Total Fat 28g, Saturated Fat 7g, Total Carbs 13g, Net Carbs 1g, Protein 36g, Sugar 9g, Fiber 2g, Sodium 111mg, Potassium 943g

342. Almond Crusted Salmon

Preparation time: 10 minutes

Cooking time: 15 minutes

Servings: 4

INGREDIENTS

- ½ cup sliced walnuts
- 1tsp smoked paprika
- ½ tsp onion powder
- ½ tsp garlic powder
- 1Tbsp apple cider vinegar
- 1tsp coconut aminos
- 2Tbsp butter
- 24oz salmon filets

DIRECTIONS:

1. Preheat your air fryer to 400 degrees F and line the air fryer tray with foil.
2. In a large bowl, combine the almonds, paprika, onion powder, garlic powder, vinegar and coconut aminos.
3. Place the salmon on the prepared tray and spoon the walnut mix over the top of the fish.
4. Place the tray in the fridge and let cool for 2 hours.
5. Remove the tray from the fridge and dot the butter throughout the tray, dispersing it around the fish.
6. Place in the air fryer and bake for 15 minutes
7. Servings hot!

NUTRITION: Calories 402, Total Fat 28g, Saturated Fat 7g, Total Carbs 8g, Net Carbs 6g, Protein 36g, Sugar 7g, Fiber 2g, Sodium 111mg, Potassium 943g

343. Maple Walnut Flounder

Preparation time: 10 minutes

Cooking time: 15 minutes

Servings: 4

INGREDIENTS

- ½ cup chopped walnuts
- 1tsp smoked paprika
- ½ tsp onion powder
- ½ tsp garlic powder
- 3Tbsp keto maple syrup
- 1Tbsp apple cider vinegar
- 1tsp coconut aminos
- 2Tbsp butter
- 24oz flounder filets

DIRECTIONS:

1. Preheat your air fryer to 400 degrees F and line the air fryer tray with foil.
2. In a large bowl, combine the walnuts, paprika, onion powder, garlic powder, keto syrup, vinegar and coconut aminos.
3. Place the flounder on the prepared tray and spoon the walnut mix over the top of the fish.
4. Place the tray in the fridge and let cool for 2 hours.
5. Remove the tray from the fridge and dot the butter throughout the tray, dispersing it around the fish.
6. Place in the air fryer and bake for 15 minutes
7. Servings hot!

NUTRITION: Calories 432, Total Fat 25g, Saturated Fat 6g, Total Carbs 13g, Net Carbs 1g, Protein 34g, Sugar 9g, Fiber 2g, Sodium 111mg, Potassium 943g

344. Sesame Walnut Tuna

Preparation time: 10 minutes

Cooking time: 20 minutes

Servings: 4

INGREDIENTS

- ½ cup chopped walnuts
- 1tsp smoked paprika
- ½ tsp onion powder
- ½ tsp garlic powder
- 1Tbsp sesame seeds
- 1Tbsp apple cider vinegar
- 2tsp coconut aminos
- 2Tbsp butter
- 24oz Tuna Steaks

DIRECTIONS:

1. Preheat your air fryer to 400 degrees F and line the air fryer tray with foil.
2. In a large bowl, combine the walnuts, paprika, onion powder, garlic powder, sesame seeds, vinegar and coconut aminos.

3. Place the tuna on the prepared tray and spoon the walnut mix over the top of the fish.
4. Place the tray in the fridge and let cool for 2 hours.
5. Remove the tray from the fridge and dot the butter throughout the tray, dispersing it around the fish.
6. Place in the air fryer and bake for 15 minutes
7. Servings hot!

NUTRITION: Calories 451, Total Fat 30g, Saturated Fat 7g, Total Carbs 9g, Net Carbs 1g, Protein 34g, Sugar 6g, Fiber 2g, Sodium 111mg, Potassium 872g

345. Spicy Cod Fish Sticks

Preparation time: 10 minutes

Cooking time: 10 minutes

Servings: 4

INGREDIENTS

- 1pound cod
- ¼ cup mayonnaise
- 2bsp mustard
- ½ tsp salt
- ½ tsp ground cayenne pepper
- 1½ cups ground pork rinds
- 2Tbsp whole milk

DIRECTIONS:

1. Preheat your air fryer to 400 degrees F and line your air fryer tray with foil and spray with cooking grease.
2. Dry the cod filets by patting with a paper towel. Cut the fish into strips about 1 inch wide and two inches long.
3. In a small bowl, combine the mustard, mayo and milk and stir together well.
4. In a separate bowl, combine the ground pork rinds, salt and cayenne pepper.
5. Dip the fish strips into the mayonnaise mix and then into the pork rind mix, coating the fish completely. Place it on the prepared tray when done and repeat with the remaining fish sticks.
6. Place the tray in the air fryer and bake the fish for 5 minutes, flip and bake for another 5 minutes Servings while hot!

NUTRITION: Calories 264, Total Fat 16g, Saturated Fat 5g, Total Carbs 1g, Net Carbs 0g, Protein 26g, Sugar 0g, Fiber 1g, Sodium 679mg, Potassium 68g

346. Italian Fish Sticks

Preparation time: 10 minutes

Cooking time: 10 minutes

Servings: 4

INGREDIENTS

- 1pound cod
- ¼ cup mayonnaise
- 2Tbsp mustard
- ½ tsp salt
- 1tsp Italian seasoning
- ½ tsp ground black pepper
- 1½ cups ground pork rinds
- 2Tbsp whole milk

DIRECTIONS:

1. Preheat your air fryer to 400 degrees F and line your air fryer tray with foil and spray with cooking grease.
2. Dry the cod filets by patting with a paper towel. Cut the fish into strips about 1 inch wide and two inches long.
3. In a small bowl, combine the mustard, mayo and milk and stir together well.
4. In a separate bowl, combine the ground pork rinds, salt, Italian seasoning and pepper.

5. Dip the fish strips into the mayonnaise mix and then into the pork rind mix, coating the fish completely. Place it on the prepared tray when done and repeat with the remaining fish sticks.
6. Place the tray in the air fryer and bake the fish for 5 minutes, flip and bake for another 5 minutes Servings while hot!

NUTRITION: Calories 283, Total Fat 16g, Saturated Fat 5g, Total Carbs 1g, Net Carbs 0g, Protein 26g, Sugar 0g, Fiber 1g, Sodium 683mg, Potassium 68g

347. Lemon Pepper Fish Sticks

Preparation time: 10 minutes

Cooking time: 10 minutes

Servings: 4

INGREDIENTS

- 1 pound cod
- ¼ cup mayonnaise
- 2 Tbsp mustard
- ½ tsp salt
- 1 tsp lemon pepper seasoning
- 1½ cups ground pork rinds
- 2 Tbsp whole milk

DIRECTIONS:

1. Preheat your air fryer to 400 degrees F and line your air fryer tray with foil and spray with cooking grease.
2. Dry the cod filets by patting with a paper towel. Cut the fish into strips about 1 inch wide and two inches long.
3. In a small bowl, combine the mustard, mayo and milk and stir together well.
4. In a separate bowl, combine the ground pork rinds, lemon pepper and salt.
5. Dip the fish strips into the mayonnaise mix and then into the pork rind mix, coating the fish completely. Place it on the prepared tray when done and repeat with the remaining fish sticks.
6. Place the tray in the air fryer and bake the fish for 5 minutes, flip and bake for another 5 minutes Servings while hot!

NUTRITION: Calories 265, Total Fat 16g, Saturated Fat 5g, Total Carbs 1g, Net Carbs 0g, Protein 26g, Sugar 0g, Fiber 1g, Sodium 682mg, Potassium 69g

348. Salmon Fish Sticks

Preparation time: 10 minutes

Cooking time: 10 minutes

Servings: 4

INGREDIENTS

- 1 pound salmon filets
- ¼ cup mayonnaise
- 2 Tbsp mustard
- ½ tsp salt
- ½ tsp ground black pepper
- 1½ cups ground pork rinds
- 2 Tbsp whole milk

DIRECTIONS:

1. Preheat your air fryer to 400 degrees F and line your air fryer tray with foil and spray with cooking grease.
2. Dry the salmon filets by patting with a paper towel. Cut the fish into strips about 1 inch wide and two inches long.
3. In a small bowl, combine the mustard, mayo and milk and stir together well.
4. In a separate bowl, combine the ground pork rinds, salt and pepper.
5. Dip the fish strips into the mayonnaise mix and then into the pork rind mix, coating the fish completely. Place it on the prepared tray when done and repeat with the remaining fish sticks.

6. Place the tray in the air fryer and bake the fish for 5 minutes, flip and bake for another 5 minutes Servings while hot!

NUTRITION: Calories 282, Total Fat 18g, Saturated Fat 5g, Total Carbs 1g, Net Carbs 0g, Protein 27g, Sugar 0g, Fiber 1g, Sodium 664mg, Potassium 68g

349. Cajun Salmon Fish Sticks

Preparation time: 10 minutes

Cooking time: 10 minutes

Servings: 4

INGREDIENTS

- 1 pound salmon
- ¼ cup mayonnaise
- 2 Tbsp mustard
- ½ tsp salt
- 1 tsp Cajun seasoning
- 1½ cups ground pork rinds
- 2 Tbsp whole milk

DIRECTIONS:

1. Preheat your air fryer to 400 degrees F and line your air fryer tray with foil and spray with cooking grease.
2. Dry the salmon filets by patting with a paper towel. Cut the fish into strips about 1 inch wide and two inches long.
3. In a small bowl, combine the mustard, mayo and milk and stir together well.
4. In a separate bowl, combine the ground pork rinds, Cajun seasoning, and salt.
5. Dip the fish strips into the mayonnaise mix and then into the pork rind mix, coating the fish completely. Place it on the prepared tray when done and repeat with the remaining fish sticks.
6. Place the tray in the air fryer and bake the fish for 5 minutes, flip and bake for another 5 minutes Servings while hot!

NUTRITION: Calories 288, Total Fat 18g, Saturated Fat 5g, Total Carbs 1g, Net Carbs 0g, Protein 27g, Sugar 0g, Fiber 1g, Sodium 676mg, Potassium 68g

350. Bacon Wrapped Fish Sticks

Preparation time: 10 minutes

Cooking time: 18 minutes

Servings: 4

INGREDIENTS

- 1 pound cod
- ¼ cup mayonnaise
- 2 Tbsp mustard
- ½ tsp salt
- ½ tsp ground black pepper
- 1½ cups ground pork rinds
- 2 Tbsp whole milk
- ½ pound bacon, uncooked, strips

DIRECTIONS:

1. Preheat your air fryer to 400 degrees F and line your air fryer tray with foil and spray with cooking grease.
2. Dry the cod filets by patting with a paper towel. Cut the fish into strips about 1 inch wide and two inches long.
3. In a small bowl, combine the mustard, mayo and milk and stir together well.
4. In a separate bowl, combine the ground pork rinds, salt and pepper.
5. Dip the fish strips into the mayonnaise mix and then into the pork rind mix, coating the fish completely. Place it on the prepared tray when done and repeat with the remaining fish sticks.
6. Wrap each fish stick in the bacon and place back onto the tray.
7. Place the tray in the air fryer and bake the fish for 10 minutes, flip and bake for

another 8 minutes or until the bacon is brown and crispy. Serve while hot!

NUTRITION: Calories 310, Total Fat 24g, Saturated Fat 5g, Total Carbs 1g, Net Carbs 0g, Protein 34g, Sugar 0g, Fiber 1g, Sodium 899mg, Potassium 112g

351. Keto Tuna Melt Cups

Preparation time: 10 minutes

Cooking time: 20 minutes

Servings: 7

INGREDIENTS

- 5oz canned tuna, drained
- 2 eggs
- ¼ cup sour cream
- ¼ cup mayonnaise
- ¾ cup shredded cheddar cheese
- ¾ cup pepper jack cheese
- ¼ tsp salt
- ¼ tsp ground black pepper
- 1 Tbsp parsley, chopped

DIRECTIONS:

1. Preheat your air fryer to 325 degrees F and grease a muffin tin or individual muffin cups- whichever option fits in your air fryer better.
2. In a large bowl, combine the tuna, mayonnaise, sour cream, both kinds of grated cheese, parsley, salt and pepper.
3. Scoop the mix into the prepared muffin tin, filling each cup to the top.
4. Bake in the air fryer for 20 minutes or until the tops are golden brown.
5. Place on a slice of keto bread, serve with keto crackers or enjoy plain with a spoon!

NUTRITION: Calories 160, Total Fat 13g, Saturated Fat 3, Total Carbs 1g, Net Carbs 1g, Protein 9g, Sugar 1g, Fiber 0g, Sodium 321mg, Potassium 197g

352. Garlic Shrimp Bacon Bake

Preparation time: 10 minutes

Cooking time: 8 minutes

Servings: 4

INGREDIENTS

- ¼ cup butter
- 2 Tbsp minced garlic
- 1 pound shrimp, peeled and cleaned
- ¼ tsp ground black pepper
- ½ cup cooked, chopped bacon
- 1/3 cup heavy cream
- ¼ cup parmesan cheese

DIRECTIONS:

1. Preheat your air fryer to 400 degrees F and grease an 8x8 inch baking pan.
2. Add the butter and shrimp to the pan and place in the air fryer for 3 minutes. Remove the pan from the air fryer.
3. Add the remaining ingredients to the pan and return to the air fryer to cook for another 5 minutes. The mix should be bubbling and the shrimp should be pink.
4. Serve with zucchini noodles or enjoy plain.

NUTRITION: Calories 350, Total Fat 27g, Saturated Fat 15g, Total Carbs 3g, Net Carbs 3g, Protein 36g, Sugar 0g, Fiber 0g, Sodium 924mg, Potassium 16g

353. Gruyere Shrimp Bacon Bake

Preparation time: 10 minutes

Cooking time: 10 minutes

Servings: 4

INGREDIENTS

- ¼ cup butter

- 2 Tbsp minced garlic
- 1 pound shrimp, peeled and cleaned
- ¼ tsp ground black pepper
- ½ cup cooked, chopped bacon
- 1/3 cup heavy cream
- ¼ cup parmesan cheese
- ½ cup gruyere cheese, grated

DIRECTIONS:

1. Preheat your air fryer to 400 degrees F and grease an 8x8 inch baking pan.
2. Add the butter and shrimp to the pan and place in the air fryer for 3 minutes. Remove the pan from the air fryer.
3. Add the remaining ingredients to the pan and return to the air fryer to cook for another 5 minutes. The mix should be bubbling and the shrimp should be pink.
4. Sprinkle the gruyere over the shrimp and return to the air fryer for another 2 minutes to brown the top of the cheese.
5. Serve with zucchini noodles or enjoy plain.

NUTRITION: Calories 410, Total Fat 32g, Saturated Fat 18g, Total Carbs 4g, Net Carbs 3g, Protein 38g, Sugar 0g, Fiber 0g, Sodium 988mg, Potassium 24g

354. Cajun Shrimp Bacon Bake

Preparation time: 10 minutes

Cooking time: 10 minutes

Servings: 4

INGREDIENTS

- ¼ cup butter
- 2 Tbsp minced garlic
- 1 pound shrimp, peeled and cleaned
- ½ tsp Cajun seasoning
- ½ cup cooked, chopped bacon
- 1/3 cup heavy cream
- ¼ cup parmesan cheese

DIRECTIONS:

1. Preheat your air fryer to 400 degrees F and grease an 8x8 inch baking pan.
2. Add the butter and shrimp to the pan and place in the air fryer for 3 minutes. Remove the pan from the air fryer.
3. Add the remaining ingredients to the pan and return to the air fryer to cook for another 5 minutes. The mix should be bubbling and the shrimp should be pink.
4. Serve with zucchini noodles or enjoy plain.

NUTRITION: Calories 352, Total Fat 27g, Saturated Fat 15g, Total Carbs 3g, Net Carbs 3g, Protein 36g, Sugar 0g, Fiber 0g, Sodium 930mg, Potassium 18g

355. Garlic Shrimp Prosciutto Bake

Preparation time: 10 minutes

Cooking time: 10 minutes

Servings: 4

INGREDIENTS

- ¼ cup butter
- 2 Tbsp minced garlic
- 1 pound shrimp, peeled and cleaned
- ¼ tsp ground black pepper
- 2 oz thinly sliced, shredded prosciutto
- 1/3 cup heavy cream
- ¼ cup parmesan cheese

DIRECTIONS:

1. Preheat your air fryer to 400 degrees F and grease an 8x8 inch baking pan.
2. Add the butter and shrimp to the pan and place in the air fryer for 3 minutes. Remove the pan from the air fryer.
3. Add the remaining ingredients to the pan and return to the air fryer to cook for another 5 minutes. The mix should be bubbling and the shrimp should be pink.

4. Serve with zucchini noodles or enjoy plain.

NUTRITION: Calories 358, Total Fat 27g, Saturated Fat 15g, Total Carbs 3g, Net Carbs 3g, Protein 36g, Sugar 0g, Fiber 0g, Sodium 1026mg, Potassium 16g

356. Garlic Shrimp Tuna Bake

Preparation time: 10 minutes

Cooking time: 10 minutes

Servings: 4

INGREDIENTS

- ¼ cup butter
- 2Tbsp minced garlic
- 1pound shrimp, peeled and cleaned
- ¼ tsp ground black pepper
- 1tin canned tuna, drained well
- 1/3 cup heavy cream
- ¼ cup parmesan cheese

DIRECTIONS:

1. Preheat your air fryer to 400 degrees F and grease an 8x8 inch baking pan.
2. Add the butter and shrimp to the pan and place in the air fryer for 3 minutes. Remove the pan from the air fryer.
3. Add the remaining ingredients to the pan and return to the air fryer to cook for another 5 minutes. The mix should be bubbling and the shrimp should be pink.
4. Serve with zucchini noodles or enjoy plain.

NUTRITION: Calories 376, Total Fat 30g, Saturated Fat 15g, Total Carbs 3g, Net Carbs 3g, Protein 43g, Sugar 0g, Fiber 0g, Sodium 924mg, Potassium 16g

357. Jalapeno Tuna Melt Cups

Preparation time: 10 minutes

Cooking time: 20 minutes

Servings: 7

INGREDIENTS

- 5oz canned tuna, drained
- 2eggs
- ¼ cup sour cream
- ¼ cup mayonnaise
- ¾ cup shredded cheddar cheese
- ¾ cup pepper jack cheese
- ¼ tsp salt
- ¼ tsp ground black pepper
- 1Tbsp parsley, chopped
- ½ cup jalapeno slices

DIRECTIONS:

1. Preheat your air fryer to 325 degrees F and grease a muffin tin or individual muffin cups- whichever option fits in your air fryer better.
2. In a large bowl, combine the tuna, mayonnaise, sour cream, both kinds of grated cheese, parsley, jalapeno slices, salt, and pepper.
3. Scoop the mix into the prepared muffin tin, filling each cup to the top.
4. Bake in the air fryer for 20 minutes or until the tops are golden brown.
5. Place on a slice of keto bread, serve with keto crackers or enjoy plain with a spoon!

NUTRITION: Calories 167, Total Fat 13g, Saturated Fat 3, Total Carbs 2g, Net Carbs 1g, Protein 9g, Sugar 2g, Fiber 0g, Sodium 321mg, Potassium 197g

358. Herbed Tuna Melt Cups

Preparation time: 10 minutes

Cooking time: 20 minutes

Servings: 7

INGREDIENTS

- 5oz canned tuna, drained
- 2 eggs
- ¼ cup sour cream
- ¼ cup mayonnaise
- ¾ cup shredded cheddar cheese
- ¾ cup pepper jack cheese
- ¼ tsp salt
- ¼ tsp ground black pepper
- 1 Tbsp parsley, chopped
- 1 tsp fresh chopped rosemary
- 1 tsp fresh chopped basil

DIRECTIONS:

1. Preheat your air fryer to 325 degrees F and grease a muffin tin or individual muffin cups- whichever option fits in your air fryer better.
2. In a large bowl, combine the tuna, mayonnaise, sour cream, both kinds of grated cheese, parsley, rosemary, basil, salt, and pepper.
3. Scoop the mix into the prepared muffin tin, filling each cup to the top.
4. Bake in the air fryer for 20 minutes or until the tops are golden brown.
5. Place on a slice of keto bread, serve with keto crackers or enjoy plain with a spoon!

NUTRITION: Calories 163, Total Fat 13g, Saturated Fat 3, Total Carbs 1g, Net Carbs 1g, Protein 9g, Sugar 1g, Fiber 0g, Sodium 325mg, Potassium 197g

359. Cajun Tuna Melt Cups

Preparation time: 10 minutes

Cooking time: 20 minutes

Servings: 7

INGREDIENTS

- 5oz canned tuna, drained
- 2 eggs
- ¼ cup sour cream
- ¼ cup mayonnaise
- ¾ cup shredded cheddar cheese
- ¾ cup pepper jack cheese
- ¼ tsp salt
- ½ tsp Cajun seasoning
- 1 Tbsp parsley, chopped

DIRECTIONS:

1. Preheat your air fryer to 325 degrees F and grease a muffin tin or individual muffin cups- whichever option fits in your air fryer better.
2. In a large bowl, combine the tuna, mayonnaise, sour cream, both kinds of grated cheese, parsley, Cajun seasoning, salt, and pepper.
3. Scoop the mix into the prepared muffin tin, filling each cup to the top.
4. Bake in the air fryer for 20 minutes or until the tops are golden brown.
5. Place on a slice of keto bread, serve with keto crackers or enjoy plain with a spoon!

NUTRITION: Calories 161, Total Fat 13g, Saturated Fat 3, Total Carbs 1g, Net Carbs 1g, Protein 9g, Sugar 1g, Fiber 0g, Sodium 321mg, Potassium 197g

360. Cheddar Tuna Melt Cups

Preparation time: 10 minutes

Cooking time: 20 minutes

Servings: 7

INGREDIENTS

- 5oz canned tuna, drained
- 2 eggs
- ¼ cup sour cream
- ¼ cup mayonnaise
- 1½ cups shredded cheddar cheese
- ¼ tsp salt

- ¼ tsp ground black pepper
- 1 Tbsp parsley, chopped

DIRECTIONS

1. Preheat your air fryer to 325 degrees F and grease a muffin tin or individual muffin cups- whichever option fits in your air fryer better.
2. In a large bowl, combine the tuna, mayonnaise, sour cream, cheese, parsley, salt and pepper.
3. Scoop the mix into the prepared muffin tin, filling each cup to the top.
4. Bake in the air fryer for 20 minutes or until the tops are golden brown.
5. Place on a slice of keto bread, serve with keto crackers or enjoy plain with a spoon!

NUTRITION: Calories 160, Total Fat 13g, Saturated Fat 3, Total Carbs 1g, Net Carbs 1g, Protein 9g, Sugar 1g, Fiber 0g, Sodium 321mg, Potassium 197g

361. Sesame Tuna Melt Cups

Preparation time: 10 minutes

Cooking time: 20 minutes

Servings: 7

INGREDIENTS

- 5oz canned tuna, drained
- 2 eggs
- ¼ cup sour cream
- ¼ cup mayonnaise
- 1 Tbsp sesame seeds
- 1 Tbsp coconut aminos
- ¾ cup shredded cheddar cheese
- ¾ cup pepper jack cheese
- ¼ tsp salt
- ¼ tsp ground black pepper
- 1 Tbsp parsley, chopped

DIRECTIONS:

1. Preheat your air fryer to 325 degrees F and grease a muffin tin or individual muffin cups- whichever option fits in your air fryer better.
2. In a large bowl, combine the tuna, mayonnaise, sour cream, sesame seeds, coconut aminos, both kinds of grated cheese, parsley, salt and pepper.
3. Scoop the mix into the prepared muffin tin, filling each cup to the top.
4. Bake in the air fryer for 20 minutes or until the tops are golden brown.
5. Place on a slice of keto bread, serve with keto crackers or enjoy plain with a spoon!

NUTRITION: Calories 172, Total Fat 16g, Saturated Fat 3, Total Carbs 4g, Net Carbs 2g, Protein 9g, Sugar 1g, Fiber 2g, Sodium 327mg, Potassium 202g

362. Asian Style Crunchy Flounder

Preparation time: 10 minutes

Cooking time: 10 minutes

Servings: 4

INGREDIENTS

- 1 pound flounder filets
- ½ cup pork rinds, crushed
- ¼ tsp black pepper
- ½ tsp salt
- ¼ tsp garlic powder
- 2 tsp fresh minced garlic
- 1 Tbsp melted butter
- 1 Tbsp coconut aminos

DIRECTIONS:

1. Preheat your air fryer to 450 degrees F and line your air fryer tray with foil.
2. Place the flounder filets on the foil lined tray.

3. In a small bowl or food processor, combine the remaining ingredients and mix well.
4. Press the pork rind mix onto the salmon filets, coating the whole top evenly and packing the crust into the fish filets.
5. Bake the filets in the preheated oven for 10 minutes. The top crust should be nicely browned.
6. Serve while hot.

NUTRITION: Calories 323, Total Fat 21g, Saturated Fat 10g, Total Carbs 2g, Net Carbs 1g, Protein 40g, Sugar 0g, Fiber 1g, Sodium 482mg, Potassium 199g

363. Prosciutto Wrapped Cod

Preparation time: 5 minutes

Cooking time: 15 minutes

Servings: 2

INGREDIENTS

- 1pound cod fillets
- ¼ tsp salt
- ¼ tsp ground black pepper
- 2oz prosciutto de parma, very thinly sliced
- 2Tbsp olive oil
- 1tsp minced garlic
- 4cups baby spinach
- 2tsp lemon juice

DIRECTIONS:

1. Preheat your air fryer to 325 degrees F and line your air fryer tray with foil.
2. Dry the cod fillets by patting with a paper towel the sprinkle with salt and pepper.
3. Wrap the filets in the prosciutto, enclosing them as fully as possible.
4. Place the wrapped filets on the prepared tray.
5. Toss the spinach with the olive oil, garlic and lemon juice and place on the tray as well, around the wrapped cod.
6. Place in the air fryer and bake for 12 minutes. The spinach should be nicely wilted and the fish 145 degrees F internally.
7. Serve hot!

NUTRITION: Calories 416, Total Fat 19g, Saturated Fat 3g, Total Carbs 11g, Net Carbs 9g, Protein 49g, Sugar 3g, Fiber 2g, Sodium 482mg, Potassium 582g

364. Prosciutto Wrapped Salmon

Preparation time: 5 minutes

Cooking time: 16 minutes

Servings: 2

INGREDIENTS

- 1pound salmon fillets
- ¼ tsp salt
- ¼ tsp ground black pepper
- 2oz prosciutto de parma, very thinly sliced
- 2Tbsp olive oil
- 1tsp minced garlic
- 4cups baby spinach
- 2tsp lemon juice

DIRECTIONS:

1. Preheat your air fryer to 325 degrees F and line your air fryer tray with foil.
2. Dry the salmon fillets by patting with a paper towel the sprinkle with salt and pepper.
3. Wrap the filets in the prosciutto, enclosing them as fully as possible.
4. Place the wrapped filets on the prepared tray.
5. Toss the spinach with the olive oil, garlic and lemon juice and place on the tray as well, around the wrapped salmon.

6. Place in the air fryer and bake for 12 minutes. The spinach should be nicely wilted and the fish 145 degrees F internally.
7. Serve hot!

NUTRITION: Calories 464, Total Fat 22g, Saturated Fat 5g, Total Carbs 11g, Net Carbs 9g, Protein 49g, Sugar 3g, Fiber 2g, Sodium 482mg, Potassium 582g

365. Fast Seared Scallops

Preparation time: 5 minutes

Cooking time: 5 minutes

Servings: 4

INGREDIENTS

- 1pound jumbo scallops
- 2Tbsp butter
- ¼ tsp salt
- ¼ tsp ground black pepper

DIRECTIONS:

1. Preheat your air fryer to 400 degrees F and line your air fryer tray with foil.
2. Place the butter on the air fryer tray and place inside the air fryer for one minute to melt.
3. Remove the tray and add the scallops and seasonings, toss together and return to the air fryer for 5 minutes. The bottom of the scallops should be golden brown.
4. Serve hot.

NUTRITION: Calories 160, Total Fat 9g, Saturated Fat 4g, Total Carbs 3g, Net Carbs 2g, Protein 13g, Sugar 0g, Fiber 1g, Sodium 640mg, Potassium 232g

366. Lemon Scallops

Preparation time: 5 minutes

Cooking time: 5 minutes

Servings: 4

INGREDIENTS

- 1pound jumbo scallops
- 2Tbsp butter
- 1tsp lemon zest
- ¼ tsp salt
- ¼ tsp ground black pepper

DIRECTIONS:

1. Preheat your air fryer to 400 degrees F and line your air fryer tray with foil.
2. Place the butter on the air fryer tray and place inside the air fryer for one minute to melt.
3. Remove the tray and add the scallops and seasonings, toss together and return to the air fryer for 5 minutes. The bottom of the scallops should be golden brown.
4. Serve hot.

NUTRITION: Calories 163, Total Fat 9g, Saturated Fat 4g, Total Carbs 3g, Net Carbs 2g, Protein 13g, Sugar 0g, Fiber 1g, Sodium 640mg, Potassium 232g

367. Dijon Baked Salmon

Preparation time: 5 minutes

Cooking time: 18 minutes

Servings: 5

INGREDIENTS

- 1½ pounds salmon
- ¼ cup parsley, freshly chopped
- ¼ cup Dijon mustard
- 1Tbsp olive oil
- 1Tbsp fresh squeezed lemon juice
- 1Tbsp minced garlic
- ¼ tsp salt
- ¼ tsp ground black pepper

DIRECTIONS:

1. Preheat your air fryer to 375 degrees F line your air fryer tray with a piece of parchment paper.
2. Place the salmon on the parchment lined tray.
3. In a small bowl, mix together the remaining ingredients and then spread over the top of the salmon.
4. Place the salmon in the air fryer and bake for 18 minutes. Slice and serve hot!

NUTRITION: Calories 250, Total Fat 13g, Saturated Fat 2g, Total Carbs 2g, Net Carbs 1g, Protein 31g, Sugar 0g, Fiber 1g, Sodium 371mg, Potassium 42g

368. Garlic Dijon Baked Salmon

Preparation time: 5 minutes

Cooking time: 18 minutes

Servings: 5

INGREDIENTS

- 1½ pounds salmon
- ¼ cup parsley, freshly chopped
- ¼ cup Dijon mustard
- 1Tbsp olive oil
- 1Tbsp fresh squeezed lemon juice
- 3Tbsp minced garlic
- ¼ tsp salt
- ¼ tsp ground black pepper

DIRECTIONS:

1. Preheat your air fryer to 375 degrees F line your air fryer tray with a piece of parchment paper.
2. Place the salmon on the parchment lined tray.
3. In a small bowl, mix together the remaining ingredients and then spread over the top of the salmon.
4. Place the salmon in the air fryer and bake for 18 minutes. Slice and serve hot!

NUTRITION: Calories 272, Total Fat 13g, Saturated Fat 2g, Total Carbs 3g, Net Carbs 1g, Protein 31g, Sugar 1g, Fiber 1g, Sodium 371mg, Potassium 42g

369. Crispy Salmon Fillets

Preparation Time: 20 minutes

Servings: 4

INGREDIENTS

- 4salmon fillets, skinless
- ½ cup coconut flakes
- 1tbsp. parmesan; grated
- 1tsp. mustard
- Cooking spray
- A pinch of salt and black pepper

DIRECTIONS

1. Take a bowl and mix the parmesan with the other ingredients except the fish and cooking spray and stir well.
2. Coat the fish in this mix, grease it with cooking spray and arrange in the air fryer's basket.
3. Cook at 400°F for 15 minutes, divide between plates and serve with a side salad

NUTRITION: Calories: 240; Fat: 13g; Fiber: 3g; Carbs: 6g; Protein: 15g

370. Tilapia and Tomato

Preparation Time: 25 minutes

Servings: 4

INGREDIENTS

- 4tilapia fillets; boneless and halved
- ¼ cup tomato paste

- 1cup tomatoes; cubed
- 1cup roasted peppers; chopped.
- 2tbsp. olive oil
- 1tbsp. lemon juice
- 1tsp. oregano; dried
- 1tsp. garlic powder
- Salt and black pepper to taste.

DIRECTIONS

1. In a baking dish that fits your air fryer, mix the fish with all the other ingredients, toss.
2. Introduce in your air fryer and cook at 380°F for 20 minutes. Divide into bowls and serve

NUTRITION: Calories: 250; Fat: 9g; Fiber: 2g; Carbs: 5g; Protein: 14g

371. Cod and Spring Onions Sauce

Preparation Time: 20 minutes

Servings: 2

INGREDIENTS

- 2cod fillets; boneless
- 3tbsp. ghee; melted
- 1bunch spring onions; chopped.
- Salt and black pepper to taste.

DIRECTIONS

1. In a pan that fits the air fryer, combine all the ingredients, toss gently, introduce in the air fryer and cook at 360°F for 15 minutes
2. Divide the fish and sauce between plates and serve.

NUTRITION: Calories: 240; Fat: 12g; Fiber: 2g; Carbs: 5g; Protein: 11g

372. Sesame Crusted Tuna Steak

Preparation Time: 13 minutes

Servings: 2

INGREDIENTS

- 2(6-oz.tuna) steaks
- 1tbsp. coconut oil; melted
- 2tsp. black sesame seeds
- ½ tsp. garlic powder.
- 2tsp. white sesame seeds

DIRECTIONS

1. Brush each tuna steak with coconut oil and sprinkle with garlic powder
2. Take a large bowl, mix sesame seeds and then press each tuna steak into them, covering the steak as completely as possible. Place tuna steaks into the air fryer basket
3. Adjust the temperature to 400 Degrees F and set the timer for 8 minutes. Flip the steaks halfway through the cooking time. Steaks will be well-done at 145 Degrees F internal temperature. Serve warm.

NUTRITION: Calories: 280; Protein: 42.7g; Fiber: 0.8g; Fat: 10.0g; Carbs: 2.0g

373. Mustard Crusted Cod

Preparation Time: 24 minutes

Servings: 4

INGREDIENTS

- 4cod fillets; boneless
- 1cup parmesan; grated
- 1tbsp. mustard
- Salt and black pepper to taste.

DIRECTIONS

1. Take a bowl and mix the parmesan with salt, pepper and the mustard and stir
2. Spread this over the cod, arrange the fish in the air fryer's basket and cook at 370°F for 7 minutes on each side.

3. Divide between plates and serve with a side salad

NUTRITION: Calories: 270; Fat: 14g; Fiber: 3g; Carbs: 5g; Protein: 12g

374. Italian Style Shrimp

Preparation Time: 15 minutes

Servings: 4

INGREDIENTS

- 2lb. shrimp; peeled and deveined
- 8garlic cloves, crushed
- ¼ cup chicken stock
- 1tsp. red pepper flakes, crushed
- 1tbsp. Italian seasoning
- A drizzle of olive oil
- Salt and black pepper to taste.

DIRECTIONS

1. Grease a pan that fits your air fryer with the oil, add the shrimp and the rest of the ingredients, toss.
2. Introduce the pan in the fryer and cook at 390°F for 10 minutes. Divide into bowls and serve.

NUTRITION: Calories: 261; Fat: 12g; Fiber: 6g; Carbs: 7g; Protein: 12g

375. Rosemary Tomatoes and Shrimp

Preparation Time: 17 minutes

Servings: 4

INGREDIENTS

- 1lb. shrimp; peeled and deveined
- 4garlic cloves; minced
- 1cup cherry tomatoes; halved
- 2tbsp. ghee; melted
- 1tbsp. rosemary; chopped.
- Salt and black pepper to taste.

DIRECTIONS

1. In a pan that fits the air fryer, mix all the ingredients, toss.
2. Put the pan in the fryer and cook at 380°F for 12 minutes. Divide into bowls and serve hot

NUTRITION: Calories: 220; Fat: 14g; Fiber: 2g; Carbs: 6g; Protein: 15g

376. Shrimp and Lemon Vinaigrette

Preparation Time: 17 minutes

Servings: 4

INGREDIENTS

- 1½ lb. shrimp; peeled and deveined
- Zest of ½ lemon; grated
- Juice of ½ lemon
- 2tbsp. parsley; chopped.
- 2tbsp. olive oil
- 2tbsp. mustard
- A pinch of salt and black pepper

DIRECTIONS

1. Take a bowl and mix all the ingredients and toss well.
2. Put the shrimp in your air fryer's basket and reserve the lemon vinaigrette
3. Cook at 350°F for 12 minutes, flipping the shrimp halfway, divide between plates and serve with reserved vinaigrette drizzled on top.

NUTRITION: Calories: 202; Fat: 8g; Fiber: 2g; Carbs: 5g; Protein: 14g

377. Shrimp and Chives

Preparation Time: 17 minutes

Servings: 4

INGREDIENTS

- 1lb. shrimp; peeled and deveined
- ¼ cup coconut cream
- 1tbsp. parsley; chopped.
- 1tbsp. ghee; melted
- 1tbsp. chives; chopped.
- A pinch of red pepper flakes
- A pinch of salt and black pepper

DIRECTIONS

1. In a pan that fits the fryer, combine all the ingredients except the parsley, put the pan in the fryer and cook at 360°F for 12 minutes
2. Divide the mix into bowls, sprinkle the parsley on top and serve.

NUTRITION: Calories: 195; Fat: 11g; Fiber: 2g; Carbs: 4g; Protein: 11g

378. Tilapia and Capers

Preparation Time: 25 minutes

Servings: 4

INGREDIENTS

- 4tilapia fillets; boneless
- 2tbsp. lemon juice
- 2tbsp. capers
- 3tbsp. ghee; melted
- 1tsp. garlic powder
- ½ tsp. smoked paprika
- ½ tsp. oregano; dried
- A pinch of salt and black pepper

DIRECTIONS

1. Take a bowl and mix all the ingredients except the fish and toss.
2. Arrange the fish in a pan that fits the air fryer, pour the capers mix all over, put the pan in the air fryer and cook 360°F for 20 minutes, shaking halfway
3. Divide between plates and serve hot.

NUTRITION: Calories: 224; Fat: 10g; Fiber: 0g; Carbs: 2g; Protein: 18g

379. Pesto Almond Salmon

Preparation Time: 17 minutes

Servings: 2

INGREDIENTS

- 2(1 ½-inch-thicksalmon fillets (about 4 oz. each
- ¼ cup sliced almonds, roughly chopped
- ¼ cup pesto
- 2tbsp. unsalted butter; melted.

DIRECTIONS

1. In a small bowl, mix pesto and almonds. Set aside. Place fillets into a 6-inch round baking dish
2. Brush each fillet with butter and place half of the pesto mixture on the top of each fillet. Place dish into the air fryer basket. Adjust the temperature to 390 Degrees F and set the timer for 12 minutes
3. Salmon will easily flake when fully cooked and reach an internal temperature of at least 145 Degrees F. Serve warm.

NUTRITION: Calories: 433; Protein: 23.3g; Fiber: 2.4g; Fat: 34.0g; Carbs: 6.1g

380. Glazed Cod Fillets

Preparation Time: 19 minutes

Servings: 4

INGREDIENTS

- 4cod fillets; boneless
- 1/3 cup stevia
- 2tbsp. coconut aminos

- A pinch of salt and black pepper

DIRECTIONS

1. In a pan that fits the air fryer, combine all the ingredients and toss gently.
2. Introduce the pan in the fryer and cook at 350°F for 14 minutes, flipping the fish halfway. Divide everything between plates and serve

NUTRITION: Calories: 267; Fat: 18g; Fiber: 2g; Carbs: 5g; Protein: 20g

381. Lemongrass Sea Bass

Preparation Time: 20 minutes

Servings: 4

INGREDIENTS

- 4 sea bass fillets; boneless
- 1-inch ginger; grated
- 4 lemongrass; chopped.
- 4 small chilies; minced
- 1 cup veggie stock
- 1 bunch coriander; chopped.
- 4 garlic cloves; minced
- Juice of 1 lime
- 1 tbsp. black peppercorns, crushed
- A pinch of salt and black pepper

DIRECTIONS

1. In a blender, combine all the ingredients except the fish and pulse well.
2. Pour the mix in a pan that fits the air fryer, add the fish, toss, introduce in the fryer and cook at 380°F for 15 minutes. Divide between plates and serve

NUTRITION: Calories: 271; Fat: 12g; Fiber: 4g; Carbs: 6g; Protein: 12g

382. Baked Black Sea Bass

Preparation Time: 25 minutes

Servings: 4

INGREDIENTS

- 1 lb. broccoli florets
- 4 black sea bass fillets; boneless
- 4 tbsp. butter; melted
- ½ tsp. red pepper flakes, crushed
- 1 tsp. lemon zest; grated
- A pinch of salt and black pepper

DIRECTIONS

1. In a pan that fits your air fryer, mix the broccoli with the other ingredients except the fish and half of the butter, toss,
2. Put the pan in the fryer and cook at 380°F for 8 minutes.
3. Add the fish greased with the rest of the butter, cook at 380°F for 12 minutes more, divide between plates and serve.

NUTRITION: Calories: 251; Fat: 15g; Fiber: 4g; Carbs: 6g; Protein: 12g

383. Roasted Red Snapper

Preparation Time: 20 minutes

Servings: 4

INGREDIENTS

- 4 red snapper fillets; boneless
- 2 garlic cloves; minced
- 1 tbsp. hot chili paste
- 2 tbsp. olive oil
- 2 tbsp. coconut aminos
- 2 tbsp. lime juice
- A pinch of salt and black pepper

DIRECTIONS

1. Take a bowl and mix all the ingredients except the fish and whisk well
2. Rub the fish with this mix, place it in your air fryer's basket and cook at 380°F for 15 minutes

3. Serve with a side salad.

NUTRITION: Calories: 220; Fat: 13g; Fiber: 4g; Carbs: 6g; Protein: 11g

384. Tuna Kabobs

Preparation Time: 17 minutes

Servings: 4

INGREDIENTS

- 1lb. tuna steaks; boneless and cubed
- 4green onions; chopped.
- 1chili pepper; minced
- 2tbsp. lime juice
- A drizzle of olive oil
- Salt and black pepper to taste.

DIRECTIONS

1. In a bowl mix all the ingredients and toss them.
2. Thread the tuna cubes on skewers, arrange them in your air fryer's basket and cook at 370°F for 12 minutes.
3. Divide between plates and serve with a side salad

NUTRITION: Calories: 226; Fat: 12g; Fiber: 2g; Carbs: 4g; Protein: 15g

385. Catfish Fillet and Avocado

Preparation Time: 20 minutes

Servings: 4

INGREDIENTS

- 4catfish fillets
- 1avocado; peeled and cubed
- ½ cup spring onions; chopped.
- 2tbsp. cilantro; chopped.
- 2tbsp. lemon juice
- 2tsp. olive oil
- 2tsp. oregano; dried
- 2tsp. cumin, ground
- 2tsp. sweet paprika
- A pinch of salt and black pepper

DIRECTIONS

1. Take a bowl and mix all the ingredients except the fish and toss.
2. Arrange this in a baking pan that fits the air fryer, top with the fish, introduce the pan in the machine and cook at 360°F for 15 minutes, flipping the fish halfway
3. Divide between plates and serve

NUTRITION: Calories: 280; Fat: 14g; Fiber: 3g; Carbs: 5g; Protein: 14g

386. Shrimp and Okra

Preparation Time: 15 minutes

Servings: 4

INGREDIENTS

- 1lb. shrimp; peeled and deveined
- 1½ cups okra
- ½ cup chicken stock
- 2tbsp. coconut aminos
- 3tbsp. balsamic vinegar
- 1tbsp. parsley; chopped.
- A pinch of salt and black pepper

DIRECTIONS

1. In a pan that fits your air fryer, mix all the ingredients, toss, introduce in the fryer and cook at 380°F for 10 minutes. Divide into bowls and serve.

NUTRITION: Calories: 251; Fat: 10g; Fiber: 3g; Carbs: 4g; Protein: 8g

387. Chives Salmon

Preparation Time: 17 minutes

Servings: 4

INGREDIENTS

- 4 salmon fillets; boneless
- ¼ cup chives; chopped.
- 4 cilantro springs; chopped.
- 3 tbsp. olive oil
- Juice of ½ lemon
- Salt and black pepper to taste.

DIRECTIONS

1. Take a bowl and mix the salmon with all the other ingredients and toss
2. Put the fillets in your air fryer's basket and cook at 370°F for 12 minutes, flipping the fish halfway.
3. Divide everything between plates and serve with a side salad

NUTRITION: Calories: 240; Fat: 12g; Fiber: 5g; Carbs: 6g; Protein: 14g

388. Basil Swordfish Fillets

Preparation Time: 17 minutes

Servings: 4

INGREDIENTS

- 4 swordfish fillets; boneless
- 2 tbsp. butter; melted
- 1 tbsp. olive oil
- 2 tsp. basil; dried
- ¾ tsp. sweet paprika
- Juice of 1 lemon

DIRECTIONS

1. Take a bowl and mix the oil with the other ingredients except the fish fillets and whisk
2. Brush the fish with this mix, place it in your air fryer's basket and cook for 6 minutes on each side
3. Divide between plates and serve with a side salad.

NUTRITION: Calories: 216; Fat: 11g; Fiber: 3g; Carbs: 6g; Protein: 12g

389. Shrimp and Pesto

Preparation Time: 17 minutes

Servings: 4

INGREDIENTS

- 1½ lb. shrimp; peeled and deveined
- 1/3 cup pine nuts
- ½ cup olive oil
- ½ cup basil leaves
- ¼ cup parmesan; grated
- ½ cup parsley leaves
- 2 tbsp. lemon juice
- ¼ tsp. lemon zest; grated
- A pinch of salt and black pepper

DIRECTIONS

1. In a blender, combine all the ingredients except the shrimp and pulse well. Take a bowl and mix the shrimp with the pesto and toss
2. Put the shrimp in your air fryer's basket and cook at 360°F for 12 minutes, flipping the shrimp halfway.
3. Divide the shrimp into bowls and serve.

NUTRITION: Calories: 240; Fat: 10g; Fiber: 1g; Carbs: 4g; Protein: 12g

POULTRY

390. Chicken and Tabasco Sauce Mix

Preparation time: 10 minutes

Cooking time: 20 minutes

Servings: 4

INGREDIENTS:

- 2 pounds chicken breast, skinless, boneless and cubed
- 2 teaspoons Tabasco sauce
- 1 tablespoon ginger, grated
- 4 garlic cloves, minced
- 1 cup tomato sauce
- Salt and black pepper to the taste
- 1 teaspoon olive oil
- ¼ cup parsley, chopped

DIRECTIONS:

1. In the air fryer's pan, mix the chicken with the Tabasco sauce and the other ingredients, introduce in the air fryer and cook at 370 degrees F for 20 minutes.
2. Divide between plates and serve.

NUTRITION: Calories 281, Fat 11, Fiber 12, Carbs 22, Protein 16

391. Chicken, Leeks and Coriander Mix

Preparation time: 10 minutes

Cooking time: 20 minutes

Servings: 4

INGREDIENTS

- 2 pounds chicken breast, skinless, boneless and halved
- 2 leeks, sliced
- 2 tablespoons coriander, chopped
- 1 tablespoon turmeric powder
- 1 tablespoon sweet paprika
- Salt and black pepper to the taste
- 2 tablespoons olive oil
- 1 tablespoon chives, chopped

DIRECTIONS

1. In the air fryer's pan, mix the chicken with the leeks and the other ingredients, cook at 370 degrees F for 20 minutes, divide between plates and serve.

NUTRITION: Calories 270, Fat 11, Fiber 11, Carbs 17, Protein 11

392. Turkey Stew

Preparation time: 10 minutes

Cooking time: 20 minutes

Servings: 4

INGREDIENTS

- 1 tablespoon avocado oil
- 2 pounds turkey breast, skinless, boneless and cubed
- 1 cup chicken stock
- ½ cup tomato sauce
- 1 yellow onion, chopped
- 1 teaspoon red pepper flakes, crushed
- 2 tablespoons chives, chopped
- Salt and black pepper to the taste

DIRECTIONS

1. In the air fryer's pan, mix the turkey with the stock and the other ingredients, transfer the pan to your air fryer and cook at 370 degrees F for 20 minutes.
2. Divide into bowls and serve.

NUTRITION: Calories 280, Fat 11, Fiber 13, Carbs 27, Protein 16

393. Mozzarella Chicken Mix

Preparation time: 10 minutes

Cooking time: 20 minutes

Servings: 6

INGREDIENTS

- 2pounds chicken breast, skinless, boneless and halved
- 1cup mozzarella, shredded
- 1tablespoon olive oil
- ½ teaspoon turmeric powder
- Salt and black pepper to the taste
- 1teaspoon oregano, dried
- 1tablespoon cilantro, chopped
- 1teaspoon garlic powder

DIRECTIONS

1. In the air fryer's pan, mix the chicken with the oil, turmeric and the other ingredients, toss, cook at 370 degrees F for 20 minutes, divide between plates and serve.

NUTRITION: Calories 270, Fat 10, Fiber 16, Carbs 16, Protein 18

394. Chicken with Peppers and Zucchinis

Preparation time: 10 minutes

Cooking time: 30 minutes

Servings: 4

INGREDIENTS

- 2pounds chicken breast, skinless, boneless and cubed
- 2red bell peppers, chopped
- 2zucchinis, cubed
- 2tablespoons avocado oil
- 3garlic cloves, minced
- 1cup chicken stock
- 1teaspoon sage, dried
- Salt and black pepper to the taste

DIRECTIONS

1. In a pan that fits your air fryer, mix the chicken with the peppers and the other ingredients, toss, introduce in the fryer and cook at 360 degrees F for 30 minutes.
2. Divide everything between plates and serve.

NUTRITION: Calories 292, Fat 12, Fiber 16, Carbs 19, Protein 15

395. Maple Chicken Mix

Preparation time: 10 minutes

Cooking time: 30 minutes

Servings: 4

INGREDIENTS

- 2pounds chicken breast, skinless, boneless and cubed
- 2tablespoons maple syrup
- Salt and black pepper to the taste
- 4spring onions, chopped
- 2tablespoons olive oil

DIRECTIONS

1. In the air fryer's basket, mix the chicken with the maple syrup and the other ingredients, toss cook at 360 degrees F for 30 minutes, divide between plates and serve.

NUTRITION: Calories 271, Fat 8, Fiber 12, Carbs 26, Protein 17

396. Whole Chicken Mix

Preparation time: 10 minutes

Cooking time: 35 minutes

Servings: 8

INGREDIENTS

- 1-2 pounds whole chicken, cut into medium pieces
- 3 tablespoons olive oil
- 1 cup chicken stock
- ½ teaspoon sweet paprika
- 1 tablespoon ginger, grated
- Salt and black pepper to the taste

DIRECTIONS

1. In the air fryer's basket, mix the whole chicken with the oil and the other ingredients, rub and cook at 380 degrees F for 35 minutes.
2. Divide between plates and serve with a side salad.

NUTRITION: Calories 220, Fat 10, Fiber 8, Carbs 20, Protein 16

397. Chicken with Cauliflower Rice

Preparation time: 10 minutes

Cooking time: 30 minutes

Servings: 4

INGREDIENTS

- 1 cup cauliflower rice
- 1 cup chicken stock
- 2 pounds chicken thighs, boneless, skinless and cubed
- ¼ cup tomato sauce
- 3 garlic cloves, minced
- Salt and black pepper to the taste
- 1 tablespoon olive oil
- 1 tablespoon parsley, chopped

DIRECTIONS

1. In a pan that fits your air fryer, mix the chicken with the cauliflower rice and the other ingredients, introduce the pan in the fryer, cook at 370 degrees F for 30 minutes, divide between plates and serve.

NUTRITION: Calories 280, Fat 12, Fiber 12, Carbs 16, Protein 13

398. Chicken and Pineapple Mix

Preparation time: 10 minutes

Cooking time: 25 minutes

Servings: 4

INGREDIENTS

- 2 pounds chicken breast, skinless, boneless and cubed
- 1 cup pineapple, peeled and cubed
- 2 tablespoons avocado oil
- 1 tablespoon rosemary, chopped
- Salt and black pepper to the taste
- ½ teaspoon chili powder
- 2 tablespoons honey

DIRECTIONS

1. In the air fryer's pan, mix the chicken with the pineapple and the other ingredients, toss, cook at 390 degrees F for 25 minutes, divide between plates and serve.

NUTRITION: Calories 281, Fat 11, Fiber 12, Carbs 28, Protein 19

399. Chicken and Veggies

Preparation time: 10 minutes

Cooking time: 25 minutes

Servings: 4

INGREDIENTS:

- 2pounds chicken breast, skinless, boneless and cubed
- 1cup cherry tomatoes, halved
- 1cup zucchinis, cubed
- 1cup kalamata olives, pitted and halved
- Juice of 1 lemon
- 1teaspoon basil, dried
- 3garlic cloves, minced
- Salt and black pepper to the taste

DIRECTIONS

1. In a pan that fits your air fryer, mix the chicken with the tomatoes and the other ingredients, toss, introduce in your air fryer, cook at 380 degrees F for 25 minutes, divide between plates and serve.

NUTRITION: Calories 280, Fat 8, Fiber 12, Carbs 20, Protein 15

400. Chicken and Figs

Preparation time: 10 minutes

Cooking time: 20 minutes

Servings: 4

INGREDIENTS

- 2pounds chicken breast, skinless, boneless and cubed
- 1cup figs, halved
- 1tablespoon olive oil
- ¼ teaspoon sweet paprika
- Salt and black pepper to the taste
- ½ cup red wine
- 1tablespoon chives, chopped

DIRECTIONS

1. In the air fryer's pan, mix the chicken with the figs and the other ingredients, cook at 380 degrees F for 20 minutes, divide between plates and serve.

NUTRITION: Calories 246, Fat 12, Fiber 4, Carbs 22, Protein 16

401. Pepper Chicken Mix

Preparation time: 10 minutes

Cooking time: 25 minutes

Servings: 4

INGREDIENTS:

- 2pounds chicken breasts, skinless and boneless
- 1teaspoon red pepper flakes, crushed
- 1teaspoon cayenne pepper
- 2tablespoons lemon juice
- Salt and black pepper to the taste
- ½ teaspoon lemon pepper
- 1tablespoon olive oil

DIRECTIONS

1. In the air fryer's pan, mix the chicken with the red pepper flakes and the other ingredients, transfer this to your air fryer, cook at 360 degrees F for 25 minutes, divide between plates and serve with a side salad.

NUTRITION: Calories 240, Fat 7, Fiber 1, Carbs 17, Protein 18

402. Chicken and Pears Mix

Preparation time: 10 minutes

Cooking time: 25 minutes

Servings: 4

INGREDIENTS

- 1pound chicken breasts, skinless, boneless and halved
- 2pears, cored and cubed
- 1cup white wine
- 2tablespoons balsamic vinegar
- 2garlic cloves, minced
- 1tablespoon chives, chopped
- Salt and black pepper to the taste
- 1teaspoon sweet paprika

DIRECTIONS

1. In the air fryer's pan, mix the chicken with the pears and the other ingredients, and cook at 370 degrees F for 25 minutes.
2. Divide everything between plates and serve.

NUTRITION: Calories 271, Fat 12, Fiber 3, Carbs 17, Protein 15

403. Chicken and Chili Sauce

Preparation time: 10 minutes

Cooking time: 25 minutes

Servings: 4

INGREDIENTS

- 2pounds chicken breast, skinless, boneless and cubed
- 1tablespoon chili paste
- 1red chili, minced
- ½ teaspoon smoked paprika
- 1teaspoon mustard powder
- Salt and black pepper to the taste
- ½ cup chicken stock

DIRECTIONS

1. In the air fryer's pan, mix the chicken with the chili paste and the other ingredients, cook at 370 degrees F for 25 minutes, divide everything between plates and serve.

NUTRITION: Calories 283, Fat 13, Fiber 7, Carbs 19, Protein 17

404. Chicken with Apples and Dates

Preparation time: 10 minutes

Cooking time: 25 minutes

Servings: 4

INGREDIENTS

- 2pounds chicken breast skinless, boneless and cubed
- 1cup apples, cored and cubed
- 1cup dates
- 1/3 cup white wine
- salt and black pepper to the taste
- 1tablespoon avocado oil

DIRECTIONS

1. In the air fryer's pan, mix the chicken with the apples and the other ingredients, and cook at 370 degrees F for 25 minutes.
2. Divide the mix between plates and serve.

NUTRITION: Calories 270, Fat 14, Fiber 3, Carbs 15, Protein 20

405. Chicken with Carrots and Celery

Preparation time: 10 minutes

Cooking time: 30 minutes

Servings: 4

INGREDIENTS

- 2pounds chicken breast, skinless, boneless and cubed
- 1cup carrots, peeled and sliced
- 1cup celery, chopped

- 1 tablespoon avocado oil
- 1 tablespoon balsamic vinegar
- Salt and black pepper to the taste
- 2 tablespoon chives, chopped

DIRECTIONS

1. In the air fryer's pan, mix the chicken with the carrots and the other ingredients, put it in your air fryer and cook at 350 degrees F for 30 minutes.
2. Divide the mix between plates and serve.

NUTRITION: Calories 237, Fat 10, Fiber 4, Carbs 19, Protein 16

406. Ginger Turkey and Yogurt mix

Preparation time: 10 minutes

Cooking time: 25 minutes

Servings: 4

INGREDIENTS

- 2 pounds turkey breast, skinless, boneless and cubed
- 1 cup Greek yogurt
- 2 tablespoons ginger, grated
- Salt and black pepper to the taste
- 1 teaspoon chili powder
- 2 teaspoons olive oil
- 1 tablespoon cilantro, chopped

DIRECTIONS

1. In the air fryer's pan, mix the turkey with the yogurt and the other ingredients, toss and cook at 400 degrees F for 25 minutes.
2. Divide everything between plates and serve.

NUTRITION: Calories 245, Fat 4, Fiber 5, Carbs 17, Protein 16

407. Pesto Chicken Wings

Preparation time: 10 minutes

Cooking time: 35 minutes

Servings: 4

INGREDIENTS

- 2 pounds chicken wings
- 3 tablespoons basil pesto
- Salt and black pepper to the taste
- ¼ cup butter, melted
- 4 garlic cloves, minced
- 1 teaspoon turmeric powder

DIRECTIONS

1. In the fryer's basket, mix the chicken wings with the pesto and the other ingredients, rub well and at 400 degrees F for 35 minutes.
2. Divide the chicken between plates, and serve.

NUTRITION: Calories 274, Fat 11, Fiber 3, Carbs 19, Protein 15

408. Spicy Tomato and Chicken Mix

Preparation time: 10 minutes

Cooking time: 20 minutes

Servings: 4

INGREDIENTS

- 2 pounds chicken legs, skinless and boneless
- 1 teaspoon hot paprika
- 1 cup canned tomatoes, crushed
- 1 tablespoon tomato paste
- ½ teaspoon apple vinegar
- A pinch of salt and black pepper

DIRECTIONS

1. In the air fryer's pan, mix the chicken with the paprika and the other ingredients and cook at 370 degrees F for 20 minutes..
2. Divide the mix between plates and serve.

NUTRITION: Calories 274, Fat 11, Fiber 3, Carbs 22, Protein 13

409. Turkey and Oyster Sauce

Preparation time: 10 minutes

Cooking time: 30 minutes

Servings: 4

INGREDIENTS

- 2pounds turkey breasts, boneless, skinless and cubed
- 2red chilies, chopped
- 1red onion, chopped
- 1tablespoon avocado oil
- 1tablespoon oyster sauce
- 1cup chicken stock
- 1tablespoon chives, chopped

DIRECTIONS

1. In the air fryer's pan, mix the turkey with the chilies and the other ingredients, introduce the pan in the air fryer and cook at 380 degrees F for 30 minutes
2. Divide everything between plates and serve.

NUTRITION: Calories 280, Fat 12, Fiber 5, Carbs 16, Protein 14

410. Chicken Stew

Preparation time: 10 minutes

Cooking time: 40 minutes

Servings: 4

INGREDIENTS

- 2pounds chicken breast, skinless, boneless and cubed
- 1cup canned tomatoes, crushed
- 1tablespoon olive oil
- 2carrots, peeled and sliced
- 1parsnip, peeled and sliced
- 1tablespoon ginger, grated
- 1chili pepper, minced
- 1cup chicken stock
- Salt and black pepper to the taste

DIRECTIONS

1. In the air fryer's pan, mix the chicken with the tomatoes and the other ingredients, toss, cook at 400 degrees F for 40 minutes, divide into bowls and serve

NUTRITION: Calories 270, Fat 8, Fiber 4, Carbs 20, Protein 17

411. Parmesan Chicken

Preparation time: 10 minutes

Cooking time: 30 minutes

Servings: 4

INGREDIENTS:

- 2pounds chicken breast, skinless, boneless and cubed
- 1cup parmesan, grated
- ¼ cup butter, melted
- 1teaspoon garam masala
- Salt and black pepper to the taste
- 1tablespoon chives, chopped

DIRECTIONS

1. In the air fryer's pan, mix the chicken with the parmesan and the other ingredients, cook at 380 degrees F for 30 minutes, divide between plates and serve.

NUTRITION: Calories 271, Fat 9, Fiber 4, Carbs 19, Protein 15

412. Chicken, Sweet Potatoes and Radishes

Preparation time: 10 minutes

Cooking time: 30 minutes

Servings: 4

INGREDIENTS

- 1pound chicken breast, skinless, boneless and cubed
- 1cup radishes, halved
- 2sweet potatoes, peeled and cubed
- 2tablespoons olive oil
- 1teaspoon turmeric powder
- Salt and black pepper to the taste
- 1tablespoon parsley, chopped

DIRECTIONS

1. In the air fryer's pan, mix the chicken with the radishes and the other ingredients, toss and cook at 360 degrees F for 30 minutes.
2. Divide everything between plates and serve.

NUTRITION: Calories 290, Fat 13, Fiber 4, Carbs 10, Protein 16

413. Balsamic Chicken and Beets

Preparation time: 10 minutes

Cooking time: 20 minutes

Servings: 4

INGREDIENTS

- 2pounds chicken breasts, skinless, boneless and sliced
- ¼ cup balsamic vinegar
- 2beets, peeled and cubed
- 2teaspoons olive oil
- Salt and black pepper to the taste
- ¼ cup chives, chopped
- ¼ teaspoon garlic powder

DIRECTIONS

1. In the air fryer's pan, mix the chicken with the vinegar and the other ingredients, toss, introduce the pan in the air fryer and cook at 400 degrees F for 20 minutes.
2. Divide between plates and serve.

NUTRITION: Calories 280, Fat 11, Fiber 2, Carbs 19, Protein 16

414. Lemongrass Turkey

Preparation time: 10 minutes

Cooking time: 20 minutes

Servings: 4

INGREDIENTS:

- ½ cup lemongrass, trimmed and chopped
- 2pounds turkey breast, skinless, boneless and roughly cubed
- 1tablespoon balsamic vinegar
- 1cup coconut cream
- Salt and black pepper to the taste
- 1tablespoon chives, chopped
- 1tablespoon lemon juice

DIRECTIONS

1. In the air fryer's pan, mix the turkey with the lemongrass and the other ingredients, toss, introduce the pan in the fryer and cook at 380 degrees F for 25 minutes.
2. Divide everything between plates and serve.

NUTRITION: Calories 251, Fat 8, Fiber 14, Carbs 19, Protein 6

415. Chicken and Coriander Sauce

Preparation time: 10 minutes

Cooking time: 25 minutes

Servings: 4

INGREDIENTS

- 2pounds chicken breast, skinless, boneless and sliced
- 1cup cilantro, chopped
- Juice of 1 lime
- ½ cup heavy cream
- 1tablespoon olive oil
- ½ teaspoon cumin, ground
- 1teaspoon sweet paprika
- 5garlic cloves, chopped
- 1cup chicken stock
- A pinch of salt and black pepper

DIRECTIONS

1. In a blender, mix the cilantro with the lime juice and the other ingredients except the chicken and the stock and pulse well.
2. Put the chicken, stock and sauce in the air fryer's pan, toss, introduce the pan in the fryer and cook at 380 degrees F for 25 minutes.
3. Divide the mix between plates and serve

NUTRITION: Calories 261, Fat 12, Fiber 7, Carbs 15, Protein 25

416. Turkey Chili

Preparation time: 10 minutes

Cooking time: 25 minutes

Servings: 4

INGREDIENTS

- 1pound turkey breast, skinless, boneless and cubed
- 1red onion, chopped
- 1red chili pepper, minced
- 1cup tomato sauce
- 1teaspoon chili powder
- Salt and black pepper to the taste
- 1teaspoon cumin, ground
- 1cup chicken stock

DIRECTIONS

1. In a pan that fits your air fryer, mix the turkey with the onion and the other ingredients, stir, introduce in the fryer and cook at 380 degrees F for 25 minutes.
2. Divide into bowls and serve.

NUTRITION: Calories 251, Fat 8, Fiber 8, Carbs 15, Protein 17

417. Chicken and Chickpeas

Preparation time: 10 minutes

Cooking time: 25 minutes

Servings: 4

INGREDIENTS:

- 1pound chicken breast, skinless, boneless and cubed
- 1cup canned chickpeas, drained
- 1cup tomato sauce
- Salt and black pepper to the taste
- 2teaspoons olive oil
- ½ teaspoon garlic powder
- ½ teaspoon coriander, ground
- 1teaspoon basil, dried
- 1tablespoon parsley, chopped

DIRECTIONS

1. In the air fryer's pan, mix the chicken with the chickpeas and the other ingredients, toss, introduce the pan in the fryer and cook at 370 degrees F for 25 minutes.
2. Divide the mix into bowls and serve.

NUTRITION: Calories 261, Fat 8, Fiber 6, Carbs 16, Protein 16

418. Turkey and Lentils

Preparation time: 10 minutes

Cooking time: 20 minutes

Servings: 4

INGREDIENTS

- 2pounds turkey breast, skinless, boneless and cubed
- 1cup canned lentils, drained
- ½ cup chicken stock
- ½ teaspoon sweet paprika
- Salt and black pepper to the taste
- 4garlic cloves, minced
- ½ cup cilantro, chopped

DIRECTIONS

1. In a pan that fits your air fryer, mix the turkey with the lentils and the other ingredients, toss, introduce in the fryer and cook at 380 degrees F for 20 minutes.
2. Divide everything between plates and serve.

NUTRITION: Calories 261, Fat 7, Fiber 5, Carbs 15, Protein 16

419. Meatballs and Sauce

Preparation time: 10 minutes

Cooking time: 20 minutes

Servings: 4

INGREDIENTS

- 1pound chicken breast, skinless, boneless and ground
- 2eggs, whisked
- 1red onion, chopped
- 1tablespoon cilantro, chopped
- 1tablespoon chives, chopped
- ½ cup almond flour
- 4garlic cloves, minced
- Salt and black pepper to the taste
- 1cup tomato sauce
- 1teaspoon oregano, dried

DIRECTIONS

1. In a bowl, mix the chicken with the eggs, onion, and the other ingredients except the oregano and tomato sauce, stir and shape medium meatballs out of this mix.
2. In the air fryer's pan, mix the meatballs with the remaining ingredients, and cook at 380 degrees F for 20 minutes.
3. Divide the mix between plates and serve.

NUTRITION: Calories 261, Fat 7, Fiber 6, Carbs 15, Protein 18

420. Ground Turkey Mix

Preparation time: 10 minutes

Cooking time: 20 minutes

Servings: 4

INGREDIENTS

- 2pounds turkey breast, skinless, boneless and ground
- 1red bell pepper, chopped
- 1green bell pepper, chopped
- 4spring onions, chopped
- 1yellow onion, sliced
- 1teaspoon basil, dried

- 1cup tomato sauce
- 1tablespoon soy sauce
- Salt and black pepper to the taste
- 1tablespoon parsley, chopped

DIRECTIONS

1. In the air fryer's pan, mix the turkey with the peppers and the other ingredients, introduce the pan in the fryer and cook at 370 degrees F for 20 minutes.
2. Divide into bowls and serve hot.

NUTRITION: Calories 281, Fat 8, Fiber 5, Carbs 15, Protein 20

421. Chicken and Bacon Mix

Preparation time: 10 minutes

Cooking time: 25 minutes

Servings: 4

INGREDIENTS

A. 2pounds chicken breast, skinless, boneless and cubed
B. 1cup bacon, cooked and chopped
C. 1cup cherry tomatoes, halved
D. 1tablespoon olive oil
E. 1tablespoon balsamic vinegar
F. 2scallions, chopped
G. ½ teaspoon oregano, dried
H. 1teaspoon sweet paprika
I. Salt and black pepper to the taste
J. 1tablespoon cilantro, chopped

DIRECTIONS

1. Heat up a pan that fits your air fryer with the oil over medium heat, add the scallions and the meat and brown for 5 minutes.
2. Add the rest of the ingredients, toss, introduce the pan in the fryer and cook at 380 degrees F for 20 minutes.
3. Divide everything between plates and serve.

Nutrition: Calories 281, Fat 11, Fiber 5, Carbs 17, Protein 20

422. Turkey and Mango Mix

Preparation time: 10 minutes

Cooking time: 30 minutes

Servings: 4

INGREDIENTS

- 2pounds turkey breast, skinless, boneless and cubed
- 1cup mango, peeled and cubed
- 2tablespoons butter, melted
- 1teaspoon chili powder
- 1teaspoon turmeric powder
- Salt and black pepper to the taste
- 1yellow onion, chopped
- 1tablespoon cilantro, chopped

DIRECTIONS

1. In the air fryer's pan, mix the turkey with the mango and the other ingredients, transfer the pan to your air fryer and cook at 380 degrees F for 30 minutes.
2. Divide everything between plates and serve.

NUTRITION: Calories 291, Fat 12, Fiber 7, Carbs 20, Protein 22

423. Herbed Turkey

Preparation time: 10 minutes

Cooking time: 30 minutes

Servings: 6

INGREDIENTS

- 1 pound turkey breast, skinless, boneless and sliced
- 1 tablespoon basil, chopped
- 1 tablespoon coriander, chopped
- 1 tablespoon oregano, chopped
- 1 tablespoon olive oil
- ½ cup chicken stock
- Juice of 1 lime
- Salt and black pepper to the taste

DIRECTIONS

1. In the air fryer's pan, mix the turkey with the basil and the other ingredients and cook at 370 degrees F for 30 minutes.
2. Divide the mix between plates and serve.

NUTRITION: Calories 281, Fat 7, Fiber 8, Carbs 20, Protein 28

424. Chicken Wings and Sprouts

Preparation time: 10 minutes

Cooking time: 25 minutes

Servings: 4

INGREDIENTS

- 2 pounds chicken wings, halved
- 1 cup Brussels sprouts, trimmed and halved
- 1 cup tomato sauce
- 1 teaspoon hot sauce
- Salt and black pepper to the taste
- 1 teaspoon coriander, ground
- 1 teaspoon cumin, ground
- 1 tablespoon cilantro, chopped

DIRECTIONS

1. In the air fryer's pan, mix the chicken with the sprouts and the other ingredients, toss, cook at 380 degrees F for 25 minutes, divide between plates and serve.

NUTRITION: Calories 271, Fat 7, Fiber 6, Carbs 14, Protein 20

425. Thyme Turkey

Preparation time: 10 minutes

Cooking time: 30 minutes

Servings: 4

INGREDIENTS

- 2 pounds turkey breast, skinless, boneless and cubed
- 2 tablespoons thyme, chopped
- Juice of 1 lime
- 1 teaspoon olive oil
- Salt and black pepper to the taste
- 2 tablespoons tomato paste
- ½ cup chicken stock
- 1 tablespoon chives, chopped

DIRECTIONS

1. In the air fryer's pan, mix the turkey with the thyme and the other ingredients, introduce the pan in the air fryer and cook at 380 degrees F for 30 minutes.
2. Divide the mix between plates and serve.

NUTRITION: Calories 271, Fat 11, Fiber 7, Carbs 17, Protein 20

426. Cumin Chicken

Preparation time: 10 minutes

Cooking time: 30 minutes

Servings: 4

INGREDIENTS

- 1 tablespoon olive oil

- 1 pound chicken breast, skinless, boneless and cubed
- Salt and black pepper to the taste
- 1 teaspoon cumin, ground
- 3 spring onions, chopped
- ½ cup tomato sauce
- 1 cup chicken stock
- ½ tablespoon chives, chopped

DIRECTIONS:

1. In the air fryer's pan, mix the chicken with the oil and the other ingredients and toss.
2. Introduce the pan in the air fryer and cook at 380 degrees F for 30 minutes.
3. Divide everything between plates and serve.

NUTRITION: Calories 261, Fat 11, Fiber 6, Carbs 19, Protein 17

427. Ground Chicken and Chilies

Preparation time: 10 minutes

Cooking time: 30 minutes

Servings: 4

INGREDIENTS

- 2 pounds chicken breast, skinless, boneless and ground
- 1 yellow onion, minced
- 1 teaspoon chili powder
- 1 teaspoon sweet paprika
- Salt and black pepper to the taste
- 1 tablespoon olive oil
- 4 ounces canned green chilies, chopped
- A handful parsley, chopped

DIRECTIONS

1. In the air fryer's pan, mix the chicken with the onion, chili powder and the other ingredients, introduce the pan in the air fryer and cook at 370 degrees F for 30 minutes.
2. Divide into bowls and serve.

428. Chopped Chicken Olive Tomato Sauce

Preparation time: 10 minutes

Cooking time: 30 minutes

Servings: 4

INGREDIENTS

- 500 g chicken cutlet
- 2 minced shallots +1 degermed garlic clove
- 75 g of tomato sauce + 15 g of 30% liquid cream
- 1 bay leaf+salt+pepper+1 tsp Provence herbs
- 20 pitted green and black olives

DIRECTION:

1. Cut the chicken cutlets into strips and put them in the fryer basket with the garlic and the shallots. Do not put oil. Salt/pepper.
2. Set the timer and the temperature to 10-12 minutes at 200°C
3. Add the tomato sauce, the cream, the olives, the bay leaf, and the Provence herbs. Salt if necessary. Mix with a wooden spoon.
4. Close the air fryer and program 20 minutes at 180°C.
5. Eat hot with rice or pasta.

NUTRITION: Calories 220.2 Fat 7.0 g Carbohydrate 8.5 g Sugars 4.5 g Protein 28.9 g Cholesterol 114.8 mg

429. Chicken Thighs in Coconut Sauce, Nuts

Preparation time: 10 minutes

Cooking time: 30 minutes

Servings: 4

INGREDIENTS

- 8skinless chicken thighs
- 2chopped onions
- 25ml of coconut cream + 100 ml of coconut milk
- 4tbsp coconut powder + 1 handful of dried fruit mix+ 5 dried apricots, diced + a few cashew nuts and almonds
- Fine salt + pepper

DIRECTION:

1. Put the onions, chopped with the chicken thighs, in the air fryer (without oil). Add salt and pepper. Program 10 minutes at 200°C.
2. Stir alone with a wooden spoon.
3. Add coconut cream and milk, coconut powder, dried fruits, and apricots. Get out if necessary. Continue cooking by programming 20 minutes at 200°C. You don't have anything to do; it cooks alone, without any problem.
4. With the tongs, remove the bowl and serve hot with rice, vegetables, Chinese noodles............... A delight. Perfect kitchen

NUTRITION: Calories 320.4 Fat 11.6 g Carbohydrate 9.0 g Sugars 2.1 g Protein44.0 g Cholesterol 102.7 mg

430. Forest Guinea Hen

Preparation time: about 15 minutes

Cooking time: 1 h 15 - 1 h 30

Servings: 4

INGREDIENTS

- A beautiful guinea fowl farm weighing 1 to 1.5 kilos
- 100g of dried or fresh porcini mushrooms according to the season
- 8large potatoes Béa
- 1plate
- 2cloves of garlic
- 1shallot
- Chopped parsley
- A pinch of butter
- Vegetable oil
- Salt and pepper

DIRECTION:

1. Put the dried mushrooms in water to rehydrate them or simply clean them if they are fresh porcini mushrooms. Peel the potatoes and cut them finely. Chop the garlic and parsley and set aside.
2. Prepare the guinea fowl by cutting the neck and removing all the giblets inside. Garnish with stuffed dough, garlic cloves and parsley.
3. Place guinea fowls in the air fryer at 2000C without oil of sufficient capacity. Simply add the butter knob and a tablespoon of cooking oil. Allow approximately one hour of cooking per kilo, so you will have to check after a certain period.
4. When the guinea fowl is ready, prepare the porcini mushrooms in the oil-free fryer by adding the shallot. This preparation is very fast, and you should not forget salt and pepper.
5. When everything is ready, place each of the preparations in the air fryer, sprinkle with the cooking juices and cook for another 15 minutes.
6. Serve hot to enjoy all the flavors of the dish.

NUTRITION: Calories 110 Fat 2.5g Carbohydrate 0g Sugars 0g Protein 21g Cholesterol 63mg

431. Fried and Crispy Chicken

Preparation time: 15 minutes

Cooking time: 35-40 minutes

Servings: 4

INGREDIENTS

- 4chicken breasts
- 1tbsp olive oil
- 1tbsp breadcrumbs
- 1tbsp of a spice mixture
- Salt
- 250g of potatoes per person

DIRECTION:

2. Cut chicken breasts into 4 slices
3. Mix them with the other ingredients so that the chicken is perfectly covered with the preparation.
4. Peel and cut the potatoes in the same way as the fries, trying to make a regular cut to cook better.
5. Place the strips in the air fryer without oil and cook at 2000C for 15 to 20 minutes to get a crispy chicken.
6. For French fries, wait 30 minutes to cook.

NUTRITION: Calories 227 Carbohydrates 23g Fat 18g Sugars 0g Protein 12g Cholesterol 63mg

432. Orange Turkey Bites

Preparation time: 10-20

Cooking time: 15-30

Servings: 8

INGREDIENTS

- 750 g turkey
- 1shallot
- 2oranges
- Thyme to taste
- 1tsp oil
- Salt and pepper to taste

DIRECTION:

2. Cut the turkey into pieces and peel the oranges, cutting the skin into strips.
3. Put the chopped shallot, the orange peel, the thyme, and the oil in the basket of the preheated air fryer at 150 for 5 minutes. Brown all for 4 min.
4. Add ½ glass of water, lightly floured turkey, salt, and pepper; simmer for 6 more minutes.
5. Then add the orange juice and cook at 2000C for 15 minutes until a thick juice is obtained.
6. Serve garnished with some thyme leaves and slices of orange.

NUTRITION: Calories 80 Fat 5g Carbohydrates 1g Sugar 0g Protein 7g Cholesterol 25mg

433. Chicken Thighs with Potatoes

Preparation time: 0-10

Cooking time: 45-60

Servings: 6

INGREDIENTS

- 1kg chicken thighs
- 800g of potatoes in pieces
- Salt to taste
- Pepper to taste
- Rosemary at ease
- 1clove garlic

DIRECTION:

2. Preheat the air fryer at 1800C for 15 minutes.
3. Place the chicken thighs in the basket and add the previously peeled and washed potatoes, add a clove of garlic, rosemary sprigs, salt, and pepper.
4. Set the temperature 2000C and cook everything for 50 min. Mix 3-4 times during cooking (when they are well browned on the surfaceand chicken 1-2 times.

NUTRITION: Calories 419.4 Fat 9.5 g Carbohydrate 44.8 g Sugars 2.0 g Protein 39.1 g Cholesterol 115.8 mg

434. Chicken Blanquette With Soy

Preparation time: 10-20

Cooking time: 15-30

Servings:

INGREDIENTS

- 600g Chicken breast
- 300g Potatoes
- 100g Bean sprouts
- 150g Broth
- 50g Onion
- 1tsp Olive oil
- 25g Soy sauce

DIRECTION:

1. Cut the meat and potatoes into pieces.
2. Pour the sliced oil and onion into the bottom of the tank, close the lid.
3. Set the air fryer at 1500C to brown for 5 minutes.
4. Add the floured chicken, potatoes, broth, salt, and pepper and cook for another 13 minutes.
5. Then pour the sprouts and the soy sauce and cook for another 10 minutes.

NUTRITION: Calories 250 Carbohydrates 19g Fat 11g Sugars 7g Protein 16g Cholesterol 0mg

435. Fish Sticks

Cooking time: 15-30

Servings: 6

INGREDIENTS

- 18pieces Fish patties

DIRECTION:

1. Remove the mixing paddle from the tank.
2. Heat the air fryer at 1500C for 5 minutes
3. Cook everything for 20 min.

NUTRITION: Calories 281 Total Fat 15 g Carbohydrates 23.9 g Sugars 2.8 g Protein 12.5 g Cholesterol 36 mg

436. Vegetarian Curry with Pumpkin and Chickpeas

Preparation time: 20-30

Cooking time: 15-30

Servings: 6

INGREDIENTS

- 600g pumpkin, cleaned
- 300g chicken weights already cooked
- 1tsp oil
- 1tsp paprika
- 1tsp curry
- ½ onion
- 1clove garlic
- 1tsp tomato puree
- 200 ml of broth
- 1tsp turmeric
- 480g basmati rice

DIRECTION:

1. Remove the skin of the pumpkin and the seeds inside. Cut it into small pieces, the same size as the chickpeas to have the same cooking time.
2. Pour the chopped onion and garlic, oil, and spices (paprika - curry - turmeric - saffronin the basket.
3. Set the temperature to 1500C and brown all for 4 min.
4. Add the pumpkin and brown for 6 min. additional.

5. Then pour the chickpeas, tomato puree, broth and cook for 10 min. additional.
6. Meanwhile, boil basmati rice in saltwater, drain and serve with vegetarian curry.

NUTRITION: Calories 249.6 Fat 11.7 g Carbohydrate 27.8 g Sugars9.6 g Protein8.1 g Cholesterol 0.0 mg

437. Turkey Diced with Ginger, Apples and Vegetables

Preparation time: 10-20

Cooking time: 30-45

Servings: 4

INGREDIENTS

- 600g turkey breast
- 150g carrots
- 100g of celery
- 50g onion
- 200g of potatoes
- Ginger to taste
- Flour at discretion
- 200ml broth
- 1tsp olive oil
- Leave at discretion
- Black pepper to taste
- 1apple

DIRECTION:

1. Preheat the air fryer at 1500C for 5 minutes.
2. Cut the meat and vegetables into small pieces.
3. Pour the sliced oil and onion into the bottom of the basket and cook for 5 minutes.
4. Add carrots, celery, potatoes, and broth, then cook for another 15 minutes.
5. Add the floured turkey, salt, and pepper, then cook for another 15 minutes (if necessary, add some water).
6. Add the apple pieces and ginger at the end and continue cooking for another 5 minutes.

NUTRITION: Fat 13.6g Carbohydrates 2.3g Sugars 0g Protein 42.4g Cholesterol 124.9mg Value (Amount per Serving):

438. Ligurian Rabbit

Preparation time: 10-20Minutes

Cooking time: 45-60, 6 people, Calories: 440

INGREDIENTS

- 1kg of rabbit pieces
- 150g green olives
- 2tbsp pine nuts
- 100ml broth
- 1shallot
- 1clove garlic
- 1rosemary branch
- 1glass of red wine
- 1tsp olive oil
- 2-3 bay leaves
- Salt to taste

DIRECTION:

1. Put the chopped onion, oil, and garlic in the basket. Set the temperature to 2000C and brown for 2 min.
2. Add meat, red wine and cook for another 8 min.
3. Finally add the green olives, pine nuts, broth, herbs, salt and pepper and simmer for another 50 min. (until the rabbit becomes tender, the meat should easily detach from the boneturning 2-3 times (if the bottom is too dry, add the broth).

NUTRITION: Calories 795 Fat 8g Carbohydrates 0g Sugars 0g Protein 20.8g Cholesterol 82mg

439. Frozen Chicken Nuggets

Cooking time: 15-30

Servings: 8

INGREDIENTS

- 750 g of frozen chicken nuggets
- Fine salt to taste

DIRECTION:

1. Pour the chicken nuggets in the basket
2. Cook for 18 min at 2000C.
3. Salt and serve.

NUTRITION: Calories 33 Fat 1g Carbohydrates 2.8g Sugar 0g Protein 3.3g Cholesterol 9mg

440. Chicken with Cacciatore (Chicken Hunter

Preparation time: 10-20Minutes

Cooking time: 30-45

Servings: 6

INGREDIENTS

- 1kg of chicken pieces
- 1onion:
- 2carrots
- 3celery stalks
- 1clove garlic
- 1glass of red wine
- 400 g peeled tomatoes
- 50 g of olives
- Salt, pepper, parsley to taste

DIRECTION:

1. Clean the chicken and place it inside the basket previously greased with the cooking spray.
2. Set the temperature to 1800C and cook the chicken pieces for 15 minutes.
3. Add the celery mince, carrots, onions, garlic, red wine, salt, pepper, and simmer for an additional 5 minutes.
4. Then pour the tomato and olives and finish simmering for additional 20 minutes stirring chicken and sauce.
5. Once cooked, add a handful of chopped parsley, and serve hot with mash or polenta.

NUTRITION: Calories 233 Fat 7g 10g carbohydrates Sugars 2.2g Protein 34.7g Cholesterol 98.5mg

441. Devil Chicken

Preparation time: 10-20Minutes

Cooking time: 45-60

Servings: 4

INGREDIENTS

- 1kg of whole chicken
- Salt to taste
- Black pepper to taste
- Chili pepper

DIRECTION:

1. Thoroughly clean the chicken and cut it along the white. Flatten it well on the work surface and then massage with oil and spices.
2. Cook the chicken for 35 minutes at 2000C.
3. Turn the chicken and cook another 25 minutes.

NUTRITION: Calories 429.7 Fat 17.3 g Carbohydrate 19.5 g Sugars5.1 g Protein51.1 g Cholesterol 155.0 mg

442. Chicken with Pineapple

Preparation time: 10 - 20Minutes

Cooking time: 15 – 30

Servings: 6

INGREDIENTS

- 600g chicken breast
- 350 g canned pineapple
- 50 ml pineapple juice
- 1 tbsp of starch
- ½ tbsp ginger
- ½ tbsp curry
- 15ml soy sauce
- Salt to taste
- Pepper to taste
- Flour (sufficient quantity

DIRECTION:

2. The floured chicken cut into small pieces, salt, and pepper in the basket previously greased.
3. Simmer for 8 minutes at 1800C (If, at the end of cooking, the chicken pieces stick together, separate them with a wooden spoon).
4. Add the pineapple into small pieces, ginger and curry and simmer for added 3 minutes.
5. Finally, add water, soy sauce and diluted starch to pineapple juice. Simmer for another 6 minutes until the sauce has thickened.
6. Ideal accompanied with basmati rice.

NUTRITION: Calories 222 Fat 7.1g Carbohydrates 11g Sugars 9.7g Protein 27g Cholesterol 85mg

443. Chicken Curry

Preparation time: 10-20Minutes

Cooking time: 15-30

Servings: 6

INGREDIENTS

- 600g chicken breast
- 1 onion
- 2 carrots
- 150 ml
- 200 ml of fresh cream
- 100 ml of milk
- Salt to taste
- 2 spoons of curry
- Flour 00 (sufficient quantity

DIRECTION:

2. Chop the onion in a food processor and cut the carrots into cubes or slices.
3. Spray the basket and distribute the onion and carrots evenly in the basket.
4. Brown for 5 minutes at 1500C.
5. Add the floured chicken, cut into small pieces, the broth, salt, and simmer for another 5 min.
6. Finally pour the fresh cream, the milk and finish cooking for another 15 min. Ideal accompanied with basmati rice.

NUTRITION: Calories 243 Fat 11g Carbohydrates 7.5g Sugars 2g Protein 28g Cholesterol 74mg

444. Chicken with Yogurt and Mustard

Preparation time: 10 - 20Minutes

Cooking time: 15 – 30

Servings: 6

INGREDIENTS

- 500 g chicken breast
- 100 g of white yogurt
- 40 g mustard
- 1 shallot
- Salt to taste
- Pepper to taste

DIRECTION:

2. Place the chopped shallot inside the basket previously greased.
3. Brown for 3 minutes at 1500C
4. Add the chicken pieces, salt, pepper and cook for another 15 minutes at 1800C.

5. Then pour the mustard and yogurt and cook for another 5 minutes.

NUTRITION: Calories 287.1 Fat 8.9g Carbohydrate 4.3 g Sugars 1.7 g Protein43.6 g Cholesterol 99.9 mg

445. Almond Chicken

Preparation time: 10 - 20Minutes

Cooking time: 15 – 30

Servings: 6

INGREDIENTS

- 500 g chicken breast
- 130g crushed almonds
- ½ onion
- 1tbsp grated fresh ginger
- 60 g of soy sauce
- Water (sufficient quantity

DIRECTION:

1. Pour the almonds into the basket.
2. Roast the almonds for 5 minutes at 1500C.
3. Remove the almonds and pour the chopped onion and ginger, the oil into the tank and brown for about 2 minutes.
4. Add lightly floured chicken, salt, pepper and cook for additional 13 minutes.
5. Pour the soy sauce, a ladle of hot water, the roasted almonds and simmer for additional 5 minutes.

NUTRITION: Calories 458 Fat 34g Carbohydrates 22g Sugars 7.3g Protein 20g Cholesterol 24mg

446. Mushroom Chicken

Preparation time: 10-20Minutes

Cooking time: 15-30

Servings: 6

INGREDIENTS:

- 500 g chicken breast
- Mushroom 300g
- 100 g of fresh cream
- 1shallot

DIRECTION:

1. Cut the chicken into pieces and sliced mushrooms. Spray the basket and chopped shallot into the basket. Set the temperature to 1500C and lightly brown for 5 minutes.
2. Add the mushrooms and cook for additional 6 minutes.
3. Finally pour the chicken, salt, pepper, and simmer for another 10 minutes.
4. Then add the fresh cream and cook for 5 min. until the sauce has thickened.

NUTRITION: Calories 220 Fat 14g Carbohydrates 11g Sugar 4g Protein 12g Cholesterol 50mg

447. Pepper Chicken

Preparation time: 10-20

Cooking time: 45-60

Servings: 6

INGREDIENTS

- 1kg of chicken pieces
- 500 g of red and yellow peppers
- salt to taste
- 50g onion

DIRECTION:

1. Pour the chopped onion into the bowl with the chopped peppers and chicken. Add salt and pepper.
2. Set the temperature to 1500C.
3. Cook everything for about 50 minutes, mixing 3 to 4 times during cooking, both meat and peppers.

NUTRITION: Calories 281 Fat 12g Carbohydrates 21g Sugars 3.4g Protein 23g Cholesterol 102mg

448. Stuffed Chicken and Baked Potatoes

Preparation time: 10-20Minutes

Cooking time: 45-60

Servings: 4

INGREDIENTS

- 800 g boneless chicken
- 300 g minced meat
- 150 g sausage
- 80 g French toast
- 1tbsp chopped parsley

DIRECTION:

1. Bone the chicken (or bone directly by the butcher).
2. Prepare the filling:
3. Put in a food processor the meat, the sausage, the French toast bathed in milk to soften it, the parsley, the eggs, the grated cheese, the salt, the pepper and mix until obtaining a homogeneous and compact mixture.
4. Fill the boneless chicken and tie it well with a kitchen rope so that the filling does not come out.
5. Place the chicken inside the bowl, add the chopped potatoes, oil, salt, and pepper.
6. Set the air fryer to 1600C. Cook everything for 60 minutes over mix the potatoes 2-3 times to cook evenly and turn the chicken about once in the middle of cooking.

NUTRITION: Calories 223.8 Fat 6.5 g Carbohydrate 19.8 g Sugars 1.9 g Protein 21.2 g Cholesterol 48.8 mg

449. Tandoori Chicken

Preparation time: more than 30Minutes

Cooking time: 15 – 30

Servings: 4

INGREDIENTS

- 600 g chicken pieces
- 125 g whole yogurt
- 1tbsp curry
- 3tsp of spices for roasted meats

DIRECTION:

1. Place all ingredients in a bowl, flame well and let stand for 1 hour in the refrigerator.
2. Place the pieces of meat in the basket and set the temperature to 1600C
3. Cook the meat for 30 minutes, turning it 1-2 times to brown the chicken on both sides.

NUTRITION: Calories 263 Fat 12g Carbohydrates 6.1g Sugars 3.7g Protein 31g Cholesterol 135mg

450. Crispy Chicken Fillets in Brine in Pickle Juice

Preparation time: 10 minutes

Cooking time: 12 minutes

Servings: 4

INGREDIENTS

- 12chicken offers (1 ¼ pounds in total
- 1¼ cups pickled dill juice
- 1large egg
- 1large egg white
- ½ tsp kosher salt
- Freshly ground black pepper
- ½ cup seasoned breadcrumbs, regular or gluten free
- ½ cup seasoned breadcrumbs, regular or gluten free
- Olive oil spray

DIRECTION:

1. Place the chicken in a shallow bowl and cover with the pickle juice (enough to cover completely). Cover and marine for 8 hours in the refrigerator.
2. Drain the chicken and dry it completely with a paper towel (discard the marinade). In a medium bowl, beat the whole egg, egg white, salt, and pepper. In a shallow arch, combine the breadcrumbs.
3. Dip the chicken in the egg mixture, piece by piece, then in the breadcrumbs, pressing lightly. Remove excess breadcrumbs and place it on a work surface. Spray generously both sides of the chicken with oil.
4. Preheat the fryer to 400°F.
5. Working in batches, place a single layer of chicken in the fryer basket. Cook 10 to 12 minutes, turning halfway through cooking, until cooked, crispy and golden brown. (For a toaster-style air fryer, the temperature stays the same; cook for about 10 minutes.

NUTRITION: Calories: 244kcal Carbohydrates 10g Protein: 37g Fat: 6g Cholesterol 150mg Sugar 1g

451. Turkey and Rosemary Butter

Preparation Time: 29 minutes

Servings: 4

INGREDIENTS

- 1turkey breast, skinless; boneless and cut into 4 pieces
- 2tbsp. rosemary; chopped
- 2tbsp. butter; melted
- Juice of 1 lemon
- A pinch of salt and black pepper

DIRECTIONS

1. Take a bowl and mix the butter with the rosemary, lemon juice, salt and pepper and whisk really well.
2. Brush the turkey pieces with the rosemary butter, put them your air fryer's basket, cook at 380°F for 12 minutes on each side. Divide between plates and serve with a side salad

NUTRITION: Calories: 236; Fat: 12g; Fiber: 4g; Carbs: 6g; Protein: 13g

452. Spiced Chicken Breasts

Preparation Time: 25 minutes

Servings: 4

INGREDIENTS

- 4chicken breasts, skinless and boneless
- 1tbsp. parsley; chopped
- 1tsp. smoked paprika
- 1tsp. garlic powder
- 1tsp. chili powder
- A drizzle of olive oil
- A pinch of salt and black pepper

DIRECTIONS

1. Season chicken with salt and pepper and rub it with the oil and all the other ingredients except the parsley
2. Put the chicken breasts in your air fryer's basket and cook at 350°F for 10 minutes on each side
3. Divide between plates, sprinkle the parsley on top and serve

NUTRITION: Calories: 222; Fat: 11g; Fiber: 4g; Carbs: 6g; Protein: 12g

453. Chicken and Pepperoni Pizza Bake

Preparation Time: 25 minutes

Servings: 4

INGREDIENTS

- 20slices pepperoni
- 2cups cubed cooked chicken
- 1cup shredded mozzarella cheese
- ¼ cup grated Parmesan cheese.
- 1cup low-carb, sugar-free pizza sauce

DIRECTIONS

2. In a 4-cup round baking dish add chicken, pepperoni and pizza sauce. Stir so meat is completely covered with sauce.
3. Top with mozzarella and grated Parmesan. Place dish into the air fryer basket. Adjust the temperature to 375 Degrees F and set the timer for 15 minutes
4. Dish will be brown and bubbling when cooked. Serve immediately.

NUTRITION: Calories: 353; Protein: 34.4g; Fiber: 1.0g; Fat: 17.4g; Carbs: 7.5g

454. Ginger Chicken Breasts

Preparation Time: 25 minutes

Servings: 4

INGREDIENTS

- 4chicken breasts, skinless; boneless and halved
- ¼ cup chicken stock
- 2tbsp. stevia
- 1tbsp. ginger, grated
- 4tbsp. coconut aminos
- 1tsp. olive oil
- Salt and black pepper to taste.

DIRECTIONS

1. In a pan that fits the air fryer, combine the chicken with the ginger and all the ingredients and toss.
2. Put the pan in your air fryer and cook at 4380°F for 20, shaking the fryer halfway
3. Divide between plates and serve with a side salad.

NUTRITION: Calories: 256; Fat: 12g; Fiber: 4g; Carbs: 6g; Protein: 14g

455. Creamy Chicken Wings

Preparation Time: 35 minutes

Servings: 4

INGREDIENTS

- 2lb. chicken wings
- ¼ cup parmesan, grated
- ½ cup heavy cream
- 3garlic cloves; minced
- 3tbsp. butter; melted
- ½ tsp. oregano; dried
- ½ tsp. basil; dried
- Salt and black pepper to taste.

DIRECTIONS

1. In a baking dish that fits your air fryer, mix the chicken wings with all the ingredients except the parmesan and toss
2. Put the dish to your air fryer and cook at 380°F for 30 minutes. Sprinkle the cheese on top, leave the mix aside for 10 minutes, divide between plates and serve

NUTRITION: Calories: 270; Fat: 12g; Fiber: 3g; Carbs: 6g; Protein: 17g

456. Jalapeño Popper Hasselback Chicken

Preparation Time: 40 minutes

Servings: 2

INGREDIENTS

- 4slices sugar-free bacon; cooked and crumbled

- 2 (6-oz. boneless, skinless chicken breasts
- 2oz. full-fat cream cheese; softened.
- ¼ cup sliced pickled jalapeños
- ½ cup shredded sharp Cheddar cheese, divided.

DIRECTIONS

1. Take a medium bowl, place cooked bacon, then fold in cream cheese, half of the Cheddar and the jalapeño slices.
2. Use a sharp knife to make slits in each of the chicken breasts about ¾ of the way across the chicken, being careful not to cut all the way through.
3. Depending on the size of the chicken breast, you'll likely have 6–8 slits per breast
4. Spoon the cream cheese mixture into the slits of the chicken.
5. Sprinkle remaining shredded cheese over chicken breasts and place into the air fryer basket.
6. Adjust the temperature to 350 Degrees F and set the timer for 20 minutes
7. Servings warm.

NUTRITION: Calories: 501; Protein: 53.8g; Fiber: 0.2g; Fat: 25.3g; Carbs: 1.6g

457. Thyme Duck Legs

Preparation Time: 35 minutes

Servings: 4

INGREDIENTS

- 4 duck legs
- 2 tbsp. olive oil
- 4 tsp. thyme; dried
- 3 tsp. fennel seeds, crushed
- A pinch of salt and black pepper

DIRECTIONS

1. Take a bowl and mix the duck legs with all the other ingredients and toss well.
2. Put the duck legs in your air fryer's basket and cook at 380°F for 15 minutes on each side. Divide between plates and serve

NUTRITION: Calories: 274; Fat: 11g; Fiber: 4g; Carbs: 6g; Protein: 14g

458. Chicken Enchiladas

Preparation Time: 30 minutes

Servings: 4

INGREDIENTS

- ½ lb. medium-sliced deli chicken
- 1 medium avocado; peeled, pitted and sliced
- 1 cup shredded medium Cheddar cheese.
- ½ cup shredded Monterey jack cheese
- ⅓ cup low-carb enchilada sauce, divided.
- ½ cup full-fat sour cream.
- 1½ cups shredded cooked chicken

DIRECTIONS

1. Take a large bowl, mix shredded chicken and half of the enchilada sauce. Lay slices of deli chicken on a work surface and spoon 2 tbsp. shredded chicken mixture onto each slice
2. Sprinkle 2 tbsp. of Cheddar onto each roll. Gently roll closed
3. In a 4-cup round baking dish, place each roll, seam side down. Pour remaining sauce over rolls and top with Monterey jack. Place dish into the air fryer basket. Adjust the temperature to 370 Degrees F and set the timer for 10 minutes.
4. Enchiladas will be golden on top and bubbling when cooked. Serve warm with sour cream and sliced avocado.

NUTRITION: Calories: 416; Protein: 34.2g; Fiber: 2.3g; Fat: 25.2g; Carbs: 6.5g

459. Crispy Chicken Tenders

Preparation Time: 25 minutes

Servings: 4

INGREDIENTS

- 9oz. coconut flakes
- 4 chicken breasts, skinless; boneless and cut into tenders
- 1/3 cup almond flour
- 2 eggs, whisked
- A pinch of salt and black pepper

DIRECTIONS

1. Season the chicken tenders with salt and pepper, dredge them in almond flour, then dip in eggs and roll in coconut flakes.
2. Put the chicken tenders in your air fryer's basket and cook at 400°F for 10 minutes on each side.
3. Divide between plates and serve with a side salad.

NUTRITION: Calories: 250; Fat: 12g; Fiber: 4g; Carbs: 6g; Protein: 15g

460. Chicken Cheese Sticks

Preparation Time: 13 minutes

Servings: 2

INGREDIENTS

- 1 cup shredded cooked chicken
- 1 large egg.
- ¼ cup crumbled feta
- 1 cup shredded mozzarella cheese
- ¼ cup buffalo sauce

DIRECTIONS

1. Take a large bowl, mix all ingredients except the feta. Cut a piece of parchment to fit your air fryer basket and press the mixture into a ½-inch-thick circle
2. Sprinkle the mixture with feta and place into the air fryer basket. Adjust the temperature to 400 Degrees F and set the timer for 8 minutes
3. After 5 minutes, flip over the cheese mixture. Allow to cool 5 minutes before cutting into sticks. Serve warm.

NUTRITION: Calories: 369; Protein: 35.7g; Fiber: 0.0g; Fat: 21.5g; Carbs: 2.2g

461. Marinated Drumsticks

Preparation Time: 40 minutes

Servings: 4

INGREDIENTS

- 2lb. chicken drumsticks
- 1½ cups tomato sauce
- 1 tbsp. coconut aminos
- 1 tsp. onion powder
- ½ tsp. chili powder
- A pinch of salt and black pepper

DIRECTIONS

1. In bowl, mix the chicken drumsticks with all the other ingredients, toss and keep in the fridge for 10 minutes.
2. Drain the drumsticks, put them in your air fryer's basket and cook at 380°F for 15 minutes on each side. Divide everything between plates and serve

NUTRITION: Calories: 254; Fat: 14g; Fiber: 4g; Carbs: 6g; Protein: 15g

462. Mustard Turkey Bites

Preparation Time: 25 minutes

Servings: 4

INGREDIENTS

- 1 big turkey breast, skinless; boneless and cubed
- 4 garlic cloves; minced
- 1 tbsp. mustard
- 1½ tbsp. olive oil
- Salt and black pepper to taste.

DIRECTIONS

1. Take a bowl and mix the chicken with the garlic and the other ingredients and toss.
2. Put the turkey in your air fryer's basket, cook at 360°F for 20 minutes, divide between plates and serve with a side salad

NUTRITION: Calories: 240; Fat: 12g; Fiber: 4g; Carbs: 6g; Protein: 15g

463. Lemon Pepper Drumsticks

Preparation Time: 30 minutes

Servings: 8 drumsticks

INGREDIENTS

- 8 chicken drumsticks
- 1 tbsp. lemon pepper seasoning
- 4 tbsp. salted butter; melted.
- 2 tsp. baking powder.
- ½ tsp. garlic powder.

DIRECTIONS

1. Sprinkle baking powder and garlic powder over drumsticks and rub into chicken skin. Place drumsticks into the air fryer basket.
2. Adjust the temperature to 375 Degrees F and set the timer for 25 minutes
3. Use tongs to turn drumsticks halfway through the cooking time. When skin is golden and internal temperature is at least 165 Degrees F, remove from fryer
4. Take a large bowl, mix butter and lemon pepper seasoning. Add drumsticks to the bowl and toss until coated. Serve warm.

NUTRITION: Calories: 532; Protein: 48.3g; Fiber: 0.0g; Fat: 32.3g; Carbs: 1.2g

464. Chives Chicken Tenders

Preparation Time: 25 minutes

Servings: 4

INGREDIENTS

- 1 lb. chicken tenders, boneless, skinless
- 1 tbsp. chives; chopped
- A drizzle of olive oil
- Juice of 1 lemon
- A pinch of salt and black pepper

DIRECTIONS

1. Take a bowl and mix the chicken tenders with all ingredients except the chives, toss, put the meat in your air fryer's basket and cook at 370°F for 10 minutes on each side
2. Divide between plates and serve with chives sprinkled on top.

NUTRITION: Calories: 230; Fat: 13g; Fiber: 4g; Carbs: 6g; Protein: 16g

465. Cinnamon Duck Breasts

Preparation Time: 25 minutes

Servings: 2

INGREDIENTS

- 2 duck breasts; boneless and skin scored
- 4 tbsp. stevia
- 3 tbsp. balsamic vinegar
- ¼ tsp. cinnamon powder
- A pinch of salt and black pepper

DIRECTIONS

1. Take a bowl and mix the duck breasts with the rest of the ingredients and rub well.
2. Put the duck breasts in your air fryer's basket and cook at 380°F for 10 minutes on each side. Divide everything between plates and serve

NUTRITION: Calories: 294; Fat: 12g; Fiber: 4g; Carbs: 6g; Protein: 15g

466. Cheddar Turkey Bites

Preparation Time: 25 minutes

Servings: 4

INGREDIENTS:

- 1big turkey breast, skinless; boneless and cubed
- 1tbsp. olive oil
- ¼ cup cheddar cheese, grated
- ¼ tsp. garlic powder
- Salt and black pepper to taste.

DIRECTIONS

1. Rub the turkey cubes with the oil, season with salt, pepper and garlic powder and dredge in cheddar cheese.
2. Put the turkey bits in your air fryer's basket and cook at 380°F for 20 minutes. Divide between plates and serve with a side salad

NUTRITION: Calories: 240; Fat: 11g; Fiber: 2g; Carbs: 5g; Protein: 12g

467. Crispy Chicken Wings

Preparation Time: 35 minutes

Servings: 4

INGREDIENTS

- 2lb. chicken wings
- ¼ cup olive oil
- Zest of 1 lemon, grated
- 2garlic cloves; minced
- Juice of 2 lemons
- A pinch of salt and black pepper

DIRECTIONS

1. Take a bowl and mix the chicken wings with the rest of the ingredients and toss well
2. Put the chicken wings in your air fryer's basket and cook at 400°F for 30 minutes, shaking halfway. Divide between plates and serve with a side salad

NUTRITION: Calories: 263; Fat: 14g; Fiber: 4g; Carbs: 6g; Protein: 15g

468. Mozzarella Chicken Breasts

Preparation Time: 29 minutes

Servings: 6

INGREDIENTS

- 1lb. mozzarella; sliced
- 2tomatoes; sliced
- 2cups baby spinach
- 6chicken breasts, skinless; boneless and halved
- 2tbsp. olive oil
- 1tbsp. basil; chopped
- 1tsp. Italian seasoning
- A pinch of salt and black pepper

DIRECTIONS

1. Make slits in each chicken breast halves, season with salt, pepper and Italian seasoning and stuff with mozzarella, spinach and tomatoes.

2. Drizzle the oil over stuffed chicken, put it in your air fryer's basket and cook at 370°F for 12 minutes on each side. Divide between plates and serve with basil sprinkled on top.

NUTRITION: Calories: 285; Fat: 12g; Fiber: 4g; Carbs: 7g; Protein: 15g

469. Smoked Chicken Wings

Preparation Time: 35 minutes

Servings: 4

INGREDIENTS

- 2lb. chicken wings
- 1tbsp. olive oil
- 1tbsp. lime juice
- 1tsp. red pepper flakes, crushed
- 2tsp. smoked paprika
- Salt and black pepper to taste.

DIRECTIONS:

1. Take a bowl and mix the chicken wings with all the other ingredients and toss well
2. Put the chicken wings in your air fryer's basket and cook at 380°F for 15 minutes on each side. Divide between plates and serve with a side salad.

NUTRITION: Calories: 280; Fat: 13g; Fiber: 3g; Carbs: 6g; Protein: 14g

470. Mediterranean Chicken

Preparation Time: 40 minutes

Servings: 4

INGREDIENTS

- 1lb. chicken thighs; boneless and skinless
- ½ lb. asparagus, trimmed and halved
- 1 zucchini; halved lengthwise and sliced into half-moons
- 3 garlic cloves; minced
- Juice of 1 lemon
- 2tbsp. olive oil
- 1tsp. oregano; dried
- A pinch of salt and black pepper

DIRECTIONS

1. Take a bowl and mix the chicken with all the ingredients except the asparagus and the zucchinis, toss and leave aside for 15 minutes
2. Add the zucchinis and the asparagus, toss, put everything into a pan that fits the air fryer and cook at 380°F for 25 minutes. Divide everything between plates and serve.

NUTRITION: Calories: 280; Fat: 11g; Fiber: 4g; Carbs: 6g; Protein: 17g

471. Lemon-Oregano Chicken BBQ

Servings: 6

Cooking Time: 40 minutes

INGREDIENTS

- 1 tablespoon grated lemon zest
- 2 tablespoons fresh lemon juice
- 2 tablespoons oregano, chopped
- 3 pounds chicken breasts
- 4 cloves of garlic, minced
- Salt and pepper to taste

DIRECTIONS:

1. Preheat the air fryer to 3900F.
2. Place the grill pan accessory in the air fryer.
3. Season the chicken with oregano, garlic, lemon zest, lemon juice, salt and pepper.
4. Grill for 40 minutes and flip every 10 minutes to cook evenly.

NUTRITION: Calories: 388; Carbs: 1.9g; Protein: 47.5g; Fat: 21.2g

472. Chicken BBQ Recipe from Peru

Servings: 4

Cooking Time: 40 minutes

INGREDIENTS

- ½ teaspoon dried oregano
- 1 teaspoon paprika
- 1/3 cup soy sauce
- 2½ pounds chicken, quartered
- 2 tablespoons fresh lime juice
- 2 teaspoons ground cumin
- 5 cloves of garlic, minced

DIRECTIONS:

- Place all Ingredients in a Ziploc bag and shake to mix everything.
- Allow to marinate for at least 2 hours in the fridge.
- Preheat the air fryer to 3900F.
- Place the grill pan accessory in the air fryer.
- Grill the chicken for 40 minutes making sure to flip the chicken every 10 minutes for even grilling.

NUTRITION: Calories: 377; Carbs: 7.9g; Protein: 59.7g; Fat: 11.8g

472. Turmeric and Lemongrass Chicken Roast

Servings: 6

Cooking Time: 40 minutes

INGREDIENTS

- 1 teaspoon turmeric
- 2 lemongrass stalks
- 2 tablespoons fish sauce
- 3 cloves of garlic, minced
- 3 pounds whole chicken
- 3 shallots, chopped
- Salt and pepper to taste

DIRECTIONS:

- Place all Ingredients in a Ziploc bag and allow to marinate for at least 2 hours in the fridge.
- Preheat the air fryer to 3900F.
- Place the grill pan accessory in the air fryer.
- Grill the chicken for 40 minutes making sure to flip every 10 minutes for even grilling.

NUTRITION: Calories: 495; Carbs: 49.1g; Protein: 38.5g; Fat: 16.1g

473. Roast Chicken Recipe from Africa

Servings: 6

Cooking Time: 45 minutes

INGREDIENTS

- ¼ cup fresh lemon juice
- ½ cup piri piri sauce
- 1 large shallots, quartered
- 1-inch fresh ginger, peeled and sliced thinly
- 3 cloves of garlic, minced
- 3 pounds chicken breasts
- Salt and pepper to taste

DIRECTIONS:

1. Preheat the air fryer to 3900F.
2. Place the grill pan accessory in the air fryer.
3. On a large foil, place the chicken top with the rest of the Ingredients.
4. Fold the foil and crimp the edges.
5. Grill for 45 minutes.

NUTRITION: Calories: 395; Carbs: 3.4g; Protein: 47.9g; Fat: 21.1g

474. Shishito Pepper Rubbed Wings

Servings: 6

Cooking Time: 30 minutes

INGREDIENTS

- 1½ cups shishito peppers, pureed
- 2 tablespoons sesame oil
- 3 pounds chicken wings
- Salt and pepper to taste

DIRECTIONS:

- Place all Ingredients in a Ziploc bowl and allow to marinate for at least 2 hours in the fridge.
- Preheat the air fryer to 390OF.
- Place the grill pan accessory in the air fryer.
- Grill for at least 30 minutes flipping the chicken every 5 minutes and basting with the remaining sauce.

NUTRITION: Calories: 321; Carbs: 1.7g; Protein: 50.2g; Fat: 12.6g

475. Grilled Chicken Recipe from Korea

Servings: 4

Cooking Time: 30 minutes

INGREDIENTS

- ½ cup gochujang
- ½ teaspoon fresh ground black pepper
- 1 scallion, sliced thinly
- 1 teaspoon salt
- 2 pounds chicken wings

DIRECTIONS:

- Place in a Ziploc bag the chicken wings, salt, pepper, and gochujang sauce.
- Allow to marinate in the fridge for at least 2 hours.
- Preheat the air fryer to 390OF.
- Place the grill pan accessory in the air fryer.
- Grill the chicken wings for 30 minutes making sure to flip the chicken every 10 minutes.
- Top with scallions and serve with more gochujang.

NUTRITION: Calories: 278; Carbs: 0.8g; Protein: 50.1g; Fat: 8.2g

476. Lemon-Parsley Chicken Packets

Servings: 4

Cooking Time: 45 minutes

INGREDIENTS

- ¼ cup smoked paprika
- ½ cup parsley leaves
- ½ teaspoon liquid smoke seasoning
- 1½ tablespoon cayenne pepper
- 2 pounds chicken thighs
- 4 lemons, halved
- Salt and pepper to taste

DIRECTIONS:

1. Preheat the air fryer to 390OF.
2. Place the grill pan accessory in the air fryer.
3. In a large foil, place the chicken and season with paprika, liquid smoke seasoning, salt, pepper, and cayenne pepper.
4. Top with lemon and parsley.
5. Place on the grill and cook for 45 minutes.

NUTRITION: Calories: 551; Carbs: 10.4g; Protein: 39.2g; Fat: 39.1g

477. Grilled Chicken Wings with Curry-Yogurt Sauce

Servings: 4

Cooking Time: 35 minutes

INGREDIENTS

- ½ cup plain yogurt
- 1 tablespoons curry powder
- 2 pounds chicken wings
- Salt and pepper to taste

DIRECTIONS:

- Season the chicken wings with yogurt, curry powder, salt and pepper. Toss to combine everything.
- Allow to marinate in the fridge for at least 2 hours.
- Preheat the air fryer to 390°F.
- Place the grill pan accessory in the air fryer.
- Grill the chicken for 35 minutes and make sure to flip the chicken halfway through the cooking time.

NUTRITION: Calories: 301; Carbs: 3.3g; Protein: 51.3g; Fat: 9.2g

478. Tomato, Eggplant 'n Chicken Skewers

Servings: 4

Cooking Time: 25 minutes

INGREDIENTS

- ¼ teaspoon cayenne pepper
- ¼ teaspoon ground cardamom
- 1½ teaspoon ground turmeric
- 1 can coconut milk
- 1 cup cherry tomatoes
- 1 medium eggplant, cut into cubes
- 1 onion, cut into wedges
- 1-inch ginger, grated
- 2 pounds boneless chicken breasts, cut into cubes
- 2 tablespoons fresh lime juice
- 2 tablespoons tomato paste
- 3 teaspoons lime zest
- 4 cloves of garlic, minced
- Salt and pepper to taste

DIRECTIONS:

- Place in a bowl the garlic, ginger, coconut milk, lime zest, lime juice, tomato paste, salt, pepper, turmeric, cayenne pepper, cardamom, and chicken breasts. Allow to marinate in the fridge for at least for 2 hours.
- Preheat the air fryer to 390°F.
- Place the grill pan accessory in the air fryer.
- Skewer the chicken cubes with eggplant, onion, and cherry tomatoes on bamboo skewers.
- Place on the grill pan and cook for 25 minutes making sure to flip the chicken every 5 minutes for even cooking.

NUTRITION: Calories: 485; Carbs: 19.7 g; Protein: 55.2g; Fat: 20.6g

479. Garam Masala 'n Yogurt Marinated Chicken

Servings: 3

Cooking Time: 40 minutes

INGREDIENTS

- ½ cup whole milk yogurt
- ½ teaspoon ground cumin
- 1½ pounds skinless chicken thighs
- 1½ teaspoon garam masala
- 1 tablespoon ground coriander
- 1 tablespoon smoked paprika
- 1-inch ginger, peeled and chopped
- 2 tablespoons prepared mustard
- 3 tablespoons fresh lime juice
- 4 cloves of garlic, minced
- 7 dried chilies, seeds removed and broken into pieces
- Salt and pepper to taste

DIRECTIONS:

1. Place all ingredients in a Ziploc bag and give a good shake to combine everything.
2. Allow to marinate for at least 2 hours in the fridge.
3. Preheat the air fryer to 390OF.
4. Place the grill pan accessory in the air fryer.
5. Grill for at least 40 minutes.
6. Make sure to flip the chicken every 10 minutes.

NUTRITION: Calories: 589; Carbs: 25.5g; Protein:54.6 g; Fat: 29.8g

481. Grilled Chicken Pesto

Servings: 8

Cooking Time: 30 minutes

INGREDIENTS

- 1¾ cup commercial pesto
- 8chicken thighs
- Salt and pepper to taste

DIRECTIONS:

1. Place all Ingredients in the Ziploc bag and allow to marinate in the fridge for at least 2 hours.
2. Preheat the air fryer to 390OF.
3. Place the grill pan accessory in the air fryer.
4. Grill the chicken for at least 30 minutes.
5. Make sure to flip the chicken every 10 minutes for even grilling.

NUTRITION: Calories: 477; Carbs: 3.8g; Protein: 32.6g; Fat: 36.8g

482. Quick 'n Easy Garlic Herb Wings

Servings: 4

Cooking Time: 35 minutes

INGREDIENTS

- ¼ cup chopped rosemary
- 2pounds chicken wings
- 6medium garlic cloves , grated
- salt and pepper to taste

DIRECTIONS:

1. Season the chicken with garlic, rosemary, salt and pepper.
2. Preheat the air fryer to 390OF.
3. Place the grill pan accessory in the air fryer.
4. Grill for 35 minutes and make sure to flip the chicken every 10 minutes.

NUTRITION: Calories: 287; Carbs: 2.9g; Protein: 50.4g; Fat: 8.2g

483. Lemon-Aleppo Chicken

Servings: 4

Cooking Time: 1 hour

INGREDIENTS

- ¼ cup Aleppo-style pepper
- ¼ cup fresh lemon juice
- ¼ cup oregano
- 1cup green olives, pitted and cracked
- 14 cup chopped rosemary
- 2pounds whole chicken, backbones removed and butterflied
- 6cloves of garlic, minced
- Salt and pepper to taste

DIRECTIONS:

1. Place the chicken breast side up and slice through the breasts. Using your palms, press against the breastbone to flatten the breasts or you may remove the bones altogether.
2. Once the bones have been removed, season the chicken with salt, pepper,

garlic, pepper, rosemary, lemon juice, and oregano.
3. Allow to marinate in the fridge for at least 12 hours.
4. Preheat the air fryer to 3900F.
5. Place the grill pan accessory in the air fryer.
6. Place the chicken on the grill pan and place the olives around the chicken.
7. Grill for 1 hour and make sure to flip the chicken every 10 minutes for even grilling.

NUTRITION: Calories: 502; Carbs: 50.4 g; Protein: 37.6 g; Fat: 16.6g

484. Drunken Chicken Jerk Spiced

Servings: 8

Cooking Time: 60 minutes

INGREDIENTS

- ¾ ground cloves
- ¾ malt vinegar
- ¾ soy sauce
- 1½ teaspoons ground nutmeg
- 2½ teaspoons ground allspice
- 2 tablespoons rum
- 2 tablespoon salt
- 4 habanero chilies
- 5 cloves of garlic, minced
- 8 pieces chicken legs

DIRECTIONS:

1. Place all Ingredients in a Ziploc bag and give a good shake. Allow to marinate in the fridge for at least 2 hours.
2. Preheat the air fryer to 3900F.
3. Place the grill pan accessory in the air fryer.
4. Grill the chicken for 60 minutes and flip the chicken every 10 minutes for even grilling.

NUTRITION: Calories: 193; Carbs: 1.2g; Protein: 28.7 g; Fat: 8.1g

485. Honey, Lime, And Garlic Chicken BBQ

Servings: 4

Cooking Time: 40 minutes

INGREDIENTS

- ¼ cup lime juice, freshly squeezed
- ½ cup cilantro, chopped finely
- ½ cup honey
- 1 tablespoon olive oil
- 2 cloves of garlic, minced
- 2 pounds boneless chicken breasts
- 2 tablespoons soy sauce
- Salt and pepper to taste

DIRECTIONS:

1. Place all Ingredients in a Ziploc bag and give a good shake. Allow to marinate in the fridge for at least 2 hours.
2. Preheat the air fryer to 3900F.
3. Place the grill pan accessory in the air fryer.
4. Grill the chicken for 40 minutes making sure to flip the chicken every 10 minutes to grill evenly on all sides.

NUTRITION: Calories: 458; Carbs: 38.9g; Protein: 52.5 g; Fat: 10.2g

486. Chicken in Packets Southwest Style

Servings: 4

Cooking Time: 40 minutes

INGREDIENTS

- 1 can black beans, rinsed and drained
- 1 cup cilantro, chopped
- 1 cup commercial salsa
- 1 cup corn kernels, frozen
- 1 cup Mexican cheese blend, shredded

- 4 chicken breasts
- 4 lime wedges
- 4 teaspoons taco seasoning
- Salt and pepper to taste

DIRECTIONS:

1. Preheat the air fryer to 390°F.
2. Place the grill pan accessory in the air fryer.
3. On a big aluminum foil, place the chicken breasts and season with salt and pepper to taste.
4. Add the corn, commercial salsa beans, and taco seasoning.
5. Close the foil and crimp the edges.
6. Place on the grill pan and cook for 40 minutes.
7. Before serving, top with cheese, cilantro and lime wedges.

NUTRITION: Calories: 837; Carbs: 47.5g; Protein: 80.1g; Fat: 36.2g

487. Cheese Stuffed Chicken

Servings: 4

Cooking Time: 30 minutes

INGREDIENTS

- 1 tablespoon creole seasoning
- 1 tablespoon olive oil
- 1 teaspoon garlic powder
- 1 teaspoon onion powder
- 4 chicken breasts, butterflied and pounded
- 4 slices Colby cheese
- 4 slices pepper jack cheese

DIRECTIONS:

1. Preheat the air fryer to 390°F.
2. Place the grill pan accessory in the air fryer.
3. Create the dry rub by mixing in a bowl the creole seasoning, garlic powder, and onion powder. Season with salt and pepper if desired.
4. Rub the seasoning on to the chicken.
5. Place the chicken on a working surface and place a slice each of pepper jack and Colby cheese.
6. Fold the chicken and secure the edges with toothpicks.
7. Brush chicken with olive oil.
8. Grill for 30 minutes and make sure to flip the meat every 10 minutes.

NUTRITION: Calories: 727; Carbs: 5.4 g; Protein: 73.1g; Fat: 45.9g

488. Cilantro-Lime 'n Liquid Smoke Chicken Grill

Servings: 4

Cooking Time: 40 minutes

INGREDIENTS

- 1½ teaspoon honey
- 1 tablespoon lime zest
- 1 teaspoon liquid smoke
- 1/3 cup chopped cilantro
- 1/3 cup fresh lime juice
- 2 tablespoons olive oil
- 3 cloves of garlic, minced
- 4 chicken breasts, halved
- Salt and pepper to taste

DIRECTIONS:

1. Place all Ingredients in a bowl and allow to marinate in the fridge for at least 2 hours.
2. Preheat the air fryer to 390°F.
3. Place the grill pan accessory in the air fryer.
4. Grill in the chicken for 40 minutes and make sure to flip the chicken every 10 minutes for even grilling.

NUTRITION: Calories: 571; Carbs: 6.1g; Protein: 60.9g; Fat: 33.6g

489. Chicken BBQ on Kale Salad

Servings: 4

Cooking Time: 30 minutes

INGREDIENTS

- ¼ cup Greek yogurt
- ¼ cup parmesan cheese, grated
- ½ cup cherry tomatoes, halved
- ½ teaspoon Worcestershire sauce
- 1 clove of garlic, minced
- 1 large bunch Tuscan kale, cleaned and torn
- 3 tablespoons extra virgin olive oil
- 4 large chicken breasts, pounded
- Juice from 2 lemons, divided
- Salt and pepper to taste

DIRECTIONS:

1. Place all Ingredients in a bowl except for the kale and tomatoes. Allow to marinate in the fridge for at least 2 hours.
2. Preheat the air fryer to 3900F.
3. Place the grill pan accessory in the air fryer.
4. Grill the chicken for 30 minutes.
5. Once cooked, slice the chicken and toss together with the kale and tomatoes.

NUTRITION: Calories: 500; Carbs: 5.9g; Protein: 82.3g; Fat: 16.3g

490. Sriracha-vinegar Marinated Chicken

Servings: 4

Cooking Time: 40 minutes

INGREDIENTS

- ¼ cup Thai fish sauce
- ¼ cups sriracha sauce
- ½ cup rice vinegar
- 1 tablespoons sugar
- 2 garlic cloves, minced
- 2 pounds chicken breasts
- Juice from 1 lime, freshly squeezed
- Salt and pepper to taste

DIRECTIONS:

1. Place all Ingredients in a Ziploc bag except for the corn. Allow to marinate in the fridge for at least 2 hours.
2. Preheat the air fryer to 3900F.
3. Place the grill pan accessory in the air fryer.
4. Grill the chicken for 40 minutes and make sure to flip the chicken to grill evenly.
5. Meanwhile, place the marinade in a saucepan and heat over medium flame until it thickens.
6. Brush the chicken with the glaze and serve with cucumbers if desired.

NUTRITION: Calories: 427; Carbs: 6.7g; Protein: 49.1g; Fat: 22.6g

491. Chicken BBQ Recipe from Italy

Servings: 2

Cooking Time: 40 minutes

INGREDIENTS

- 1 tablespoon fresh Italian parsley
- 1 tablespoon minced garlic
- 1-pound boneless chicken breasts
- 2 tablespoons tomato paste
- Salt and pepper to taste

DIRECTIONS:

1. Place all Ingredients in a Ziploc bag except for the corn. Allow to marinate in the fridge for at least 2 hours.
2. Preheat the air fryer to 3900F.
3. Place the grill pan accessory in the air fryer.
4. Grill the chicken for 40 minutes.

NUTRITION: Calories: 292; Carbs: 6.6g; Protein: 52.6g; Fat: 6.1g

492. Chili, Lime & Corn Chicken BBQ

Servings: 4

Cooking Time: 40 minutes

INGREDIENTS

- ½ teaspoon cumin
- 1 tablespoon lime juice
- 1 teaspoon chili powder
- 2 chicken breasts
- 2 chicken thighs
- 2 cups barbecue sauce
- 2 teaspoon grated lime zest
- 4 ears of corn, cleaned
- Salt and pepper to taste

DIRECTIONS:

1. Place all Ingredients in a Ziploc bag except for the corn. Allow to marinate in the fridge for at least 2 hours.
2. Preheat the air fryer to 3900F.
3. Place the grill pan accessory in the air fryer.
4. Grill the chicken and corn for 40 minutes.
5. Meanwhile, pour the marinade in a saucepan over medium heat until it thickens.
6. Before serving, brush the chicken and corn with the glaze.

NUTRITION: Calories per serving:849 ; Carbs: 87.7g; Protein: 52.3g; Fat: 32.1g

493. Honey-Balsamic Orange Chicken

Servings: 3

Cooking Time: 40 minutes

INGREDIENTS

- ½ cup balsamic vinegar
- ½ cup honey
- 1½ pounds boneless chicken breasts, pounded
- 1 tablespoon orange zest
- 1 teaspoon fresh oregano, chopped
- 2 tablespoons extra virgin olive oil
- Salt and pepper to taste

DIRECTIONS:

1. Put the chicken in a Ziploc bag and pour over the rest of the Ingredients. Shake to combine everything. Allow to marinate in the fridge for at least 2 hours.
2. Preheat the air fryer to 3900F.
3. Place the grill pan accessory in the air fryer.
4. Grill the chicken for 40 minutes.

NUTRITION: Calories: 521; Carbs: 56.1g; Protein: 51.8g; Fat: 9.9g

494. Salsa Verde Over Grilled Chicken

Servings: 2

Cooking Time: 40 minutes

INGREDIENTS

- ½ red onion, chopped
- ½ teaspoon chili powder
- 1 jalapeno thinly sliced
- 1 jar salsa verde, divided
- 1-pound boneless skinless chicken breasts
- 2 cloves of garlic, minced
- 2 tablespoons chopped cilantro
- 2 tablespoons extra virgin olive oil
- 4 slices Monterey Jack cheese
- Juice from ½ lime
- Lime wedges for serving

DIRECTIONS:

1. In a Ziploc bag, add half of the salsa verde, olive oil, lime juice, garlic, chili

powder and chicken. Allow to marinate in the fridge for at least 2 hours.
2. Preheat the air fryer to 3900F.
3. Place the grill pan accessory in the air fryer.
4. Grill the chicken for 40 minutes.
5. Flip the chicken every 10 minutes to cook evenly.
6. Serve the chicken with the cheese, jalapeno, red onion, cilantro, and lime wedges.

NUTRITION: Calories: 541; Carbs: 4.5g; Protein: 65.3g; Fat: 29.1g

495. Chicken Grill Recipe from California

Servings: 4

Cooking Time: 40 minutes

INGREDIENTS

- ¾ cup balsamic vinegar
- 1teaspoon garlic powder
- 2tablespoons extra virgin olive oil
- 2tablespoons honey
- 2teaspoons Italian seasoning
- 4boneless chicken breasts
- 4slices mozzarella
- 4slices of avocado
- 4slices tomato
- Balsamic vinegar for drizzling
- Salt and pepper to taste

DIRECTIONS:

1. In a Ziploc bag, mix together the balsamic vinegar, garlic powder, honey, olive oil, Italian seasoning, salt, pepper, and chicken.
2. Allow to marinate in the fridge for at least 2 hours.
3. Preheat the air fryer to 3900F.
4. Place the grill pan accessory in the air fryer.
5. Put the chicken on the grill and cook for 40 minutes.
6. Flip the chicken every 10 minutes to grill all sides evenly.
7. Serve the chicken with mozzarella, avocado, and tomato. Drizzle with balsamic vinegar.

NUTRITION: Calories: 853; Carbs: 43.2g; Protein:69.4 g; Fat: 44.7g

496. Grilled Thighs with Honey Balsamic Sauce

Servings: 8

Cooking Time: 40 minutes

INGREDIENTS

- 1/3 cup honey
- 2tablespoons balsamic vinegar
- 2tablespoons butter
- 3cloves of garlic, minced
- 8bone-in chicken thighs
- Chopped chives for garnish
- Lemon wedges for garnish
- Salt and pepper to taste

DIRECTIONS:

1. In a mixing bowl, season the chicken with salt and pepper to taste.
2. Add the butter, balsamic vinegar, honey, and garlic.
3. Allow to marinate for 2 hours in the fridge.
4. Preheat the air fryer to 3900F.
5. Place the grill pan accessory in the air fryer.
6. Put the chicken on the grill pan and cook for 40 minutes. Flip the chicken every 10 minutes to grill evenly.
7. Meanwhile, place the remaining marinade in a saucepan and allow to simmer until thickened.

8. Once cooked, brush the chicken with the sauce and garnish with chives and lemon wedges.

NUTRITION: Calories: 524; Carbs: 32.4g; Protein: 25.1g; Fat: 32.7g

497. Chicken Roast with Pineapple Salsa

Servings: 2

Cooking Time: 45 minutes

INGREDIENTS

- ¼ cup extra virgin olive oil
- ¼ cup freshly chopped cilantro
- 1 avocado, diced
- 1-pound boneless chicken breasts
- 2 cups canned pineapples
- 2 teaspoons honey
- Juice from 1 lime
- Salt and pepper to taste

DIRECTIONS:

1. Preheat the air fryer to 390°F.
2. Place the grill pan accessory in the air fryer.
3. Season the chicken breasts with lime juice, olive oil, honey, salt, and pepper.
4. Place on the grill pan and cook for 45 minutes.
5. Flip the chicken every 10 minutes to grill all sides evenly.
6. Once the chicken is cooked, serve with pineapples, cilantro, and avocado.

NUTRITION: Calories: 744; Carbs: 57.4g; Protein: 54.7g; Fat: 32.8g

498. Sweet Lime 'n Chili Chicken Barbecue

Servings: 2

Cooking Time: 40 minutes

INGREDIENTS

- ¼ cup soy sauce
- 1 cup sweet chili sauce
- 1-pound chicken breasts
- Juice from 2 limes, freshly squeezed

DIRECTIONS:

1. In a Ziploc bag, combine all Ingredients and give a good shake. Allow to marinate for at least 2 hours in the fridge.
2. Preheat the air fryer to 390°F.
3. Place the grill pan accessory in the air fryer.
4. Place chicken on the grill and cook for 30 to 40 minutes. Make sure to flip the chicken every 10 minutes to cook evenly.
5. Meanwhile, use the remaining marinade and put it in a saucepan. Simmer until the sauce thickens.
6. Once the chicken is cooked, brush with the thickened marinade.

NUTRITION: Calories: 563; Carbs: 39.2g; Protein: 43.6g; Fat: 25.7g

499. Sticky-Sweet Chicken BBQ

Servings: 2

Cooking Time: 40 minutes

INGREDIENTS

- ½ cup balsamic vinegar
- ½ cup soy sauce
- 1-pound chicken drumsticks
- 2 cloves of garlic, minced
- 2 green onion, sliced thinly
- 2 tablespoons sesame seeds
- 3 tablespoons honey

DIRECTIONS:

1. In a Ziploc bag, combine the soy sauce, balsamic vinegar, honey, garlic, and

chicken. Allow to marinate in the fridge for at least 30 minutes.
2. Preheat the air fryer to 3300F.
3. Place the grill pan accessory in the air fryer.
4. Place on the grill and cook for 30 to 40 minutes. Make sure to flip the chicken every 10 minutes to cook evenly.
5. Meanwhile, use the remaining marinade and put it in a saucepan. Simmer until the sauce thickens.
6. Once the chicken is cooked, brush with the thickened marinade and garnish with sesame seeds and green onions.

NUTRITION: Calories: 594; Carbs: 43.7g; Protein: 48.7g; Fat: 24.9g

MEAT

500. Lime Lamb Mix

Preparation time: 5 minutes

Cooking time: 30 minutes

Servings: 4

INGREDIENTS

- 2pounds lamb chops
- Juice of 1 lime
- Zest of 1 lime, grated
- A pinch of salt and black pepper
- 1tablespoon olive oil
- 1teaspoon sweet paprika
- 1teaspoon cumin, ground
- 1tablespoon cumin, ground

DIRECTIONS

1. In the air fryer's basket, mix the lamb chops with the lime juice and the other ingredients, rub and cook at 380 degrees F for 15 minutes on each side.
2. Serve with a side salad.

NUTRITION: Calories 284, Fat 13, Fiber 3, Carbs 5, Protein 15

501. Lamb and Corn

Preparation time: 5 minutes

Cooking time: 30 minutes

Servings: 4

INGREDIENTS

- 2pounds lamb stew meat, cubed
- 1cup corn
- 1cup spring onions, chopped
- ¼ cup beef stock
- 1tablespoon olive oil
- A pinch of salt and black pepper
- 2tablespoons rosemary, chopped

DIRECTIONS

1. In the air fryer's pan, mix the lamb with the corn, spring onions and the other ingredients, toss and cook at 380 degrees F for 30 minutes.
2. Divide the mix between plates and serve.

NUTRITION: Calories 274, Fat 12, Fiber 3, Carbs 5, Protein 15

502. Herbed Beef and Squash

Preparation time: 10 minutes

Cooking time: 30 minutes

Servings: 4

INGREDIENTS

- 2pounds beef stew meat, cubed
- 1cup butternut squash, peeled and cubed
- 1tablespoon basil, chopped
- 1tablespoon oregano, chopped
- A pinch of salt and black pepper
- A drizzle of olive oil
- 2garlic cloves, minced

DIRECTIONS

1. In the air fryer's pan, mix the beef with the squash and the other ingredients, toss and cook at 380 degrees F for 30 minutes.
2. Divide between plates and serve.

NUTRITION: Calories 284, Fat 13, Fiber 3, Carbs 6, Protein 14

503. Smoked Beef Mix

Preparation time: 5 minutes

Cooking time: 20 minutes

Servings: 4

INGREDIENTS

- 1 pound beef stew meat, roughly cubed
- 1 tablespoon smoked paprika
- ½ cup beef stock
- ½ teaspoon garam masala
- 2 tablespoons olive oil
- A pinch of salt and black pepper

DIRECTIONS

1. In the air fryer's basket, mix the beef with the smoked paprika and the other ingredients, toss and cook at 390 degrees F for 20 minutes on each side.
2. Divide between plates and serve.

NUTRITION: Calories 274, Fat 12, Fiber 4, Carbs 6, Protein 17

504. Marjoram Pork Mix

Preparation time: 5 minutes

Cooking time: 25 minutes

Servings: 4

INGREDIENTS

- 2 pounds pork stew meat, roughly cubed
- 1 tablespoon marjoram, chopped
- 1 cup heavy cream
- 2 tablespoons olive oil
- Salt and black pepper to the taste
- 2 garlic cloves, minced

DIRECTIONS

1. Heat up a pan that fits the air fryer with the oil over medium-high heat, add the meat and brown for 5 minutes
2. Add the rest of the ingredients, toss, put the pan in the fryer and cook at 400 degrees F for 20 minutes more.
3. Divide between plates and serve.

NUTRITION: Calories 274, Fat 14, Fiber 3, Carbs 6, Protein 14

505. Nutmeg Lamb

Preparation time: 5 minutes

Cooking time: 30 minutes

Servings: 4

INGREDIENTS

- 1 pound lamb stew meat, cubed
- 2 teaspoons nutmeg, ground
- 1 teaspoon coriander, ground
- 1 cup heavy cream
- 2 tablespoons olive oil
- 2 tablespoons chives, chopped
- Salt and black pepper to the taste

DIRECTIONS

1. In the air fryer's pan, mix the lamb with the nutmeg and the other ingredients, put the pan in the air fryer and cook at 380 degrees F for 30 minutes.
2. Divide everything into bowls and serve.

NUTRITION: Calories 287, Fat 13, Fiber 2, Carbs 6, Protein 12

506. Greek Beef Mix

Preparation time: 5 minutes

Cooking time: 30 minutes

Servings: 4

INGREDIENTS:

- 2pounds beef stew meat, roughly cubed
- 1teaspoon coriander, ground
- 1teaspoon garam masala
- 1teaspoon cumin, ground
- A pinch of salt and black pepper
- 1cup Greek yogurt
- ½ teaspoon turmeric powder

DIRECTIONS

1. In the air fryer's pan, mix the beef with the coriander and the other ingredients, toss and cook at 380 degrees F for 30 minutes.
2. Divide between plates and serve.

NUTRITION: Calories 283, Fat 13, Fiber 3, Carbs 6, Protein 15

507. Beef and Fennel

Preparation time: 5 minutes

Cooking time: 30 minutes

Servings: 4

INGREDIENTS

- 2pounds beef stew meat, cut into strips
- 2fennel bulbs, sliced
- 2tablespoons mustard
- A pinch of salt and black pepper
- 1tablespoon black peppercorns, ground
- 2tablespoons balsamic vinegar
- 2tablespoons olive oil

DIRECTIONS

1. In the air fryer's pan, mix the beef with the fennel and the other ingredients.
2. Put the pan in the fryer and cook at 380 degrees for 30 minutes.
3. Divide everything into bowls and serve.

NUTRITION: Calories 283, Fat 13, Fiber 2, Carbs 6, Protein 17

508. Lamb and Eggplant Meatloaf

Preparation time: 5 minutes

Cooking time: 35 minutes

Servings: 4

INGREDIENTS

- 2pounds lamb stew meat, ground
- 2eggplants, chopped
- 1yellow onion, chopped
- A pinch of salt and black pepper
- ½ teaspoon coriander, ground
- Cooking spray
- 2tablespoons cilantro, chopped
- 1egg
- 2tablespoons tomato paste

DIRECTIONS

1. In a bowl, mix the lamb with the eggplants of the ingredients except the cooking spray and stir.
2. Grease a loaf pan that fits the air fryer with the cooking spray, add the mix and shape the meatloaf.
3. Put the pan in the air fryer and cook at 380 degrees F for 35 minutes.
4. Slice and serve with a side salad.

NUTRITION: Calories 263, Fat 12, Fiber 3, Carbs 6, Protein 15

509. Pork Chops with Olives and Corn

Preparation time: 10 minutes

Cooking time: 25 minutes

Servings: 4

INGREDIENTS

- 2pounds pork chops
- 1cup kalamata olives, pitted and halved
- 1cup black olives, pitted and halved
- 1cup corn
- Salt and black pepper to the taste
- 1tablespoons avocado oil
- 2tablespoons garlic powder
- 2tablespoons oregano, dried

DIRECTIONS

1. In the air fryer's pan, mix the pork chops with the olives and the other ingredients, toss, cook at 400 degrees F for 25 minutes, divide between plates and serve.

NUTRITION: Calories 281, Fat 8, Fiber 7, Carbs 17, Protein 19

510. Beef and Broccoli Mix

Preparation time: 10 minutes

Cooking time: 30 minutes

Servings: 4

INGREDIENTS

- 1pound beef stew meat, cubed
- 2cups broccoli florets
- ½ cup tomato sauce
- 1teaspoon sweet paprika
- 2teaspoons olive oil
- 1tablespoon cilantro, chopped

DIRECTIONS

1. In your air fryer, mix the beef with the broccoli and the other ingredients, toss, cook at 390 degrees F for 30 minutes, divide into bowls and serve.

NUTRITION: Calories 281, Fat 12, Fiber 7, Carbs 19, Protein 20

511. Cajun Beef Mix

Preparation time: 10 minutes

Cooking time: 30 minutes

Servings: 4

INGREDIENTS

- 2pounds beef stew meat, cubed
- 1tablespoon Cajun seasoning
- 1teaspoon sweet paprika
- 1teaspoon chili powder
- Salt and black pepper to the taste
- 1tablespoon olive oil

DIRECTIONS

1. In a baking dish that fits your air fryer, mix the beef with the seasoning and the other ingredients, toss, introduce the pan in the fryer and cook at 400 degrees F for 30 minutes.
2. Divide the mix into bowls and serve.

NUTRITION: Calories 291, Fat 8, Fiber 7, Carbs 19, Protein 20

512. Pork with Sprouts and Mushroom Mix

Preparation time: 10 minutes

Cooking time: 30 minutes

Servings: 4

INGREDIENTS

- 2pounds pork stew meat, cubed
- 1cup Brussels sprouts, trimmed and halved
- 1cup mushrooms, sliced
- Salt and black pepper to the taste
- 1tablespoon balsamic vinegar
- 1yellow onion, chopped

- 2 teaspoons olive oil

DIRECTIONS

1. In a baking dish that fits your air fryer, mix the pork with the sprouts and the other ingredients, introduce the pan in the fryer and cook at 390 degrees F for 30 minutes.
2. Divide everything between plates and serve.

NUTRITION: Calories 285, Fat 8, Fiber 2, Carbs 18, Protein 20

513. Pork Chops and Yogurt Sauce

Preparation time: 10 minutes

Cooking time: 30 minutes

Servings: 4

INGREDIENTS

- 2 tablespoons avocado oil
- 2 pounds pork chops
- 1 cup yogurt
- 2 garlic cloves, minced
- 1 teaspoon turmeric powder
- Salt and black pepper to the taste
- 2 tablespoon oregano, chopped

DIRECTIONS

1. In the air fryer's pan, mix the pork chops with the yogurt and the other ingredients, toss and cook at 400 degrees F for 30 minutes.
2. Divide the mix between plates and serve.

NUTRITION: Calories 301, Fat 7, Fiber 5, Carbs 19, Protein 22

514. Lamb and Macadamia Nuts Mix

Preparation time: 10 minutes

Cooking time: 20 minutes

Servings: 4

INGREDIENTS

- 2 pounds lamb stew meat, cubed
- 2 tablespoons macadamia nuts, peeled
- 1 cup baby spinach
- ½ cup beef stock
- 2 garlic cloves, minced
- Salt and black pepper to the taste
- 1 tablespoon oregano, chopped

DIRECTIONS

1. In the air fryer's pan, mix the lamb with the nuts and the other ingredients, cook at 380 degrees F for 20 minutes, divide between plates and serve.

NUTRITION: Calories 280, Fat 12, Fiber 8, Carbs 20, Protein 19

515. Beef, Cucumber and Eggplants

Preparation time: 10 minutes

Cooking time: 20 minutes

Servings: 4

INGREDIENTS

- 1 pound beef stew meat, cut into strips
- 2 eggplants, cubed
- 2 cucumbers, sliced
- 2 garlic cloves, minced
- 1 cup heavy cream
- 2 tablespoons olive oil
- Salt and black pepper to the taste

DIRECTIONS

1. In a baking dish that fits your air fryer, mix the beef with the eggplants and the other ingredients, toss, introduce the pan

in the fryer and cook at 400 degrees F for 20 minutes.
2. Divide everything into bowls and serve.

NUTRITION: Calories 283, Fat 11, Fiber 9, Carbs 22, Protein 14

516. Rosemary Pork and Artichokes

Preparation time: 10 minutes

Cooking time: 25 minutes

Servings: 4

INGREDIENTS

- 1pound pork stew meat, cubed
- 1cup canned artichoke hearts, drained and halved
- 2tablespoons olive oil
- 2tablespoons rosemary, chopped
- ½ teaspoon cumin, ground
- ½ teaspoon nutmeg, ground
- ½ cup sour cream
- Salt and black pepper to the taste

DIRECTIONS

1. In a pan that fits your air fryer, mix the pork with the artichokes and the other ingredients, introduce in the fryer and cook at 400 degrees F for 25 minutes.
2. Divide everything into bowls and serve.

NUTRITION: Calories 280, Fat 13, Fiber 9, Carbs 22, Protein 18

517. Nutmeg Beef Mix

Preparation time: 10 minutes

Cooking time: 30 minutes

Servings: 4

INGREDIENTS

- 2pounds beef stew meat, cubed
- 1teaspoon nutmeg, ground
- 2tablespoons avocado oil
- ½ teaspoon chili powder
- ¼ cup beef stock
- 2tablespoons chives, chopped
- Salt and black pepper to the taste

DIRECTIONS

1. In a pan that fits your air fryer, mix the beef with the nutmeg and the other ingredients, toss, introduce the pan in the fryer and cook at 400 degrees F for 30 minutes.
2. Divide the mix into bowls and serve.

NUTRITION: Calories 280, Fat 12, Fiber 2, Carbs 17, Protein 14

518. Lamb and Asparagus Mix

Preparation time: 10 minutes

Cooking time: 30 minutes

Servings: 4

INGREDIENTS

- 2tablespoons butter, melted
- 2pounds lamb chops
- 4asparagus spears, trimmed and halved
- Salt and black pepper to the taste
- 1tablespoon avocado oil
- ¼ cup beef stock
- 1tablespoon dill, chopped

DIRECTIONS

1. In the air fryer's pan, mix the melted butter with the lamb chops and the other ingredients, toss and cook at 400 degrees F for 30 minutes.
2. Divide into bowls and serve.

NUTRITION: Calories 300, Fat 11, Fiber 4, Carbs 18, Protein 22

519. Paprika Lamb Chops

Preparation time: 10 minutes

Cooking time: 25 minutes

Servings: 4

INGREDIENTS

- 1pound lamb chops
- 2tablespoons butter, melted
- 1tablespoon smoked paprika
- 1garlic clove, minced
- ½ teaspoon nutmeg, ground
- Salt and black pepper to the taste
- ¼ cup beef stock

DIRECTIONS

1. In the air fryer's pan, mix the lamb chops with the melted butter and the other ingredients, toss and cook at 380 degrees F for 25 minutes.
2. Divide everything between plates and serve.

NUTRITION: Calories 310, Fat 8, Fiber 10, Carbs 19, Protein 25

520. Lamb and Mustard Sauce

Preparation time: 10 minutes

Cooking time: 25 minutes

Servings: 4

INGREDIENTS

- 2pounds lamb chops
- 2tablespoons mustard
- 2tablespoons butter, melted
- 1cup beef stock
- 1teaspoon coriander, ground
- 1teaspoon sweet paprika
- Salt and black pepper to the taste

DIRECTIONS

1. In the air fryer's pan, mix the lamb chops with the mustard and the other ingredients, toss and cook at 400 degrees F for 25 minutes.
2. Divide the mix between plates and serve.

NUTRITION: Calories 284, Fat 14, Fiber 4, Carbs 17, Protein 28

521. Beef with Apples and Plums

Preparation time: 10 minutes

Cooking time: 30 minutes

Servings: 4

INGREDIENTS

- 2pounds beef stew meat, cubed
- 1cup apples, cored and cubed
- 1cup plums, pitted and halved
- 2tablespoons butter, melted
- Salt and black pepper to the taste
- ½ cup red wine
- 1tablespoon chives, chopped

DIRECTIONS

1. In the air fryer's pan, mix the beef with the apples and the other ingredients, toss, put the pan in the machine and cook at 390 degrees F for 30 minutes.
2. Divide the mix between plates and serve right away.

NUTRITION: Calories 290, Fat 12, Fiber 5, Carbs 19, Protein 28

522. Sage Beef

Preparation time: 10 minutes

Cooking time: 30 minutes

Servings: 4

INGREDIENTS

- 2pounds beef stew meat, cubed
- 1tablespoon sage, chopped
- 2tablespoons butter, melted
- ½ teaspoon coriander, ground
- ½ tablespoon garlic powder
- 1teaspoon Italian seasoning
- Salt and black pepper to the taste

DIRECTIONS

1. In the air fryer's pan, mix the beef with the sage, melted butter and the other ingredients, introduce the pan in the fryer and cook at 360 degrees F for 30 minutes.
2. Divide everything between plates and serve.

NUTRITION: Calories 290, Fat 11, Fiber 6, Carbs 20, Protein 29

523. Beef, Olives and Tomatoes

Preparation time: 10 minutes

Cooking time: 35 minutes

Servings: 4

INGREDIENTS

- 2pounds beef stew meat, cubed
- 1cup black olives, pitted and halved
- 1cup cherry tomatoes, halved
- 1tablespoon smoked paprika
- 3tablespoons olive oil
- 1teaspoon coriander, ground
- Salt and black pepper to the taste

DIRECTIONS

1. In the air fryer's pan, mix the beef with the olives and the other ingredients, toss and cook at 390 degrees F for 35 minutes.
2. Divide between plates and serve.

NUTRITION: Calories 291, Fat 12, Fiber 9, Carbs 20, Protein 26

524. Tarragon Beef

Preparation time: 10 minutes

Cooking time: 35 minutes

Servings: 4

INGREDIENTS

- 2pounds beef roast, sliced
- 2tablespoons tarragon, chopped
- 3tablespoons butter, melted
- Juice of 1 lime
- Salt and black pepper to the taste
- 3garlic cloves, minced
- 1tablespoon chives, chopped

DIRECTIONS

1. In the air fryer's pan, mix the roast with the tarragon and the other ingredients, put the pan your air fryer and cook at 390 degrees F for 35 minutes.
2. Divide between plates and serve.

NUTRITION: Calories 290, Fat 14, Fiber 9, Carbs 19, Protein 22

525. Beef with Celery and Peas

Preparation time: 10 minutes

Cooking time: 40 minutes

Servings: 4

INGREDIENTS

- 2pounds beef stew meat, roughly cubed
- 1cup celery, cubed
- 1cup peas
- 2tablespoons olive oil
- Salt and black pepper to the taste
- ½ cup beef stock
- ½ cup canned tomatoes, crushed

DIRECTIONS

1. In a baking dish that fits your air fryer, mix the beef with the celery and the other ingredients, toss, introduce the pan in the fryer and cook at 390 degrees F for 40 minutes.
2. Divide the mix between plates and serve.

NUTRITION: Calories 300, Fat 12, Fiber 4, Carbs 18, Protein 20

526. Lamb with Peas and Tomatoes

Preparation time: 10 minutes

Cooking time: 30 minutes

Servings: 4

INGREDIENTS

- 2pounds lamb stew meat, cubed
- 1cup peas
- 1cup canned tomatoes, crushed
- 1cup spring onions, chopped
- 2tablespoons tomato paste
- 3garlic cloves, minced
- A pinch of salt and black pepper
- ½ teaspoon coriander, ground

DIRECTIONS

1. In a pan that fits your air fryer, mix the lamb with the peas and the other ingredients, toss, introduce in the fryer and cook at 390 degrees F for 30 minutes.
2. Divide everything into bowls and serve.

NUTRITION: Calories 289, Fat 8, Fiber 12, Carbs 20, Protein 19

527. Lamb with Zucchinis and Eggplants Mix

Preparation time: 10 minutes

Cooking time: 30 minutes

Servings: 4

INGREDIENTS

- 1pound lamb stew meat, cubed
- 2zucchinis, cubed
- 2eggplants, cubed
- 4garlic cloves, minced
- 2tablespoons avocado oil
- ½ teaspoon coriander, ground
- 1teaspoon nutmeg, ground
- A pinch of salt and black pepper
- ½ cup beef stock

DIRECTIONS

1. In a pan that fits your air fryer mix the lamb with the zucchinis, eggplants and the other ingredients, introduce in the fryer and cook at 400 degrees F for 30 minutes, shaking the fryer halfway.
2. Divide everything between plates and serve.

NUTRITION: Calories 293, Fat 12, Fiber 12, Carbs 20, Protein 29

528. Beef with Beans

Preparation time: 10 minutes

Cooking time: 30 minutes

Servings: 4

INGREDIENTS

- 2pounds beef stew meat, cubed
- 1cups canned kidney beans, drained
- 1teaspoon sweet paprika
- ½ teaspoon coriander, ground
- 2tablespoons olive oil
- 1cup tomato sauce
- Salt and black pepper to the taste
- 1tablespoon chives, chopped

DIRECTIONS

1. In baking dish that fits your air fryer, mix the beef with the beans and the other ingredients, introduce the dish in the fryer and cook at 390 degrees F for 30 minutes
2. Divide everything into bowls and serve.

NUTRITION: Calories 275, Fat 3, Fiber 7, Carbs 20, Protein 18

529. Mediterranean Lamb Meatballs

Preparation time: 10 minutes

Cooking time: 40 minutes

Servings: 4

INGREDIENTS

- 454g ground lamb
- 3cloves garlic, minced
- 5g of salt
- 1g black pepper
- 2g of mint, freshly chopped
- 2g ground cumin
- 3ml hot sauce
- 1g chili powder
- 1scallion, chopped
- 8g parsley, finely chopped
- 15 ml of fresh lemon juice
- 2g lemon zest
- 10 ml of olive oil

DIRECTION:

1. Mix the lamb, garlic, salt, pepper, mint, cumin, hot sauce, chili powder, chives, parsley, lemon juice and lemon zest until well combined.
2. Create balls with the lamb mixture and cool for 30 minutes.
3. Select Preheat in the air fryer and press Start/Pause.
4. Cover the meatballs with olive oil and place them in the preheated fryer.
5. Select Steak, set the time to 10 minutes and press Start/Pause.

NUTRITION:

Calories:282Fat:23.41Carbohydrates: 0g Protein: 16.59 Sugar: 0g Cholesterol: 73gm

530. Pork Rind

Preparation time: 10 minutes

Cooking time: 1h. Serve: 4

INGREDIENTS

- 1kg of pork rinds
- Salt
- ½ tsp black pepper coffee

DIRECTION:

1. Preheat the air fryer. Set the time of 5 minutes and the temperature to 2000C.
2. Cut the bacon into cubes - 1 finger wide.
3. Season with salt and a pinch of pepper.
4. Place in the basket of the air fryer. Set the time of 45 minutes and press the power button.
5. Shake the basket every 10 minutes so that the pork rinds stay golden brown equally.
6. Once they are ready, drain a little on the paper towel so they stay dry. Transfer to a plate and serve.

NUTRITION: Calories: 172 Fat: 10.02g Carbohydrates: 0g Protein: 19.62g Sugar: 0g Cholesterol: 30 mg

531. Pork Trinoza Wrapped in Ham

Preparation time: 10 minutes

Cooking time: 20 minutes

Servings: 6

INGREDIENTS

- 6pieces of Serrano ham, thinly sliced
- 454g pork, halved, with butter and crushed
- 6g of salt
- 1g black pepper
- 227g fresh spinach leaves, divided
- 4slices of mozzarella cheese, divided
- 18g sun-dried tomatoes, divided
- 10ml of olive oil, divided

DIRECTION:

1. Place 3 pieces of ham on baking paper, slightly overlapping each other. Place 1 half of the pork in the ham. Repeat with the other half.
2. Season the inside of the pork rolls with salt and pepper.
3. Place half of the spinach, cheese, and sun-dried tomatoes on top of the pork loin, leaving a 13 mm border on all sides.
4. Roll the fillet around the filling well and tie with a kitchen cord to keep it closed.
5. Repeat the process for the other pork steak and place them in the fridge.
6. Select Preheat in the air fryer and press Start/Pause.
7. Brush 5 ml of olive oil on each wrapped steak and place them in the preheated air fryer.
8. Select Steak. Set the timer to 9 minutes and press Start/Pause.
9. Allow it to cool for 10 minutes before cutting.

NUTRITION: Calories: 250 Fat: 14.20g Carbohydrates: 35g Protein: 27.60g Sugar: 0g Cholesterol: 0g

532. Homemade Flamingos

Preparation time: 10 minutes

Cooking time: 20 minutes

Servings: 4

INGREDIENTS

- 400g of very thin sliced pork fillets c / n
- 2boiled and chopped eggs
- 100g chopped Serrano ham
- 1beaten egg
- Breadcrumbs

DIRECTION:

1. Make a roll with the pork fillets. Introduce half cooked egg and Serrano ham. So that the roll does not lose its shape, fasten with a string or chopsticks.
2. Pass the rolls through beaten egg and then through the breadcrumbs until it forms a good layer.
3. Preheat the air fryer a few minutes at 180° C.
4. Insert the rolls in the basket and set the timer for about 8 minutes at 180o C.
5. Serve right away.

NUTRITION: Calories: 424 Fat: 15.15g Carbohydrates: 37.47g Protein: 31.84g Sugar: 3.37g Cholesterol: 157mg

533. North Carolina Style Pork Chops

Preparation time: 5 minutes

Cooking time: 10 minutes

Servings: 2

INGREDIENTS

- 2 boneless pork chops
- 15ml of vegetable oil
- 25g dark brown sugar, packaged
- 6g of Hungarian paprika
- 2g ground mustard
- 2g freshly ground black pepper
- 3g onion powder
- 3g garlic powder
- Salt and pepper to taste

DIRECTION:

1. Preheat the air fryer a few minutes at 1800C.
2. Cover the pork chops with oil.
3. Put all the spices and season the pork chops abundantly, almost as if you were making them breaded.
4. Place the pork chops in the preheated air fryer.
5. Select Steak, set the time to 10 minutes.
6. Remove the pork chops when it has finished cooking. Let it stand for 5 minutes and serve.

NUTRITION: Calories: 118 Fat: 6.85g Carbohydrates: 0 Protein: 13.12g Sugar: 0g Cholesterol: 39mg

534. Beef with Sesame and Ginger

Preparation time: 10 minutes

Cooking time: 23 minutes

Servings: 4-6

INGREDIENTS

- ½ cup tamari or soy sauce
- 3 tbsp olive oil
- 2 tbsp toasted sesame oil
- 1 tbsp brown sugar
- 1 tbsp ground fresh ginger
- 3 cloves garlic, minced
- 1 to 1½ pounds skirt steak, boneless sirloin, or low loin

DIRECTION:

1. Put together the tamari sauce, oils, brown sugar, ginger, and garlic in small bowl. Add beef to a quarter-size plastic bag and pour the marinade into the bag. Press on the bag as much air as possible and seal it.
2. Refrigerate for 1 to 1½ hours, turning half the time. Remove the meat from the marinade and discard the marinade. Dry the meat with paper towels. Cook at a temperature of 350°F for 20 to 23 minutes, turning halfway through cooking.

NUTRITION: Calories: 381 Fat: 5g Carbohydrates: 9.6g Protein: 38g Sugar: 1.8g Cholesterol: 0mg

535. Katsu Pork

Preparation time: 10 minutes

Cooking time: 14 minutes

Servings: 2

INGREDIENTS

- 170g pork chops, boneless
- 56g of breadcrumbs
- 3g garlic powder
- 2g onion powder
- 6g of salt
- 1g white pepper
- 60g all-purpose flour
- 2 eggs, shakes
- Nonstick Spray Oil

DIRECTION:

1. Place the pork chops in an airtight bag or cover them with a plastic wrap.
2. Crush the pork with a meat roller or hammer until it is 13 mm thick.

3. Combine the crumbs and seasonings in a bowl. Leave aside.
4. Pass each pork chop through the flour, then soak them in the beaten eggs and finally pass them through the crumb mixture.
5. Preheat the air fryer set the temperature to 180°C.
6. Spray pork chops on each side with cooking oil and place them in the preheated air fryer.
7. Cook the pork chops at 180°C for 4 minutes.
8. Remove them from the air fryer when finished and let them sit for 5 minutes.
9. Cut them into pieces and serve them.

NUTRITION: Calories: 820 Fat: 24.75g Carbohydrates: 117g Protein: 33.75g Sugar: 0g Cholesterol: 120mg

536. Pork on A Blanket

Preparation time: 5 minutes

Cooking time: 10 minutes

Servings: 4

INGREDIENTS

- ½ puff pastry sheet, defrosted
- 16 thick smoked sausages
- 15ml of milk

DIRECTION:

1. Preheat la air fryer to 200°C and set the timer to 5 minutes.
2. Cut the puff pastry into 64 x 38 mm strips.
3. Place a cocktail sausage at the end of the puff pastry and roll around the sausage, sealing the dough with some water.
4. Brush the top (with the seam facing down of the sausages wrapped in milk and place them in the preheated air fryer.
5. Cook at 200°C for 10 minutes or until golden brown.

NUTRITION: Calories: 242 Fat: 14g Carbohydrates: 0g Protein: 27g Sugar: 0g Cholesterol: 80mg

537. Lamb Shawarma

Preparation time: 12 minutes

Cooking time: 8 minutes

Servings: 2

INGREDIENTS

- 340g ground lamb
- 2g cumin
- 2g of paprika
- 3g garlic powder
- 2g onion powder
- 1g of cinnamon
- 1g turmeric
- 1g fennel seeds
- 1g ground coriander seed
- 3g salt
- 4 bamboo skewers (229 mm

DIRECTION:

1. Put all the ingredients in a bowl and mix well.
2. Stir 85g of meat into each skewer, then place them in the fridge for 10 minutes.
3. Preheat in the air fryer to 200°C.
4. Place the skewers in the preheated air fryer, select Steak. Adjust to 8 minutes.
5. Serve with lemon yogurt dressing or alone.

NUTRITION: Calories: 562 Fat: 11.19g Carbohydrates: 76.89g Protein: 35.84g Sugar: 7.45g Cholesterol: 69mg

538. Stuffed Cabbage and Pork Loin Rolls

Preparation time: 5 minutes

Cooking time: 25 minutes

Servings: 4

INGREDIENTS

- 500g of white cabbage
- 1 onion
- 8 pork tenderloin steaks
- 2 carrots
- 4 tbsp soy sauce
- 50g of olive oil
- Salt
- 8 sheets of rice

DIRECTION:

2. Put the chopped cabbage in the Thermomix glass together with the onion and the chopped carrot.
3. Select 5 seconds, speed Add the extra virgin olive oil. Select 5 minutes, varoma temperature, left turn, spoon speed.
4. Cut the tenderloin steaks into thin strips. Add the meat to the Thermomix glass. Select 5 minutes, varoma temperature, left turn, spoon speed. Without beaker
5. Add the soy sauce. Select 5 minutes, varoma temperature, left turn, spoon speed. Rectify salt. Let it cold down.
6. Hydrate the rice slices. Extend and distribute the filling between them.
7. Make the rolls, folding so that the edges are completely closed. Place the rolls in the air fryer and paint with the oil.
8. Select 10 minutes, 1800C.

NUTRITION: Calories: 120 Fat: 3.41g Carbohydrates: 0g Protein: 20.99g Sugar: 0g Cholesterol: 65mg

539. Pork Head Chops with Vegetables

Preparation time: 5 minutes

Cooking time: 20 minutes

Servings: 2-4

INGREDIENTS

- 4 pork head chops
- 2 red tomatoes
- 1 large green pepper
- 4 mushrooms
- 1 onion
- 4 slices of cheese
- Salt
- Ground pepper
- Extra virgin olive oil

DIRECTION:

1. Put the four chops on a plate and salt and pepper.
2. Put two of the chops in the air fryer basket.
3. Place tomato slices, cheese slices, pepper slices, onion slices and mushroom slices. Add some threads of oil.
4. Take the air fryer and select 1800C, 15 minutes.
5. Check that the meat is well made and take out.
6. Repeat the same operation with the other two pork chops.

NUTRITION: Calories: 106 Fat: 5g Carbohydrates: 2g Protein: 11g Sugar: 0g Cholesterol: 0mg

540. Provencal Ribs

Preparation time: 10 minutes

Cooking time: 1h 20 minutes

Servings: 4

INGREDIENTS

- 500g of pork ribs
- Provencal herbs
- Salt
- Ground pepper
- Oil

DIRECTION:

1. Put the ribs in a bowl and add some oil, Provencal herbs, salt, and ground pepper.
2. Stir well and leave in the fridge for at least 1 hour.
3. Put the ribs in the basket of the air fryer and select 2000C, 20 minutes.
4. From time to time shake the basket and remove the ribs.

NUTRITION: Calories: 296 Fat: 22.63g Carbohydrates: 0g Protein: 21.71g Sugar: 0g Cholesterol: 90mg

541. Beef Scallops

Preparation time: 15 minutes

Cooking time: 20 minutes

Servings: 4

INGREDIENTS

- 16veal scallops
- Salt
- Ground pepper
- Garlic powder
- 2eggs
- Breadcrumbs
- Extra virgin olive oil

DIRECTION:

1. Put the beef scallops well spread and salt and pepper. Add some garlic powder.
2. In a bowl, beat the eggs.
3. In another bowl put the breadcrumbs.
4. Pass the Beef scallops for beaten egg and then for the breadcrumbs.
5. Spray with extra virgin olive oil on both sides.
6. Put a batch in the basket of the air fryer. Do not pile the scallops too much.
7. Select 1800C, 15 minutes. From time to time shake the basket so that the scallops move.
8. When finishing that batch, put the next one and so on until you finish with everyone, usually 4 or 5 scallops enter per batch.

NUTRITION: Calories: 330 Fat: 16.27g Carbohydrates: 0g Protein: 43g Sugar: 0g Cholesterol: 163mg

542. Potatoes with Loin and Cheese

Preparation time: 10 minutes

Cooking time: 30 minutes

Servings: 4

INGREDIENTS

- 1kg of potatoes
- 1large onion
- 1piece of roasted loin
- Extra virgin olive oil
- Salt
- Ground pepper
- Grated cheese

DIRECTION:

1. Peel the potatoes, cut the cane, wash, and dry.
2. Put salt and add some threads of oil, we bind well.
3. Pass the potatoes to the basket of the air fryer and select 1800C, 20 minutes.
4. Meanwhile, in a pan, put some extra virgin olive oil and add the peeled onion and cut into julienne.
5. When the onion is transparent, add the chopped loin.
6. Sauté well and pepper.
7. Put the potatoes on a baking sheet.
8. Add the onion with the loin.
9. Cover with a layer of grated cheese.
10. Bake a little until the cheese takes heat and melts.

NUTRITION: Calories: 332 Fat: 7g Carbohydrates: 41g Protein: 23g Sugar: 0g Cholesterol: 0mg

543. Potatoes with Loin and Cheese

Preparation time: 10 minutes

Cooking time: 30 minutes

Servings: 4

INGREDIENTS

- 1kg of potatoes
- 1large onion
- 1piece of roasted loin
- Extra virgin olive oil
- Salt
- Ground pepper
- Grated cheese

DIRECTION:

1. Peel the potatoes, cut the cane, wash, and dry.
2. Put salt and add some threads of oil, bind well.
3. Pass the potatoes to the basket of the air fryer and select 1800C, 20 minutes.
4. Meanwhile, in a pan, put some extra virgin olive oil and add the peeled onion and cut into julienne.
5. When the onion is transparent, add the chopped loin.
6. Sauté well and pepper.
7. Put the potatoes on a baking sheet.
8. Add the onion with the loin.
9. Cover with a layer of grated cheese.
10. Bake a little until the cheese takes heat and melts.

NUTRITION: Calories: 332 Fat: 7g Carbohydrates: 41g Protein: 23g Sugar: 0g Cholesterol: 0mg

544. Russian Steaks with Nuts and Cheese

Preparation time: 5 minutes

Cooking time: 20 minutes

Servings: 4

INGREDIENTS

- 800g of minced pork
- 200g of cream cheese
- 50g peeled walnuts
- 1onion
- Salt
- Ground pepper
- 1egg
- Breadcrumbs
- Extra virgin olive oil

DIRECTION:

1. Put the onion cut into quarters in the Thermomix glass and select 5 seconds speed
2. Add the minced meat, cheese, egg, salt, and pepper.
3. Select 10 seconds, speed 5, turn left.
4. Add the chopped and peeled walnuts and select 4 seconds, turn left, speed
5. Pass the dough to a bowl.
6. Make Russian steaks and go through breadcrumbs.
7. Paint the Russian fillets with extra virgin olive oil on both sides with a brush.
8. Put in the basket of the air fryer, without stacking the Russian fillets.
9. Select 1800C, 15 minutes.

NUTRITION: Calories: 36 Fat: 20g Carbohydrates: 6g Protein: 46g Sugar: 0g Cholesterol: 63mg

545. Potatoes with Bacon, Onion and Cheese

Preparation time: 10 minutes

Cooking time: 15 minutes

Servings: 4

INGREDIENTS

- 200g potatoes
- 150g bacon
- 1onion
- Slices of cheese
- Extra virgin olive oil
- Salt

DIRECTION:

1. Peel the potatoes, cut into thin slices, and wash them well.
2. Drain and dry the potatoes, put salt and a few strands of extra virgin olive oil.
3. Stir well and place in the basket of the air fryer.
4. Cut the onion into julienne, put a little oil, and stir, place on the potatoes.
5. Finally, put the sliced bacon on the onion.
6. Take the basket to the air fryer and select 20 minutes, 1800C.
7. From time to time, remove the basket.
8. Take all the contents of the basket to a source and when it is still hot, place the slices of cheese on top.
9. You can let the heat of the potatoes melt the cheese or you can gratin a few minutes in the oven.

NUTRITION: Calories: 125 Fat: 2g Carbohydrates: 24g Protein: 5g Sugar: 0.1g Cholesterol: 40mg

546. Pork Liver

Preparation time: 5 minutes

Cooking time: 15 minutes

Servings: 4

INGREDIENTS

- 500g of pork liver cut into steaks
- Breadcrumbs
- Salt
- Ground pepper
- 1lemon
- Extra virgin olive oil

DIRECTION:

1. Put the steaks on a plate or bowl.
2. Add the lemon juice, salt, and ground pepper.
3. Leave a few minutes to macerate the pork liver fillets.
4. Drain well and go through breadcrumbs, it is not necessary to pass the fillets through beaten egg because the liver is very moist, the breadcrumbs are perfectly glued.
5. Spray with extra virgin olive oil. If you don't have a sprayer, paint with a silicone brush.
6. Put the pork liver fillets in the air fryer basket.
7. Program 1800C, 10 minutes.
8. Take out if you see them golden to your liking and put another batch.
9. You should not pile the pork liver fillets, which are well extended so that the empanada is crispy on all sides.

NUTRITION: Calories: 134 Fat: 3.65g Carbohydrates: 2.47g Protein: 21.39g

547. Marinated Loin Potatoes

Preparation time: 10 minutes

Cooking time: 1h.

Serve: 2

INGREDIENTS

- 2medium potatoes
- 4fillets of marinated loin
- A little extra virgin olive oil
- Salt

DIRECTION:

1. Peel the potatoes and cut. Cut with match-sized mandolin, potatoes with a cane but very thin.
2. Wash and immerse in water 30 minutes.
3. Drain and dry well.
4. Add a little oil and stir so that the oil permeates well in all the potatoes.
5. Go to the basket of the air fryer and distribute well.
6. Select 1600C, 10 minutes.
7. Take out the basket, shake so that the potatoes take off. Let the potato tender. If it is not, leave 5 more minutes.
8. Place the steaks on top of the potatoes.
9. Select 1600C, 10 minutes and 180 degrees 5 minutes again.

NUTRITION: Calories: 136 Fat: 5.1g Carbohydrates: 1.9g Protein: 20.7g Sugar: 0.4g Cholesterol: 65mg

548. Pork Fritters

Preparation time: 5 minutes

Cooking time: 20 minutes

Servings: 2-4

INGREDIENTS

- Pork fillets cut into pieces
- 264g flour
- ½ tsp salt
- ½ tsp ground paprika
- A pinch of cayenne pepper
- 500 ml of sparkling water
- Flour to cover
- Nonstick cooking spray

DIRECTION:

1. Coat the pork pieces with flour, shaking off the excess.
2. Mix the flour, seasonings and carbonated water creating a dough in a medium container. Beat until smooth.
3. Preheat the air fryer to 360°F (182°C).
4. Introduce previously sprinkled pork into the dough.
5. Spray the basket of the air fryer with nonstick cooking spray
6. Place the battered pork pieces in the air fryer basket in a single layer.
7. Cook the pork for 10 to 12 minutes, turning it in the middle of the process.
8. Pork fritters will be ready when the breaded has a brown-gold color and the pork is fully cooked.

NUTRITION: Calories: 412 Fat: 18.30g Carbohydrates: 59.5g Protein: 3.10g Sugar: 35.11g Cholesterol: 11mg

549. Pork Tenderloin

Preparation time: 10 minutes

Cooking time: 45 minutes

Servings: 2-4

INGREDIENTS

- 2large eggs
- ¼ cup milk
- 2cups seasoned breadcrumbs
- Salt and pepper to taste
- Nonstick cooking spray

DIRECTION:

1. Slice the tenderloin into ½ inch slices.
2. Place the slices between two plastic sheets and tap them until each piece is ¼ inch thick.
3. In a large container, mix the eggs and milk.
4. In a separate container or dish, pour the breadcrumbs.

5. Introduce each piece of pork in the mixture of eggs and milk, letting the excess drain.
6. Then introduce the pork in the breadcrumbs, covering each side.
7. Place the covered pork on a wire rack for 30 minutes to make sure the cover adheres.
8. Preheat the air fryer to 400°F (204 °C).
9. Spray the basket of the air fryer with nonstick cooking spray. Place the covered sirloin in the basket in a single layer.
10. Cook the sirloin for 10 minutes, then take it out, turn it over and sprinkle with more nonstick spray.
11. Cook for 5-minutes more or until both sides are crispy and golden brown.

NUTRITION: Calories: 158 Fat: 7.12g Carbohydrates: 0g Protein: 22.05g Sugar: 0g Cholesterol: 67mg

550. **Cheesy Beef Paseíllo**

Preparation time: 10 minutes

Cooking time: 20 minutes

Servings: 15

INGREDIENTS

- 1-2 tbsp olive oil
- 2 pounds lean ground beef
- ½ chopped onion
- 2 cloves garlic, minced
- ½ tbsp Adobo seasoning
- 2 tsp dried oregano
- 1 packet of optional seasoning
- 2 tbsp chopped cilantro
- ¼ cup grated cheese
- 15 dough disks
- 15 slices of yellow cheese

DIRECTION:

1. In a large skillet over medium-high heat, heat the oil. Once the oil has warmed, add the meat, onions, and Adobo seasoning.
2. Brown veal, about 6-7 minutes. Drain the ground beef. Add the remaining seasonings and cilantro. Cook an additional minute. Add grated cheese, if desired. Melt the cheese.
3. On each dough disk, add a slice of cheese to the center and add 3-4 tablespoons of meat mixture over the slice of cheese. Fold over the dough disk, and with a fork, fold the edges and set it aside.
4. Preheat the air fryer to 3700C for 3 minutes.
5. Once three minutes have passed, spray the air fryer pan with cooking spray and add 3-4 cupcakes to the basket. Close the basket and set to 3700C and cook for 7 minutes. After 7 minutes, verify it. Cook up to 3 additional minutes, or the desired level of sharpness, if desired.
6. Repeat until finished.

NUTRITION: Calories: 225 Fat: 5g Carbohydrates: 10g Protein: 10g Sugar: 0g Cholesterol: 25mg

551. **Beef Patty**

Preparation time: 20 minutes

Cooking time: 30 minutes

Servings: 4

INGREDIENTS

- Prepared dough
- 300g beef
- 1 large onion
- 1 red pepper
- 2 hard-boiled eggs
- Salt
- Pepper to taste.
- 1 tsp oil

DIRECTION:

1. Remove the dough from the refrigerator 10 minutes before.
2. In a pan, place oil, 1 onion, 1 pepper, garlic, seasoning. Add ground beef until cooked well. Season with salt and pepper to taste.
3. Let the filling cool
4. Place the filling in each circle of the dough and seal with egg white at the edges.
5. Butter a refractory mold and accommodate the patty.
6. Preheat the oven to 190°C for 10 minutes by pressing the Convection button
7. Place the refractory on the metal rack and bring to the preheated oven for 30 minutes at 190°C.

NUTRITION: Calories: 263 Fat: 17.25g Carbohydrates: 20.22g Protein: 6.65g Sugar: 0.96g Cholesterol: 59mg

552. Roasted Pork

Preparation time: 5 minutes

Cooking time: 30 minutes

Servings: 2-4

INGREDIENTS

- 500-2000g Pork meat (To roast
- Salt
- Oil

DIRECTION:

1. Join the cuts in an orderly manner.
2. Place the meat on the plate
3. Varnish with a little oil.
4. Place the roasts with the fat side down.
5. Cook in air fryer at 1800C for 30 minutes.
6. Turn when you hear the beep.
7. Remove from the oven. Drain excess juice.
8. Let stand for 10 minutes on aluminum foil before serving.

NUTRITION: Calories: 820 Fat: 24.75g Carbohydrates: 117g Protein: 33.75g Sugar: 0g Cholesterol: 120mg

553. Fried Pork Chops

Preparation time: 5 minutes

Cooking time: 35 minutes

Servings: 2

INGREDIENTS

- 3cloves of ground garlic
- 2tbsp olive oil
- 1tbsp of marinade
- 4thawed pork chops

DIRECTION:

1. Mix the cloves of ground garlic, marinade, and oil. Then apply this mixture on the chops.
2. Put the chops in the air fryer at 3600C for 35 minutes.

NUTRITION: Calories: 118 Fat: 6.85g Carbohydrates: 0 Protein: 13.12gSugar: 0g Cholesterol: 39mg

554. Crispy Pork Chops

Preparation time: 5 minutes

Cooking time: 12 minutes

Servings: 4

INGREDIENTS

- Olive oil spray
- 6(3/4-inch thick central cut boneless pork chops, trimmed fat (5 oz each
- Kosher salt

- 1 large egg, beaten
- ½ cup panko crumbs (check labels for GF
- 1/3 cup crushed corn crumbs
- 2 tbsp grated Parmesan cheese (skip for vegetarians
- 1¼ tsp sweet paprika
- ½ tsp garlic powder
- ½ tsp onion powder
- ¼ tsp chili powder
- 1/8 tsp black pepper

DIRECTION:

1. Preheat the fryer with air at 4000F for 12 minutes and lightly spray the basket with oil.
2. Season the pork chops on both sides with ½ teaspoon of kosher salt.
3. Put the panko, corn crumbs, Parmesan cheese, ¾ teaspoon kosher salt, paprika, garlic powder, onion powder, chili powder and black pepper in a large, shallow bowl.
4. Place the beaten egg in another. Dip the pork in the egg, then the crumb mixture.
5. When the fryer is ready, place 3 of the chops in the prepared basket and sprinkle the top with oil.
6. Cook 12 minutes turning in half, sprinkling both sides with oil. Set aside and repeat with the rest.

NUTRITION: Calories: 378 Fat: 13g Carbohydrates: 8g Protein: 33g Sugar: 1 g Cholesterol: 121 mg

555. Pork Bondiola Chop

Preparation time: 5 minutes

Cooking time: 20 minutes

Servings: 4

INGREDIENTS

- 1kg bondiola in pieces
- Breadcrumbs
- 2 eggs
- Seasoning to taste

DIRECTION:

1. Cut the bondiola into small pieces, seasonings to taste.
2. Beat the eggs.
3. Pass the bondiola seasoned by beaten egg and then by breadcrumbs.
4. Then place in the air fryer for 20 minutes, halfway around turn and ready snacks of bondiola.

NUTRITION: Calories: 265 Fat: 20.36g Carbohydrates: 0g Protein: 19.14g Sugar: 0g Cholesterol: 146mg

556. Pork Taquitos

Preparation time: 10 minutes

Cooking time: 15 minutes

Servings: 6

INGREDIENTS

- 3 cups shredded pork loin (previously cooked
- Lemon juice
- 10 templates
- 2 cups mozzarella cheese
- Cooking spray (oil
- Sauce to taste
- Sour cream to taste

DIRECTION:

1. Preheat the fryer to 380 degrees F. Meanwhile, soften the templates in the microwave for 10 seconds.
2. On the other hand, in a bowl add the pork with a pinch of lemon.
3. Then, add the shredded pork and cheese to the template. Roll up the template and close.

4. Once ready, add spray on them and take to the air fryer for 10 minutes.

NUTRITION: Calories: 133 Fat: 4g Carbohydrates: 22g Protein: 5g Sugar: 0g Cholesterol: 0mg

557. Pork Knuckle

Preparation time: 15 minutes

Cooking time: 50 minutes

Servings: 2

INGREDIENTS

- Knuckle:
- 3potatoes
- 1head of garlic
- Water
- Extra virgin olive oil
- Salt
- Peppercorns
- 1bay leaf
- Vinaigrette
- Mustard and beer (to accompany
- For the sauerkraut:
- 1cabbage
- 100g of butter
- 1glass of white wine
- 5tbsp vinegar
- a pinch of cumin
- Some coriander seeds
- Peppercorns
- Juniper berries

DIRECTION:

1. Cook the knuckle in a quick pot with the potatoes and a little salt.
2. Add some pepper balls, a bay leaf, and a garlic head.
3. Cover with water and cook for 40 minutes.
4. When it starts to boil, lower the heat to medium heat.
5. For sauerkraut, chop the cabbage into quarters and cut into strips with the mandolin.
6. Put the cabbage in a bowl, water with a glass of white wine and a dash of vinegar and mix everything well.
7. Crush some juniper berries with a knife, add them and sprinkle with pepper, coriander, and cumin.
8. Mix the whole well, wet with a glass of water and let stand for 3 days or more.
9. Cook the cabbage for 15 minutes in a pot, drain and sauté over medium heat for 8 minutes.
10. Season and water with a dash of olive oil.
11. Pass the knuckle in the air fryer basket, dip extra virgin olive oil at 250°C for 10 minutes
12. Servings the knuckle with potatoes and sauerkraut.

NUTRITION: Calories: 333 Fat: 22g Carbohydrates: 0g Protein: 28g Sugar: 0g Cholesterol: 84mg

VEGETABLES

558. Creamy Beets

Preparation time: 5 minutes

Cooking time: 25 minutes

Servings: 4

INGREDIENTS

- 2pounds baby beets, peeled and halved
- 1cup heavy cream
- 1teaspoon turmeric powder
- A pinch of salt and black pepper
- 2tablespoons olive oil
- 2garlic cloves, minced
- Juice of 1 lime
- ½ teaspoon coriander, ground

DIRECTIONS

1. In a pan that fits your air fryer, mix the beet with the cream, turmeric and the other ingredients, toss, introduce the pan in the fryer and cook at 400 degrees F for 25 minutes.
2. Divide between plates and serve.

NUTRITION: Calories 135, Fat 3, Fiber 2, Carbs 4, Protein 6

559. Chard and Olives

Preparation time: 5 minutes

Cooking time: 20 minutes

Servings: 4

INGREDIENTS

- 2cups red chard, torn
- 1cup kalamata olives, pitted and halved
- ½ cup tomato sauce
- 1teaspoon chili powder
- 2tablespoons olive oil
- Salt and black pepper to the taste

DIRECTIONS

1. In a pan that fits the air fryer, combine the chard with the olives and the other ingredients and toss.
2. Put the pan in your air fryer, cook at 370 degrees F for 20 minutes, divide between plates and serve.

NUTRITION: Calories 154, Fat 3, Fiber 2, Carbs 4, Protein 6

560. Coconut Mushrooms Mix

Preparation time: 5 minutes

Cooking time: 20 minutes

Servings: 4

INGREDIENTS

- 1pound white mushrooms, halved
- 1teaspoon sweet paprika
- 1red onion, chopped
- 1teaspoon rosemary, dried
- Salt and black pepper to the taste
- 2tablespoons olive oil
- 1cup coconut milk

DIRECTIONS

1. In a pan that fits your air fryer, mix the mushrooms with the paprika and the other ingredients and toss.
2. Put the pan in the fryer, cook at 380 degrees F for 20 minutes, divide between plates and serve.

NUTRITION: Calories 162, Fat 4, Fiber 1, Carbs 3, Protein 5

561. Kale and Tomatoes

Preparation time: 5 minutes

Cooking time: 20 minutes

Servings: 4

INGREDIENTS:

- 2 cups baby kale
- 1 pound cherry tomatoes, halved
- 1 cup mild salsa
- 2 scallions, chopped
- 1 tablespoon olive oil
- A pinch of salt and black pepper
- 2 tablespoons chives, chopped

DIRECTIONS

1. In a pan that fits the air fryer, combine the kale with the tomatoes and the other ingredients and toss.
2. Put the pan in the air fryer and cook at 380 degrees F for 20 minutes.
3. Divide between plates and serve.

NUTRITION: Calories 140, Fat 3, Fiber 2, Carbs 3, Protein 5

562. Brussels Sprouts and Tomatoes

Preparation time: 5 minutes

Cooking time: 20 minutes

Servings: 4

INGREDIENTS

- 1 pound Brussels sprouts, trimmed
- ½ pound cherry tomatoes, halved
- 2 tablespoons tomato paste
- 1 cup chicken stock
- ½ teaspoon sweet paprika
- 1 tablespoon olive oil
- Salt and black pepper to the taste
- 1 tablespoon chives, chopped

DIRECTIONS

1. In a pan that fits the air fryer, mix the sprouts with the tomatoes and the other ingredients and toss.
2. Put the pan in the air fryer and cook at 380 degrees F for 20 minutes.
3. Divide between plates and serve.

NUTRITION: Calories 170, Fat 5, Fiber 3, Carbs 4, Protein 7

563. Italian Tomatoes

Preparation time: 5 minutes

Cooking time: 20 minutes

Servings: 4

INGREDIENTS

- 1 pound cherry tomatoes, halved
- 1 teaspoon Italian seasoning
- 1 tablespoon basil, chopped
- Juice of 1 lime
- A pinch of salt and black pepper
- 4 garlic cloves, minced
- 2 tablespoons olive oil

DIRECTIONS

1. In a pan that fits the air fryer, mix the tomatoes with the seasoning and the other ingredients, put the pan in the fryer and cook at 380 degrees F for 20 minutes.
2. Divide between plates and serve.

NUTRITION: Calories 173, Fat 6, Fiber 2, Carbs 4, Protein 5

564. Salsa Zucchini

Preparation time: 5 minutes

Cooking time: 20 minutes

Servings: 4

INGREDIENTS

- 1pound zucchinis, roughly sliced
- 1cup mild salsa
- 1red onion, chopped
- Salt and black pepper to the taste
- 2tablespoons lime juice
- 2tablespoons olive oil
- 1teaspoon coriander, ground

DIRECTIONS

1. In a pan that fits your air fryer, mix the zucchinis with the salsa and the other ingredients, toss, introduce in the fryer and cook at 390 degrees F for 20 minutes.
2. Divide the mix between plates and serve.

NUTRITION: Calories 150, Fat 4, Fiber 2, Carbs 4, Protein 5

565. Green Beans and Olives

Preparation time: 5 minutes

Cooking time: 20 minutes

Servings: 4

INGREDIENTS

- 1pound green beans, trimmed and halved
- 1cup black olives, pitted and halved
- 1cup kalamata olives, pitted and halved
- 1red onion, sliced
- 2tablespoons balsamic vinegar
- 1tablespoon olive oil
- 3garlic cloves, minced
- ½ cup tomato sauce

DIRECTIONS

1. In a pan that fits your air fryer, mix the green beans with the olives and the other ingredients, toss, put the pan in the fryer and cook at 350 degrees F for 20 minutes.
2. Divide the mix between plates and serve.

NUTRITION: Calories 180, Fat 4, Fiber 3, Carbs 5, Protein 6

566. Spicy Avocado Mix

Preparation time: 5 minutes

Cooking time: 15 minutes

Servings: 4

INGREDIENTS:

- 2small avocados, pitted, peeled and cut into wedges
- 1tablespoon olive oil
- Zest of 1 lime, grated
- Juice of 1 lime
- 1tablespoon avocado oil
- A pinch of salt and black pepper
- ½ teaspoon sweet paprika

DIRECTIONS

1. In a pan that fits the air fryer, mix the avocado with the lime juice and the other ingredients, put the pan in your air fryer and cook at 350 degrees F for 15 minutes.
2. Divide the mix between plates and serve.

NUTRITION: Calories 153, Fat 3, Fiber 3, Carbs 4, Protein 6

567. Spicy Black Beans

Preparation time: 5 minutes

Cooking time: 20 minutes

Servings: 4

INGREDIENTS

- 2cups canned black beans, drained

- 1 tablespoon olive oil
- 1 teaspoon chili powder
- 2 red chilies, minced
- A pinch of salt and black pepper
- ¼ cup tomato sauce

DIRECTIONS

1. In a pan that fits the air fryer, mix the beans with the oil and the other ingredients, toss, put the pan in the air fryer and cook at 380 degrees F for 20 minutes.
2. Divide between plates and serve.

NUTRITION: Calories 160, Fat 4, Fiber 3, Carbs 5, Protein 4

568. Cajun Tomatoes and Peppers

Preparation time: 4 minutes

Cooking time: 20 minutes

Servings: 4

INGREDIENTS

- 1 tablespoon avocado oil
- ½ pound mixed bell peppers, sliced
- 1 pound cherry tomatoes, halved
- 1 red onion, chopped
- A pinch of salt and black pepper
- 1 teaspoon sweet paprika
- ½ tablespoon Cajun seasoning

DIRECTIONS

1. In a pan that fits the air fryer, combine the peppers with the tomatoes and the other ingredients, put the pan it in your air fryer and cook at 390 degrees F for 20 minutes.
2. Divide the mix between plates and serve.

NUTRITION: Calories 151, Fat 3, Fiber 2, Carbs 4, Protein 5

569. Olives and Sweet Potatoes

Preparation time: 5 minutes

Cooking time: 25 minutes

Servings: 4

INGREDIENTS

- 1 pound sweet potatoes, peeled and cut into wedges
- 1 cup kalamata olives, pitted and halved
- 1 tablespoon olive oil
- 2 tablespoons balsamic vinegar
- A bunch of cilantro, chopped
- Salt and black pepper to the taste
- 1 tablespoon basil, chopped

DIRECTIONS

1. In a pan that fits the air fryer, combine the potatoes with the olives and the other ingredients and toss.
2. Put the pan in the air fryer and cook at 370 degrees F for 25 minutes.
3. Divide between plates and serve.

NUTRITION: Calories 132, Fat 4, Fiber 2, Carbs 4, Protein 4

570. Spinach and Sprouts

Preparation time: 5 minutes

Cooking time: 20 minutes

Servings: 4

INGREDIENTS

- 1 pound Brussels sprouts, trimmed and halved
- ½ pound baby spinach
- 1 tablespoon olive oil
- Juice of 1 lime
- Salt and black pepper to the taste
- 1 tablespoon parsley, chopped

DIRECTIONS:

1. In the air fryer's pan, mix the sprouts with the spinach and the other ingredients, toss, put the pan in the air fryer and cook at 380 degrees F for 20 minutes.
2. Transfer to bowls and serve.

NUTRITION: Calories 140, Fat 3, Fiber 2, Carbs 5, Protein 6

571. Lemon Tomatoes

Preparation time: 5 minutes

Cooking time: 20 minutes

Servings: 4

INGREDIENTS

- 2pounds cherry tomatoes, halved
- 1teaspoon sweet paprika
- 1teaspoon coriander, ground
- 2teaspoons lemon zest, grated
- 2tablespoons olive oil
- 2tablespoons lemon juice
- A handful parsley, chopped

DIRECTIONS

1. In the air fryer's pan, mix the tomatoes with the paprika and the other ingredients, toss and cook at 370 degrees F for 20 minutes.
2. Divide between plates and serve.

NUTRITION: Calories 151, Fat 2, Fiber 3, Carbs 5, Protein 5

572. Tomato and Green Beans

Preparation time: 5 minutes

Cooking time: 20 minutes

Servings: 4

INGREDIENTS

- 1pound cherry tomatoes, halved
- ½ pound green beans, trimmed and halved
- Juice of 1 lime
- 1teaspoon coriander, ground
- 1teaspoon sweet paprika
- A pinch of salt and black pepper
- 2tablespoons olive oil

DIRECTIONS

1. In a pan that fits your air fryer, mix the tomatoes with the green beans and the other ingredients, toss, put the pan in the machine and cook at 380 degrees F for 20 minutes.
2. Divide between plates and serve.

NUTRITION: Calories 151, Fat 3, Fiber 2, Carbs 4, Protein 4

573. Tomato and Onions Mix

Preparation time: 5 minutes

Cooking time: 20 minutes

Servings: 4

INGREDIENTS

- 1pound cherry tomatoes, halved
- 2red onions, sliced
- 2tablespoons avocado oil
- 1teaspoon hot paprika
- 1tablespoon olive oil
- 2teaspoons chili powder
- A pinch of salt and black pepper
- 1tablespoon chives, chopped

DIRECTIONS

1. In a pan that fits your air fryer, mix the tomatoes with the onions and the other

ingredients, put the pan in the fryer and cook at 390 degrees F for 20 minutes.
2. Divide the mix between plates and serve.

NUTRITION: Calories 173, Fat 4, Fiber 2, Carbs 4, Protein 6

574. Kale Salad

Preparation time: 5 minutes

Cooking time: 15 minutes

Servings: 4

INGREDIENTS

- 1pound kale leaves, torn
- 1cup kalamata olives, pitted and halved
- 1cup corn
- Salt and black pepper to the taste
- ¼ cup heavy cream
- 1tablespoon chives, chopped
- 1cup cherry tomatoes, halved
- Juice of 1 lime

DIRECTIONS

1. In a pan that fits your air fryer, mix the kale with the olives and the other ingredients, toss, put the pan in the fryer and cook at 390 degrees F for 15 minutes.
2. Divide into bowls and serve right away.

NUTRITION: Calories 161, Fat 2, Fiber 2, Carbs 4, Protein 6

575. Garlic Carrots

Preparation time: 5 minutes

Cooking time: 20 minutes

Servings: 4

INGREDIENTS

- 1tablespoon avocado oil
- 1pound baby carrots, peeled
- Juice of 1 lime
- ½ teaspoon sweet paprika
- 6garlic cloves, minced
- 1tablespoon balsamic vinegar
- Salt and black pepper to the taste

DIRECTIONS

1. In a pan that fits the air fryer, combine the carrots with the oil and the other ingredients, toss gently, put the pan in the air fryer and cook at 380 degrees F for 20 minutes.
2. Divide between plates and serve.

NUTRITION: Calories 121, Fat 3, Fiber 2, Carbs 4, Protein 6

576. Creamy Green Beans and Walnuts

Preparation time: 5 minutes

Cooking time: 20 minutes

Servings: 4

INGREDIENTS

- 1pound green beans, trimmed and halved
- 1cup walnuts, chopped
- 2cups cherry tomatoes, halved
- 2tablespoons olive oil
- A pinch of salt and black pepper
- 1tablespoon chives, chopped

DIRECTIONS

1. In a pan that fits the air fryer, mix the green beans with the walnuts and the other ingredients, toss, put the pan in the air fryer and cook at 380 degrees F for 20 minutes.
2. Divide between plates and serve.

NUTRITION: Calories 141, Fat 3, Fiber 2, Carbs 4, Protein 5

577. Garlic Corn

Preparation time: 5 minutes

Cooking time: 15 minutes

Servings: 4

INGREDIENTS

- 2cups corn
- 3garlic cloves, minced
- 1tablespoon olive oil
- Juice of 1 lime
- 1teaspoon sweet paprika
- Salt and black pepper to the taste
- 2tablespoons dill, chopped

DIRECTIONS

1. In a pan that fits the air fryer, mix the corn with the garlic and the other ingredients, toss, put the pan in the machine and cook at 390 degrees F for 15 minutes.
2. Divide everything between plates and serve.

NUTRITION: Calories 180, Fat 3, Fiber 2, Carbs 4, Protein 6

578. Green Beans Salad

Preparation time: 5 minutes

Cooking time: 20 minutes

Servings: 4

INGREDIENTS

- 1pound green beans, trimmed and halved
- 1cup baby spinach
- 1cup baby kale
- 2tablespoons olive oil
- 1cup corn
- 1tablespoon lime juice
- A pinch of salt and black pepper
- 1teaspoon rosemary, dried
- 1teaspoon chili powder

DIRECTIONS

1. In the air fryer's pan, combine the green beans with the spinach and the other ingredients, toss and cook at 400 degrees F for 20 minutes.
2. Divide into bowls and serve right away.

NUTRITION: Calories 151, Fat 4, Fiber 2, Carbs 4, Protein 6

579. Red Cabbage and Tomatoes

Preparation time: 5 minutes

Cooking time: 20 minutes

Servings: 4

INGREDIENTS

- 1pound red cabbage, shredded
- ½ pound cherry tomatoes, halved
- 2tablespoons olive oil
- Salt and black pepper to the taste
- ½ cup heavy cream
- 1tablespoon chives, chopped

DIRECTIONS

1. In a pan that fits the air fryer, combine the cabbage with the tomatoes and other ingredients, put the pan in the air fryer and cook at 390 degrees F for 20 minutes.
2. Divide between plates and serve.

NUTRITION: Calories 173, Fat 5, Fiber 3, Carbs 5, Protein 8

580. Savoy Cabbage Sauté

Preparation time: 5 minutes

Cooking time: 20 minutes

Servings: 4

INGREDIENTS

- 1pound Savoy cabbage, shredded
- 2scallions, chopped
- 2tablespoons avocado oil
- Juice of 1 lime
- 2spring onions, chopped
- 2tablespoons tomato sauce
- Salt and black pepper to the taste
- 1tablespoon chives, chopped

DIRECTIONS

1. In a pan that fits your air fryer, mix the cabbage with the scallions and the other ingredients, toss, put the pan in the fryer and cook at 360 degrees F for 20 minutes.
2. Divide between plates and serve.

NUTRITION: Calories 163, Fat 4, Fiber 3, Carbs 6, Protein 7

581. Turmeric Kale

Preparation time: 5 minutes

Cooking time: 20 minutes

Servings: 4

INGREDIENTS

- 1pound baby kale
- 1teaspoon turmeric powder
- 1red bell pepper, cut into strips
- 1red onion, chopped
- 2tablespoons butter, melted
- 1tablespoon dill, chopped

DIRECTIONS

1. In a pan that fits your air fryer, mix the kale with the turmeric and the other ingredients, put the pan in the fryer and cook at 370 degrees F for 20 minutes.
2. Divide everything between plates and serve.

NUTRITION: Calories 173, Fat 5, Fiber 3, Carbs 6, Protein 7

582. Lemon Fennel

Preparation time: 5 minutes

Cooking time: 15 minutes

Servings: 4

INGREDIENTS

- 3tablespoons butter, melted
- 2fennel bulbs, sliced
- 1teaspoon turmeric powder
- 1teaspoon coriander, ground
- 1tablespoon lemon zest, grated
- Apinch of salt and black pepper
- 1tablespoon lemon juice

DIRECTIONS

1. In the air fryer's pan, mix the fennel with the melted butter and the other ingredients, toss and cook at 350 degrees F for 15 minutes.
2. Divide between plates and serve.

NUTRITION: Calories 163, Fat 4, Fiber 3, Carbs 5, Protein 6

583. Balsamic Kale

Preparation time: 5 minutes

Cooking time: 15 minutes

Servings: 4

INGREDIENTS

- 2cups baby kale
- 2scallions, chopped
- Juice of 1 lime

- 1 tablespoon olive oil
- A pinch of salt and black pepper
- 2 tablespoons balsamic vinegar
- 1 tablespoon oregano, chopped

DIRECTIONS

1. In the air fryer's pan, mix the kale with the scallions and the other ingredients, toss and cook at 350 degrees F for 15 minutes.
2. Divide between plates and serve.

NUTRITION: Calories 143, Fat 4, Fiber 3, Carbs 6, Protein 7

584. Coriander Endives

Preparation time: 5 minutes

Cooking time: 15 minutes

Servings: 4

INGREDIENTS

- 2 endives, trimmed and halved
- 1 tablespoon coriander, chopped
- 1 teaspoon sweet paprika
- 2 tablespoons olive oil
- A pinch of salt and black pepper
- 2 tablespoons white vinegar
- ½ cup almonds, chopped

DIRECTIONS

1. In the air fryer's pan, mix the endives with the coriander and the other ingredients, toss, cook at 350 degrees F for 15 minutes, divide between plates and serve.

NUTRITION: Calories 154, Fat 4, Fiber 3, Carbs 6, Protein 7

585. Cheesy Beets

Preparation time: 5 minutes

Cooking time: 30 minutes

Servings: 4

INGREDIENTS

- 2 beets, peeled and roughly cut into wedges
- 1 cup mozzarella, shredded
- 1 red onion, sliced
- A pinch of salt and black pepper
- 1 tablespoon lemon juice
- 2 tablespoons chives, chopped
- 2 tablespoons olive oil

DIRECTIONS

2. In the air fryer's basket, mix the beets with the onion and the other ingredients except the cheese, toss and cook at 380 degrees F for 30 minutes.
3. Divide the corn between plates and serve with cheese on top.

NUTRITION: Calories 140, Fat 4, Fiber 3, Carbs 5, Protein 7

586. Frying Potatoes

Preparation time: 5 minutes

Cooking time: 40 minutes

Servings: 4

INGREDIENTS

- 5 to 6 medium potatoes
- Olive oil in a spray bottle if possible
- Mill salt
- Freshly ground pepper

DIRECTION:

1. Wash the potatoes well and dry them.
2. Brush with a little oil on both sides if not with the oil

3. Crush some ground salt and pepper on top.
4. Place the potatoes in the fryer basket
5. Set the cooking at 190°C for 40 minutes, in the middle of cooking turn the potatoes for even cooking on both sides.
6. At the end of cooking, remove the potatoes from the basket, cut them in half and slightly scrape the melting potato inside and add only a little butter, and enjoy!

NUTRITION: Calories 365 Fat 17g Carbohydrates 48g Sugars 0.3g Protein 4g Cholesterol 0mg

587. Avocado Fries

Preparation time: 5 minutes

Cooking time: 10 minutes

Servings: 1

INGREDIENTS:

- 1egg
- 1ripe avocado
- ½ tsp salt
- ½ cup of panko breadcrumbs

DIRECTION:

1. Preheat the air fryer to 400°F (200°Cfor 5 minutes.
2. Remove the avocado pit and cut into fries. In a small bowl, whisk the egg with the salt.
3. Enter the breadcrumbs on a plate.
4. Dip the quarters in the egg mixture, then in the breadcrumbs.
5. Put them in the fryer. Cook for 8-10 minutes.
6. Turn halfway through cooking.

NUTRITION: Calories 390 Fat 32g Carbohydrates 24g Sugars 3g Protein 4g Cholesterol 0mg

588. Crispy French Fries

Preparation time: 5 minutes

Cooking time: 10 minutes

Servings: 2

INGREDIENTS

- 2medium sweet potatoes
- 2tsp olive oil
- ½ tsp salt
- ½ tsp garlic powder
- ¼ tsp paprika
- Black pepper

DIRECTION:

1. Preheat the hot air fryer to 400°F (200°C
2. Spray the basket with a little oil.
3. Cut the sweet potatoes into potato chips about 1 cm wide.
4. Add oil, salt, garlic powder, pepper and paprika.
5. Cook for 8 minutes, without overloading the basket.
6. Repeat 2 or 3 times, as necessary.

NUTRITION: Calories 240 Fat 9g Carbohydrates 36g Sugars 1g Protein 3g Cholesterol 0mg

589. Frying Potatoes with Butter

Preparation time: 5 minutes

Cooking time: 10 minutes

Servings: 2

INGREDIENTS

- 2Russet potatoes
- Butter
- Fresh parsley (optional

DIRECTION:

1. Spray the basket with a little oil.
2. Open your potatoes along.
3. Make some holes with a fork.
4. Add the butter and parsley.
5. Transfer to the basket. If your air fryer to a temperature of 198°C (390°F).
6. Cook for 30 to 40 minutes.
7. Try about 30 minutes. Bon Appetite!

NUTRITION: Calories 365 Fat 17g Carbohydrates 48g Sugars 0.3g Protein 4g Cholesterol 0mg

590. Homemade French Fries

Preparation time: 5 minutes

Cooking time: 10 minutes

Servings: 2

INGREDIENTS

- 25 lb. sliced and sliced potato chips
- 1 tbsp olive oil
- Salt and pepper to taste
- 1 tsp salt to season or paprika

DIRECTION:

1. Put the fries in a bowl with very cold water.
2. Let it soak for at least 30 minutes.
3. Drain completely. Add the oil. Shake
4. Put them in the fryer bowl. Cook for 15 to 25 minutes. Set to 380°F (193°C).
5. Set the time according to your preferences or the power of your fryer to 23 minutes.

NUTRITION: Calories 118 Fat 7g Carbohydrates 27 Sugars 1g Protein 2 Cholesterol 0mg

591. Mini pepper/tomato/shallot/goat cheese tartlets

Preparation time: 10 minutes

Cooking time: 15 minutes

Servings: 4-6

INGREDIENTS:

- 1 pure butter puff pastry
- 3 peppers + 2 tomatoes + 1 shallot + 1 degermed garlic clove
- 1 whole egg + 2 tbsp salad seeds (squash, sunflower, sesame
- 3 tablespoons cheese in cubes + ½ goat cheese log + 50 g grated emmental cheese
- 6/8 mini silicone molds (round, square, heart ....
- Salt + pepper 5 berries

DIRECTION:

1. Put the grid / cubes in the 11 in 1 mandolin and cut all the vegetables (cleanedinto small pieces.
2. Beat the egg in an omelet and add the cut vegetables, the cubed cheese, the seeds, salt, and pepper.
3. Unroll the puff pastry and cut circles (squares of hearts ...and darken the mini molds. Prick the bottom with a fork.
4. Garnish with the egg/vegetable preparation and add a little goat cheese and grated emmental cheese on top.
5. Place the molds on the fryer grid, close the hood, and program the "15-minute pie" function at 1500C.
6. When it is well cooked, remove the grid with the tongs. Serve hot or warm with a salad.

NUTRITION: Calories 152g Fat 9g Carbohydrates 10g Sugars 10g Protein 4g Cholesterol 0mg

592. Almond Apples

Preparation time: 10 minutes

Cooking time: 45 minutes

Vegetables

Servings: 5-6

INGREDIENTS

- 600 g of peeled potatoes
- 2egg yolks
- 2eggs
- 60g of almond powder
- Salt,
- Pepper
- frying oil
- 30g of butter
- 50g of almond chips
- 50g of breadcrumbs
- 50g of flour

DIRECTION:

2. Peel the potatoes (if you feel like it, instead of throwing the husks, baked shell chips, it's a delight).
3. Cut the potatoes into cubes and cook them in salted water (starting with cold waterapproximately 15 minutes after boiling.
4. Drain and puree with a potato masher. Add salt and pepper.
5. Add the egg yolks, butter, and almond powder, mix well.
6. Place in the refrigerator for a quarter of an hour, then roll balls into the palm of your hand. Then, roll them rolling successively in flour, beaten eggs in an omelet, then in a mixture of breadcrumbs and flaked almonds.
7. Let cool for 15 minutes.
8. Put them in the air fryer at 180°C for 15 minutes. Then place the almond apples on a paper towel.

NUTRITION: Calories 284.0 Fat 19.1 g Carbohydrate 27.9 g Sugars13.8 g Protein5.0 g Cholesterol 0.0 mg

593. French fries without dry

INGREDIENTS

- 500g of French fries
- 1tbsp oil

PREPARATION:

- Peel and cut the potatoes, using a knife or a "fried cut".
- Rinse with water and dry the fries.
- Put them in a bowl and add the oil spoon, mix well.
- Preheat the air fryer to 160°C. Put the fries in the basket for 15 minutes.
- Pour the fries in the bowl, mix, and pass the fryer to more than 200°C.
- Put the fries back in the basket and cook again for about 10 minutes. Look carefully because the overhead comes quickly!

NUTRITION: Calories 118 Fat 7g Carbohydrates 27 1g Protein 2 Cholesterol 0mg

594. Bugnes Lyonnaises

Preparation: 30 minutes;

Rest: 2 hours;

Cook: 15 minutes

INGREDIENTS

- 250 g flour
- ½ packet of yeast
- 50g of powdered sugar
- 50g butter
- 2eggs
- 1tsp rum
- 1pinch of salt
- Frying oil

DIRECTION:

1. Soften the butter; beat the eggs with a fork.
2. Place the flour in a bowl; add the salt, the butter, the beaten eggs, the aroma.
3. Mix until you have a consistent paste. Form a ball and let stand at least 2 hours in the fridge.
4. Heat the fryer oil at 1500C for 15 minutes.
5. Stretch the dough to a thickness of 5 mm. Cut into strips of 10 cm by 4 cm and make an incision in the center of 5 cm.
6. Pass a corner of the strip in the incision to tie a knot or leave it as is.
7. Dip the bugnes in the fryer, flip them 1 time and drain once cooked on absorbent paper.
8. Sprinkle with icing sugar or icing sugar and serve hot.

NUTRITION: Calories 140 Carbohydrate 6 g Fat 13 g Protein 1 g Sodium 29 mg Sugar 1 g

595. Green salad with roasted pepper

Preparation time: 5 minutes

Cooking time: 10 minutes

Servings: 2

INGREDIENTS

- 1 red pepper
- 1 tbsp lemon juice
- 3 tbsp yogurt
- 2 tbsp olive oil
- Freshly ground black pepper
- 1 romaine lettuce, cut into large strips
- 50g arugula leaves

DIRECTION:

1. Preheat the Air Fryer to 200°C.
2. Place the pepper in the basket and insert it into the Air Fryer. Set the timer for 10 minutes and roast the pepper until the skin is slightly burned.
3. Then cut the pepper into quarters and remove the seeds and skin. Cut the pepper into strips.
4. Prepare vinaigrette in a bowl with 2 tablespoons of pepper juice, lemon juice, yogurt, and olive oil. Add pepper and salt according to your taste.
5. Mix the lettuce and arugula leaves in the vinaigrette and garnish the salad with the pepper strips.

NUTRITION: Calories 47.3 Fat 0.4 g Carbohydrate 10.8 g Sugars 2.0 g Protein 1.8 g Cholesterol 0.0 mg

596. Fat Free Crispy Fries

Preparation time: about 15 minutes

Cooking time: 10 to 35 minutes

Servings: 4

INGREDIENTS

- 500g of special fries
- 1 tbsp olive oil
- 1 freezer bag
- Salt + pepper

DIRECTION:

1. Peel the potatoes, cut them with a potato chip cutter, rinse them with clean water and dry them well with a cloth.

2. It is important to cut all the potatoes evenly; otherwise you may have some overcooked and not enough fries.

3. Place the sliced fries in a freezer bag, add 1 tablespoon of oil, close the bag, and stir everything.

Vegetables

4. Place the French fries in the basket, close it, and close the lid of the fryer and set to 230°C to 35 minutes.

5. At the end of cooking, remove the basket with the tongs and remove the fries. Add salt and pepper.

NUTRITION: Calories 118 Fat 7g Carbohydrates 27 Sugars 1g Protein 2 Cholesterol 0mg

597. Marinated Potatoes with Chimichurri Sauce

Preparation time: 20 minutes

Cooking time: 45 minutes

Servings: 4

INGREDIENTS

- 1kg to 1.2kg of potatoes
- 2tablespoons chimichurri sauce

DIRECTION:

1. Depending on the taste, you can peel the potatoes, but the real potatoes are prepared with the skin.
2. Wash the potatoes before cutting them.
3. Cut them in quarters to get the shape of the potatoes and place them in a freezer bag.
4. Add the sauce and use the solid closure of the sachet to keep it closed.
5. Mix everything by handling the bag in all directions. Potatoes should be well impregnated with the preparation.
6. Pour all the preparation in the air fryer without oil.
7. Set the air fryer at 1800C for 45 minutes and serve immediately after the end of cooking.

NUTRITION: Calories 367 Fat 18.4 g Carbohydrate 45 g Sugars 2.0 g Protein 5.7 g Cholesterol 0mg

598. Homemade Gluten Free Spicy Chips

Preparation time: 25 minutes

Cooking time: 30 minutes

Servings: 1

INGREDIENTS

- 500g of potatoes to choose from among those with firm meat
- 1tbsp vegetable oil
- 1pinch of salt
- 1mixture of texmex spices

DIRECTION:

1. Peel the potatoes and cut them into slices approximately 2 millimeters thick. Preferably use a mandolin for a very fine and regular cut.
2. Rinse the potatoes to get rid of their starch and let them stand for 15 minutes in a bowl of cold water.
3. Drain the potatoes and dry them with a paper towel by simply sliding them. Avoid rubbing them as they could break.
4. Pour the potatoes in the fryer and cover them with the necessary tablespoon of oil.
5. Set the air fryer at 1500C for 30 minutes.
6. Be sure to stir the fries with a wooden utensil every ten minutes to make sure they cook perfectly.
7. Wait 5 minutes before the end of cooking to add salt and spices.

NUTRITION: Calories 150 Cal 17% Carbohydrates 15g Fat 32g Protein 1g Sugars 3g Cholesterol 0mg

599. Funghetto Eggplant (Golden Neapolitan)

Preparation time: 0-10 minutes

Cooking time: 15-30 minutes

Servings:

INGREDIENTS

- 600g Eggplant
- 100g Broth
- 1 Garlic clove
- Salt
- Pepper
- 3 spoons Olive oil
- Parsley

DIRECTION:

1. Wash the eggplants, dry them, and cut them into 1.5 cm cubes.
2. Place the mixing blade in the tank
3. Pour oil and peeled garlic, close the lid.
4. Set the air fryer to 150ºC to brown for about 2 min.
5. Add eggplant, broth, salt and pepper and simmer for another 23 min.
6. Finally, before serving, sprinkle with chopped fresh parsley.

NUTRITION: Calories 142 Fat 12.9g Carbohydrate 5.20g Protein 1.9g Sugars 0g Cholesterol 0.1mg

600. Fried Bananas

Preparation time: 0-10 minutes

Cooking time: 0 – 15 minutes

Servings: 3

INGREDIENTS

- 3 Bananas
- 2 Eggs
- Breadcrumbs
- Flour at discretion
- Salt
- 1tsp Oil

DIRECTION:

1. Peel the bananas and cut them into sections of approximately 2 to 3 cm.
2. Pass them first in the flour, then in the egg beaten with salt and then in the breadcrumbs.
3. Heat the air fryer at 180ºC for 10 minutes. Then, place the breaded bananas.
4. Cook the bananas for 8 to 10 minutes, turning them 2 to 3 times during cooking to match the Dorado.
5. Serve warm.

NUTRITION: Calories 262.4 Fat 12.1 g Carbohydrate 33.9 g Sugars 20.7 g Protein 1.3 g Cholesterol 30.5 mg

601. Sautéed air mushrooms and parsley

Preparation time: 10 – 20 minutes

Cooking time: 15 – 30 minutes

Servings: 6

INGREDIENTS:

- 600 g mushrooms
- 1 clove garlic
- 1 tsp olive oil
- Parsley
- Leave at discretion
- Black pepper at discretion

DIRECTION:

1. Clean the mushrooms well and chop them.
2. Place the garlic and oil inside the basket close. Set the temperature to 150ºC.
3. Brown for 2 minutes.
4. Add the mushrooms and cook for another 15 minutes.
5. Add (at discretion) salt and pepper, parsley, and finish cooking for another 3 minutes.

NUTRITION: Calories 130 Fat 7g Carbohydrates 17g Sugars 4g Protein 4g Cholesterol 0mg

602. Cauliflowers au gratin

Preparation time: 20-30 minutes

Cooking time: 15-30 minutes

Servings: 6

INGREDIENTS:

- 800g cauliflower
- 4 slices of cheese
- ½ liter of Béchamel
- Parmesan to taste

DIRECTION:

1. Separately, cook the cauliflowers in water. Meanwhile, prepare ½ liter of bechamel (dose: 500 ml of milk, 50 g of flour, 50 g of butter, salt, and nutmeg).
2. Pour some bechamel into the basket. Arrange the cauliflower flowers, covered with the slices of cheese and cover with the béchamel sauce. Sprinkle with Parmesan cheese.
3. Set the air fryer to 1500C. Simmer for about 20 minutes or according to the degree of gratin desired.

NUTRITION: Calories 285 Fat 19g Carbohydrates 17g Sugars 2.5g Protein 14g Cholesterol 55mg

603. Peach Clafoutis

Preparation time: 20 – 30 minutes

Cooking time: 30 – 45 minutes

Servings: 10

INGREDIENTS

- 300g flour
- 150g butter
- 150g of sugar
- 4 eggs
- 1 sachet of baking powder
- 500g peaches in syrup
- 1 lemon
- 3-4 tbsp milk
- Icing sugar at discretion

DIRECTION:

1. Melt the butter in the microwave; Work the butter, sugar, and eggs in a bowl.
2. Add flour, baking powder, grated lemon peel and milk. Work everything with an electric mixer until you get a smooth and homogeneous mixture.
3. Butter and flour the tank and pour the mixture inside, smearing well.
4. Place a whole peach in the center and place the others (cut into quarters) next to each other following the circumference of the mold.
5. Set the air fryer on the lower heating temperature.
6. Bake the cake for 45 minutes.
7. Let cool and remove it from the tank; sprinkle with icing sugar.

NUTRITION: Calories 148 Carbohydrates 14g Fat 8g Sugars 6 g Protein 4g Cholesterol 102mg

604. Cauliflower Steak

Preparation Time: 12 minutes

Servings: 4

INGREDIENTS

- 1 medium head cauliflower
- ¼ cup blue cheese crumbles
- ¼ cup hot sauce
- ¼ cup full-fat ranch dressing
- 2 tbsp. salted butter; melted.

DIRECTIONS

1. Remove cauliflower leaves. Slice the head in ½-inch-thick slices.
2. In a small bowl, mix hot sauce and butter. Brush the mixture over the cauliflower.
3. Place each cauliflower steak into the air fryer, working in batches if necessary. Adjust the temperature to 400 Degrees F and set the timer for 7 minutes
4. When cooked, edges will begin turning dark and caramelized. To serve, sprinkle steaks with crumbled blue cheese. Drizzle with ranch dressing.

NUTRITION: Calories: 122; Protein: 4.9g; Fiber: 3.0g; Fat: 8.4g; Carbs: 7.7g

605. Chocolate Chip Pan Cookie

Preparation Time: 17 minutes

Servings: 4

INGREDIENTS

- ½ cup blanched finely ground almond flour.
- 1 large egg.
- ¼ cup powdered erythritol
- 2 tbsp. unsalted butter; softened.
- 2 tbsp. low-carb, sugar-free chocolate chips
- ½ tsp. unflavored gelatin
- ½ tsp. baking powder.
- ½ tsp. vanilla extract.

DIRECTIONS

1. Take a large bowl, mix almond flour and erythritol. Stir in butter, egg and gelatin until combined.
2. Stir in baking powder and vanilla and then fold in chocolate chips
3. Pour batter into 6-inch round baking pan. Place pan into the air fryer basket.
4. Adjust the temperature to 300 Degrees F and set the timer for 7 minutes
5. When fully cooked, the top will be golden brown and a toothpick inserted in center will come out clean. Let cool at least 10 minutes.

NUTRITION: Calories: 188; Protein: 5.6g; Fiber: 2.0g; Fat: 15.7g; Carbs: 16.8g

606. Mustard Greens and Green Beans

Preparation Time: 22 minutes

Servings: 4

INGREDIENTS

- 1 lb. green beans; halved
- ¼ cup tomato puree
- 3 garlic cloves; minced
- 1 bunch mustard greens, trimmed
- 2 tbsp. olive oil
- 1 tbsp. balsamic vinegar
- Salt and black pepper to taste.

DIRECTIONS

1. In a pan that fits your air fryer, mix the mustard greens with the rest of the ingredients, toss, put the pan in the fryer and cook at 350°F for 12 minutes
2. Divide everything between plates and serve.

NUTRITION: Calories: 163; Fat: 4g; Fiber: 3g; Carbs: 4g; Protein: 7g

607. Artichoke Spinach Casserole

Preparation Time: 30 minutes

Servings: 4

INGREDIENTS

- ⅓ cup full-fat mayonnaise
- 8 oz. full-fat cream cheese; softened.
- ¼ cup diced yellow onion
- ⅓ cup full-fat sour cream.

- ¼ cup chopped pickled jalapeños.
- 2cups fresh spinach; chopped
- 2cups cauliflower florets; chopped
- 1cup artichoke hearts; chopped
- 1tbsp. salted butter; melted.

DIRECTIONS

1. Take a large bowl, mix butter, onion, cream cheese, mayonnaise and sour cream. Fold in jalapeños, spinach, cauliflower and artichokes.
2. Pour the mixture into a 4-cup round baking dish. Cover with foil and place into the air fryer basket
3. Adjust the temperature to 370 Degrees F and set the timer for 15 minutes. In the last 2 minutes of cooking, remove the foil to brown the top. Serve warm.

NUTRITION: Calories: 423; Protein: 6.7g; Fiber: 5.3g; Fat: 36.3g; Carbs: 12.1g

608. Baked Egg and Veggies

Preparation Time: 20 minutes

Servings: 2

INGREDIENTS

- 1cup fresh spinach; chopped
- 1small zucchini, sliced lengthwise and quartered
- 1medium Roma tomato; diced
- ½ medium green bell pepper; seeded and diced
- 2large eggs.
- 2tbsp. salted butter
- ¼ tsp. garlic powder.
- ¼ tsp. onion powder.
- ½ tsp. dried basil
- ¼ tsp. dried oregano.

DIRECTIONS

1. Grease two (4-inchramekins with 1 tbsp. butter each.
2. Take a large bowl, toss zucchini, bell pepper, spinach and tomatoes. Divide the mixture in two and place half in each ramekin.
3. Crack an egg on top of each ramekin and sprinkle with onion powder, garlic powder, basil and oregano. Place into the air fryer basket. Adjust the temperature to 330 Degrees F and set the timer for 10 minutes
Servings immediately.

NUTRITION: Calories: 150; Protein: 8.3g; Fiber: 2.2g; Fat: 10.0g; Carbs: 6.6g

609. Mini Cheesecake

Preparation Time: 25 minutes

Servings: 2

INGREDIENTS

- 4oz. full-fat cream cheese; softened.
- ⅛ cup powdered erythritol
- 1large egg.
- ½ cup walnuts
- 2tbsp. granular erythritol.
- 2tbsp. salted butter
- ½ tsp. vanilla extract.

DIRECTIONS

1. Place walnuts, butter and granular erythritol in a food processor. Pulse until ingredients stick together and a dough form
2. Press dough into 4-inch springform pan then place the pan into the air fryer basket.
3. Adjust the temperature to 400 Degrees F and set the timer for 5 minutes. When timer beeps, remove the crust and let cool

4. Take a medium bowl, mix cream cheese with egg, vanilla extract and powdered erythritol until smooth.
5. Spoon mixture on top of baked walnut crust and place into the air fryer basket. Adjust the temperature to 300 Degrees F and set the timer for 10 minutes. Once done, chill for 2 hours before serving

NUTRITION: Calories: 531; Protein: 11.4g; Fiber: 2.3g; Fat: 48.3g; Carbs: 31.4g

610. Savoy Cabbage

Preparation Time: 20 minutes

Servings: 4

INGREDIENTS

- 1 Savoy cabbage head, shredded
- 1 tbsp. dill; chopped.
- 1½ tbsp. ghee; melted
- ¼ cup coconut cream
- Salt and black pepper to taste.

DIRECTIONS

1. In a pan that fits the air fryer, combine all the ingredients except the coconut cream, toss, put the pan in the air fryer and cook at 390°F for 10 minutes
2. Add the cream, toss, cook for 5 minutes more, divide between plates and serve

NUTRITION: Calories: 173; Fat: 5g; Fiber: 3g; Carbs: 5g; Protein: 8g

611. Spaghetti Squash Alfredo.

Preparation Time: 25 minutes

Servings: 2

INGREDIENTS

- ½ large cooked spaghetti squash
- ¼ cup grated vegetarian Parmesan cheese.
- ½ cup shredded Italian blend cheese
- ½ cup low-carb Alfredo sauce
- 2 tbsp. salted butter; melted.
- ¼ tsp. ground peppercorn
- ½ tsp. garlic powder.
- 1 tsp. dried parsley.

DIRECTIONS

1. Using a fork, remove the strands of spaghetti squash from the shell. Place into a large bowl with butter and Alfredo sauce. Sprinkle with Parmesan, garlic powder, parsley and peppercorn
2. Pour into a 4-cup round baking dish and top with shredded cheese. Place dish into the air fryer basket. Adjust the temperature to 320 Degrees F and set the timer for 15 minutes.
3. When finished, cheese will be golden and bubbling. Serve immediately

NUTRITION: Calories: 375; Protein: 13.5g; Fiber: 4.0g; Fat: 24.2g; Carbs: 24.1g

612. Vanilla Pound Cake.

Preparation Time: 35 minutes

Servings: 6

INGREDIENTS

- ½ cup full-fat sour cream.
- 1 oz. full-fat cream cheese; softened.
- 2 large eggs.
- ½ cup granular erythritol.
- 1 cup blanched finely ground almond flour.
- ¼ cup salted butter; melted.
- 1 tsp. baking powder.
- 1 tsp. vanilla extract.

DIRECTIONS

1. Take a large bowl, mix almond flour, butter and erythritol.
2. Add in vanilla, baking powder, sour cream and cream cheese and mix until well combined. Add eggs and mix.
3. Pour batter into a 6-inch round baking pan. Place pan into the air fryer basket. Adjust the temperature to 300 Degrees F and set the timer for 25 minutes.
4. When the cake is done, a toothpick inserted in center will come out clean. The center should not feel wet. Allow it to cool completely, or the cake will crumble when moved.

NUTRITION: Calories: 253; Protein: 6.9g; Fiber: 2.0g; Fat: 22.6g; Carbs: 25.2g

613. Pumpkin Spice Pecans

Preparation Time: 11 minutes

Servings: 4

INGREDIENTS

- 1cup whole pecans
- 1large egg. white
- ¼ cup granular erythritol.
- ½ tsp. pumpkin pie spice
- ½ tsp. vanilla extract.
- ½ tsp. ground cinnamon.

DIRECTIONS

1. Toss all ingredients in a large bowl until pecans are coated. Place into the air fryer basket.
2. Adjust the temperature to 300 Degrees F and set the timer for 6 minutes. Toss two to three times during cooking. Allow to cool completely. Store in an airtight container up to 3 days

NUTRITION: Calories: 178; Protein: 3.2g; Fiber: 2.6g; Fat: 17.0g; Carbs: 19.0g

614. Cream Puffs

Preparation Time: 21 minutes

Servings: 8 puffs

INGREDIENTS

- 2oz. full-fat cream cheese.
- 1large egg.
- ¼ cup powdered erythritol
- ½ cup blanched finely ground almond flour.
- ½ cup low-carb vanilla protein powder
- ½ cup granular erythritol.
- 2tbsp. heavy whipping cream.
- 5tbsp. unsalted butter; melted.
- ½ tsp. baking powder.
- ¼ tsp. ground cinnamon.
- ½ tsp. vanilla extract.

DIRECTIONS

1. Mix almond flour, protein powder, granular erythritol, baking powder, egg and butter in a large bowl until a soft dough forms.
2. Place the dough in the freezer for 20 minutes. Wet your hands with water and roll the dough into eight balls.
3. Cut a piece of parchment to fit your air fryer basket. Working in batches as necessary, place the dough balls into the air fryer basket on top of parchment.
4. Adjust the temperature to 380 Degrees F and set the timer for 6 minutes. Flip cream puffs halfway through the cooking time.
5. When the timer beeps, remove the puffs and allow to cool.
6. Take a medium bowl, beat the cream cheese, powdered erythritol, cinnamon, cream and vanilla until fluffy.
7. Place the mixture into a pastry bag or a storage bag with the end snipped. Cut a small hole in the bottom of each puff and fill with some of the cream mixture. Store

in an airtight container up to 2 days in the refrigerator.

NUTRITION: Calories: 178; Protein: 14.9g; Fiber: 1.3g; Fat: 12.1g; Carbs: 22.1g

615. Tomato and Asparagus

Preparation Time: 20 minutes

Servings: 4

INGREDIENTS

- 1lb. asparagus, trimmed
- 1 jalapeno pepper; chopped.
- 10 cherry tomatoes; halved
- 2 green onions; chopped.
- 1tbsp. olive oil
- 2tsp. chili powder
- A pinch of salt and black pepper

DIRECTIONS

1. In a pan that fits your air fryer, mix the asparagus with tomatoes and the rest of the ingredients, toss.
2. Put the pan in the fryer and cook at 390°F for 15 minutes
3. Divide the mix between plates and serve.

NUTRITION: Calories: 173; Fat: 4g; Fiber: 2g; Carbs: 4g; Protein: 6g

616. Peanut Butter Cheesecake Brownies

Preparation Time: 55 minutes

Servings: 6

INGREDIENTS

- ½ cup blanched finely ground almond flour.
- 8oz. full-fat cream cheese; softened.
- ¼ cup unsalted butter; softened.
- 2 large eggs, divided.
- 1 cup powdered erythritol, divided.
- ¼ cup heavy whipping cream.
- 2tbsp. unsweetened cocoa powder
- ½ tsp. baking powder.
- 2tbsp. no-sugar-added peanut butter
- 1tsp. vanilla extract.

DIRECTIONS

1. Take a large bowl, mix almond flour, ½ cup erythritol, cocoa powder and baking powder. Stir in butter and one egg.
2. Scoop mixture into 6-inch round baking pan. Place pan into the air fryer basket. Adjust the temperature to 300 Degrees F and set the timer for 20 minutes.
3. When fully cooked a toothpick inserted in center will come out clean. Allow 20 minutes to fully cool and firm up
4. Take a large bowl, beat cream cheese, remaining ½ cup erythritol, heavy cream, vanilla, peanut butter and remaining egg until fluffy.
5. Pour mixture over cooled brownies. Place pan back into the air fryer basket. Adjust the temperature to 300 Degrees F and set the timer for 15 minutes
6. Cheesecake will be slightly browned and mostly firm with a slight jiggle when done.
7. Allow to cool, then refrigerate 2 hours before serving.

NUTRITION: Calories: 347; Protein: 8.3g; Fiber: 2.0g; Fat: 30.9g; Carbs: 29.8g

617. BBQ Pulled Mushrooms

Preparation Time: 17 minutes

Servings: 2

INGREDIENTS:

- 4 large portobello mushrooms
- ½ cup low-carb, sugar-free barbecue sauce
- 1tbsp. salted butter; melted.
- 1tsp. paprika

- ¼ tsp. onion powder.
- ¼ tsp. ground black pepper
- 1tsp. chili powder

DIRECTIONS

1. Remove stem and scoop out the underside of each mushroom. Brush the caps with butter and sprinkle with pepper, chili powder, paprika and onion powder.
2. Place mushrooms into the air fryer basket. Adjust the temperature to 400 Degrees F and set the timer for 8 minutes.
3. When the timer beeps, remove mushrooms from the basket and place on a cutting board or work surface. Using two forks, gently pull the mushrooms apart, creating strands.
4. Place mushroom strands into a 4-cup round baking dish with barbecue sauce. Place dish into the air fryer basket.
5. Adjust the temperature to 350 Degrees F and set the timer for 4 minutes. Stir halfway through the cooking time. Serve warm.

NUTRITION: Calories: 108; Protein: 3.3g; Fiber: 2.7g; Fat: 5.9g; Carbs: 10.9g

618. Blackberry Crisp

Preparation Time: 20 minutes

Servings: 4

INGREDIENTS

- 1cup Crunchy Granola
- 2cups blackberries
- ⅓ cup powdered erythritol
- 2tbsp. lemon juice
- ¼ tsp. xanthan gum

DIRECTIONS

1. Take a large bowl, toss blackberries, erythritol, lemon juice and xanthan gum.
2. Pour into 6-inch round baking dish and cover with foil. Place into the air fryer basket.
3. Adjust the temperature to 350 Degrees F and set the timer for 12 minutes.
4. When the timer beeps, remove the foil and stir.
5. Sprinkle granola over mixture and return to the air fryer basket. Adjust the temperature to 320 Degrees F and set the timer for 3 minutes or until top is golden. Serve warm.

NUTRITION: Calories: 496; Protein: 9.2g; Fiber: 12.5g; Fat: 42.1g; Carbs: 44.0g

619. Cheese Zucchini Boats

Preparation Time: 35 minutes

Servings: 2

INGREDIENTS

- 2medium zucchini
- ¼ cup full-fat ricotta cheese
- ¼ cup shredded mozzarella cheese
- ¼ cup low-carb, no-sugar-added pasta sauce.
- 2tbsp. grated vegetarian Parmesan cheese
- 1tbsp. avocado oil
- ¼ tsp. garlic powder.
- ½ tsp. dried parsley.
- ¼ tsp. dried oregano.

DIRECTIONS

1. Cut off 1-inch from the top and bottom of each zucchini.
2. Slice zucchini in half lengthwise and use a spoon to scoop out a bit of the inside, making room for filling. Brush with oil and spoon 2 tbsp. pasta sauce into each shell

3. Take a medium bowl, mix ricotta, mozzarella, oregano, garlic powder and parsley
4. Spoon the mixture into each zucchini shell. Place stuffed zucchini shells into the air fryer basket.
5. Adjust the temperature to 350 Degrees F and set the timer for 20 minutes
6. To remove from the fryer basket, use tongs or a spatula and carefully lift out. Top with Parmesan. Serve immediately.

NUTRITION: Calories: 215; Protein: 10.5g; Fiber: 2.7g; Fat: 14.9g; Carbs: 9.3g

620. Green Beans and Lime Sauce

Preparation Time: 13 minutes

Servings: 4

INGREDIENTS

- 1lb. green beans, trimmed
- 2tbsp. ghee; melted
- 1tbsp. lime juice
- 1tsp. chili powder
- A pinch of salt and black pepper

DIRECTIONS

1. Take a bowl and mix the ghee with the rest of the ingredients except the green beans and whisk really well.
2. Mix the green beans with the lime sauce, toss
3. Put them in your air fryer's basket and cook at 400°F for 8 minutes
4. Servings right away.

NUTRITION: Calories: 151; Fat: 4g; Fiber: 2g; Carbs: 4g; Protein: 6g

621. Roasted Broccoli Salad

Preparation Time: 17 minutes

Servings: 2

INGREDIENTS

- 3cups fresh broccoli florets.
- ½ medium lemon.
- ¼ cup sliced almonds.
- 2tbsp. salted butter; melted.

DIRECTIONS

1. Place broccoli into a 6-inch round baking dish. Pour butter over broccoli. Add almonds and toss. Place dish into the air fryer basket
2. Adjust the temperature to 380 Degrees F and set the timer for 7 minutes. Stir halfway through the cooking time. When timer beeps, zest lemon onto broccoli and squeeze juice into pan. Toss. Serve warm.

NUTRITION: Calories: 215; Protein: 6.4g; Fiber: 5.0g; Fat: 16.3g; Carbs: 12.1g

622. Quiche Stuffed Peppers

Preparation Time: 20 minutes

Servings: 2

INGREDIENTS

- 2medium green bell peppers
- 3large eggs.
- ½ cup chopped broccoli
- ½ cup shredded medium Cheddar cheese.
- ¼ cup diced yellow onion
- ¼ cup full-fat ricotta cheese

DIRECTIONS

1. Cut the tops off of the peppers and remove the seeds and white membranes with a small knife. Take a medium bowl, whisk eggs and ricotta
2. Add onion and broccoli. Pour the egg and vegetable mixture evenly into each pepper. Top with Cheddar. Place peppers into a 4-cup round baking dish and place

into the air fryer basket. Adjust the temperature to 350 Degrees F and set the timer for 15 minutes
3. Eggs will be mostly firm and peppers tender when fully cooked. Serve immediately.

NUTRITION: Calories: 314; Protein: 21.6g; Fiber: 3.0g; Fat: 18.7g; Carbs: 10.8g

623. Monkey Bread

Preparation Time: 27 minutes

Servings: 6

INGREDIENTS:

- ½ cup blanched finely ground almond flour.
- 1oz. full-fat cream cheese; softened.
- 1 large egg.
- ¼ cup heavy whipping cream.
- ½ cup low-carb vanilla protein powder
- ¾ cup granular erythritol, divided
- 8tbsp. salted butter; melted and divided
- ½ tsp. vanilla extract.
- ½ tsp. baking powder

DIRECTIONS:

1. Take a large bowl, combine almond flour, protein powder, ½ cup erythritol, baking powder, 5 tbsp. butter, cream cheese and egg. A soft, sticky dough will form.
2. Place the dough in the freezer for 20 minutes. It will be firm enough to roll into balls. Wet your hands with warm water and roll into twelve balls. Place the balls into a 6-inch round baking dish
3. In a medium skillet over medium heat, melt remaining butter with remaining erythritol. Lower the heat and continue stirring until mixture turns golden, then add cream and vanilla. Remove from heat and allow it to thicken for a few minutes while you continue to stir
4. While the mixture cools, place baking dish into the air fryer basket. Adjust the temperature to 320 Degrees F and set the timer for 6 minutes
5. When the timer beeps, flip the monkey bread over onto a plate and slide it back into the baking pan. Cook an additional 4 minutes until all the tops are brown.
6. Pour the caramel sauce over the monkey bread and cook an additional 2 minutes.
7. Let cool completely before serving.

NUTRITION: Calories: 322; Protein: 20.4g; Fiber: 1.7g; Fat: 24.5g; Carbs: 33.7g

624. Broccoli Crust Pizza

Preparation Time: 27 minutes

Servings: 4

INGREDIENTS

- 3cups riced broccoli, steamed and drained well
- ½ cup shredded mozzarella cheese
- ½ cup grated vegetarian Parmesan cheese.
- 1 large egg.
- 3tbsp. low-carb Alfredo sauce

DIRECTIONS

1. Take a large bowl, mix broccoli, egg and Parmesan.
2. Cut a piece of parchment to fit your air fryer basket. Press out the pizza mixture to fit on the parchment, working in two batches if necessary. Place into the air fryer basket. Adjust the temperature to 370 Degrees F and set the timer for 5 minutes.
3. When the timer beeps, the crust should be firm enough to flip. If not, add 2 additional minutes. Flip crust.
4. Top with Alfredo sauce and mozzarella. Return to the air fryer basket and cook an

additional 7 minutes or until cheese is golden and bubbling. Serve warm.

NUTRITION: Calories: 136; Protein: 9.9g; Fiber: 2.3g; Fat: 7.6g; Carbs: 5.7g

625. Cheesy Zoodle Bake

Preparation Time: 18 minutes

Servings: 4

INGREDIENTS

- ½ cup heavy whipping cream.
- 2oz. full-fat cream cheese.
- 1 cup shredded sharp Cheddar cheese.
- 2 medium zucchini, spiralized
- ¼ cup diced white onion
- 2 tbsp. salted butter
- ½ tsp. minced garlic

DIRECTIONS

1. In a large saucepan over medium heat, melt butter. Add onion and sauté until it begins to soften, 1–3 minutes. Add garlic and sauté 30 seconds, then pour in cream and add cream cheese
2. Remove the pan from heat and stir in Cheddar. Add the zucchini and toss in the sauce, then put into a 4-cup round baking dish.
3. Cover the dish with foil and place into the air fryer basket. Adjust the temperature to 370 Degrees F and set the timer for 8 minutes
4. After 6 minutes remove the foil and let the top brown for remaining cooking time. Stir and serve.

NUTRITION: Calories: 337; Protein: 9.6g; Fiber: 1.2g; Fat: 28.4g; Carbs: 5.9g

626. Eggplant Stacks

Preparation Time: 17 minutes

Servings: 4

INGREDIENTS

- 2 large tomatoes; cut into ¼-inch slices
- ¼ cup fresh basil, sliced
- 4oz. fresh mozzarella; cut into ½-oz. slices
- 1 medium eggplant; cut into ¼-inch slices
- 2 tbsp. olive oil

DIRECTIONS

1. In a 6-inch round baking dish, place four slices of eggplant on the bottom. Place a slice of tomato on top of each eggplant round, then mozzarella, then eggplant. Repeat as necessary.
2. Drizzle with olive oil. Cover dish with foil and place dish into the air fryer basket. Adjust the temperature to 350 Degrees F and set the timer for 12 minutes.
3. When done, eggplant will be tender. Garnish with fresh basil to serve.

NUTRITION: Calories: 195; Protein: 8.5g; Fiber: 5.2g; Fat: 12.7g; Carbs: 12.7g

627. Roasted Garlic Zucchini Rolls

Preparation Time: 40 minutes

Servings: 4

INGREDIENTS

- 2 medium zucchini
- ½ cup full-fat ricotta cheese
- ¼ white onion; peeled.and diced
- 2 cups spinach; chopped
- ¼ cup heavy cream
- ½ cup sliced baby portobello mushrooms
- ¾ cup shredded mozzarella cheese, divided.
- 2 tbsp. unsalted butter.
- 2 tbsp. vegetable broth.
- ½ tsp. finely minced roasted garlic
- ¼ tsp. dried oregano.

- ⅛ tsp. xanthan gum
- ¼ tsp. salt
- ½ tsp. garlic powder.

DIRECTIONS

1. Using a mandoline or sharp knife, slice zucchini into long strips lengthwise. Place strips between paper towels to absorb moisture. Set aside
2. In a medium saucepan over medium heat, melt butter. Add onion and sauté until fragrant. Add garlic and sauté 30 seconds.
3. Pour in heavy cream, broth and xanthan gum. Turn off heat and whisk mixture until it begins to thicken, about 3 minutes.
4. Take a medium bowl, add ricotta, salt, garlic powder and oregano and mix well. Fold in spinach, mushrooms and ½ cup mozzarella
5. Pour half of the sauce into a 6-inch round baking pan. To assemble the rolls, place two strips of zucchini on a work surface. Spoon 2 tbsp. of ricotta mixture onto the slices and roll up. Place seam side down on top of sauce. Repeat with remaining ingredients
6. Pour remaining sauce over the rolls and sprinkle with remaining mozzarella. Cover with foil and place into the air fryer basket. Adjust the temperature to 350 Degrees F and set the timer for 20 minutes. In the last 5 minutes, remove the foil to brown the cheese. Serve immediately.

NUTRITION: Calories: 245; Protein: 10.5g; Fiber: 1.8g; Fat: 18.9g; Carbs: 7.1g

628. Roasted Veggie Bowl

Preparation Time: 25 minutes

Servings: 2

INGREDIENTS

- ¼ medium white onion; peeled.and sliced ¼-inch thick
- ½ medium green bell pepper; seeded and sliced ¼-inch thick
- 1 cup broccoli florets
- 1 cup quartered Brussels sprouts
- ½ cup cauliflower florets
- 1 tbsp. coconut oil
- ½ tsp. garlic powder.
- ½ tsp. cumin
- 2 tsp. chili powder

DIRECTIONS

1. Toss all ingredients together in a large bowl until vegetables are fully coated with oil and seasoning. Pour vegetables into the air fryer basket.
2. Adjust the temperature to 360 Degrees F and set the timer for 15 minutes. Shake two or three times during cooking. Serve warm.

Nutrition: Calories: 121; Protein: 4.3g; Fiber: 5.2g; Fat: 7.1g; Carbs: 13.1g

629. Espresso Mini Cheesecake

Preparation Time: 20 minutes

Servings: 2

INGREDIENTS

- ½ cup walnuts
- 4 oz. full-fat cream cheese; softened.
- 1 large egg.
- 2 tbsp. salted butter
- 2 tbsp. granular erythritol.
- 2 tbsp. powdered erythritol
- 1 tsp. espresso powder
- ½ tsp. vanilla extract.
- 2 tsp. unsweetened cocoa powder

DIRECTIONS

1. Place walnuts, butter and granular erythritol in a food processor. Pulse until ingredients stick together and a dough forms.
2. Press dough into 4-inch springform pan and place into the air fryer basket.
3. Adjust the temperature to 400 Degrees F and set the timer for 5 minutes. When timer beeps, remove crust and let cool.
4. Take a medium bowl, mix cream cheese with egg, vanilla extract, powdered erythritol, cocoa powder and espresso powder until smooth.
5. Spoon mixture on top of baked walnut crust and place into the air fryer basket. Adjust the temperature for 300 Degrees F and set the timer for 10 minutes. Once done, chill for 2 hours before serving.

NUTRITION: Calories: 535; Protein: 11.6g; Fiber: 7.2g; Fat: 48.4g; Carbs: 37.1g

SNACKS

630. Bacon Snack

Preparation Time: 15 minutes

Servings: 4

INGREDIENTS

- 1cup dark chocolate; melted
- 4bacon slices; halved
- Apinch of pink salt

DIRECTIONS

1. Dip each bacon slice in some chocolate, sprinkle pink salt over them.
2. Put them in your air fryer's basket and cook at 350°F for 10 minutes

NUTRITION: Calories: 151; Fat: 4g; Fiber: 2g; Carbs: 4g; Protein: 8g

631. Shrimp Snack

Preparation Time: 15 minutes

Servings: 4

INGREDIENTS

- 1lb. shrimp; peeled and deveined
- ¼ cup olive oil
- 3garlic cloves; minced
- ¼ tsp. cayenne pepper
- Juice of ½ lemon
- A pinch of salt and black pepper

DIRECTIONS

1. In a pan that fits your air fryer, mix all the ingredients, toss,
2. Introduce in the fryer and cook at 370°F for 10 minutes
3. Servings as a snack

NUTRITION: Calories: 242; Fat: 14g; Fiber: 2g; Carbs: 3g; Protein: 17g

632. Avocado Wraps

Preparation Time: 20 minutes

Servings: 4

INGREDIENTS

- 2avocados, peeled, pitted and cut into 12 wedges
- 1tbsp. ghee; melted
- 12bacon strips

DIRECTIONS

1. Wrap each avocado wedge in a bacon strip, brush them with the ghee.
2. Put them in your air fryer's basket and cook at 360°F for 15 minutes
3. Servings as an appetizer

NUTRITION: Calories: 161; Fat: 4g; Fiber: 2g; Carbs: 4g; Protein: 6g

633. Cheesy Meatballs

Preparation Time: 30 minutes

Servings: 16 meatballs

INGREDIENTS

- 1lb. 80/20 ground beef.
- 3oz. low-moisture, whole-milk mozzarella, cubed
- 1large egg.
- ½ cup low-carb, no-sugar-added pasta sauce.
- ¼ cup grated Parmesan cheese.
- ¼ cup blanched finely ground almond flour.

- ¼ tsp. onion powder.
- tsp. dried parsley.
- ½ tsp. garlic powder.

DIRECTIONS

1. Take a large bowl, add ground beef, almond flour, parsley, garlic powder, onion powder and egg. Fold ingredients together until fully combined
2. Form the mixture into 2-inch balls and use your thumb or a spoon to create an indent in the center of each meatball. Place a cube of cheese in the center and form the ball around it.
3. Place the meatballs into the air fryer, working in batches if necessary. Adjust the temperature to 350 Degrees F and set the timer for 15 minutes
4. Meatballs will be slightly crispy on the outside and fully cooked when at least 180 Degrees F internally.
5. When they are finished cooking, toss the meatballs in the sauce and sprinkle with grated Parmesan for serving.

NUTRITION: Calories: 447; Protein: 29.6g; Fiber: 1.8g; Fat: 29.7g; Carbs: 5.4g

634. Tuna Appetizer

Preparation Time: 15 minutes

Servings: 2

INGREDIENTS

- 1lb. tuna, skinless; boneless and cubed
- 3scallion stalks; minced
- 1chili pepper; minced
- 2tomatoes; cubed
- 1tbsp. coconut aminos
- 2tbsp. olive oil
- 1tbsp. coconut cream
- 1tsp. sesame seeds

DIRECTIONS

1. In a pan that fits your air fryer, mix all the ingredients except the sesame seeds, toss, introduce in the fryer and cook at 360°F for 10 minutes
2. Divide into bowls and serve as an appetizer with sesame seeds sprinkled on top.

NUTRITION: Calories: 231; Fat: 18g; Fiber: 3g; Carbs: 4g; Protein: 18g

635. Cheese and Leeks Dip

Preparation Time: 17 minutes

Servings: 6

INGREDIENTS

- 2spring onions; minced
- 4leeks; sliced
- ¼ cup coconut cream
- 3tbsp. coconut milk
- 2tbsp. butter; melted
- Salt and white pepper to the taste

DIRECTIONS

1. In a pan that fits your air fryer, mix all the ingredients and whisk them well.
2. Introduce the pan in the fryer and cook at 390°F for 12 minutes. Divide into bowls and serve

NUTRITION: Calories: 204; Fat: 12g; Fiber: 2g; Carbs: 4g; Protein: 14g

636. Cucumber Salsa

Preparation Time: 10 minutes

Servings: 4

INGREDIENTS

- 1½ lb. cucumbers; sliced

- 2 red chili peppers; chopped.
- 2 tomatoes cubed
- 2 spring onions; chopped.
- 1 tbsp. balsamic vinegar
- 2 tbsp. ginger; grated
- A drizzle of olive oil

DIRECTIONS

- In a pan that fits your air fryer, mix all the ingredients, toss, introduce in the fryer and cook at 340°F for 5 minutes
- Divide into bowls and serve cold as an appetizer.

NUTRITION: Calories: 150; Fat: 2g; Fiber: 1g; Carbs: 2g; Protein: 4g

637. Chicken Cubes

Preparation Time: 25 minutes

Servings: 4

INGREDIENTS

- 1lb. chicken breasts, skinless; boneless and cubed
- 2 eggs
- ¾ cup coconut flakes
- 2 tsp. garlic powder
- Cooking spray
- Salt and black pepper to taste.

DIRECTIONS

1. Put the coconut in a bowl and mix the eggs with garlic powder, salt and pepper in a second one.
2. Dredge the chicken cubes in eggs and then in coconut and arrange them all in your air fryer's basket
3. Grease with cooking spray, cook at 370°F for 20 minutes. Arrange the chicken bites on a platter and serve as an appetizer.

NUTRITION: Calories: 202; Fat: 12g; Fiber: 2g; Carbs: 4g; Protein: 7g

638. Salmon Spread

Preparation Time: 11 minutes

Servings: 4

INGREDIENTS

- 8oz. cream cheese, soft
- ½ cup coconut cream
- 4oz. smoked salmon, skinless; boneless and minced
- 2 tbsp. lemon juice
- 1 tbsp. chives; chopped.
- A pinch of salt and black pepper

DIRECTIONS

1. Take a bowl and mix all the ingredients and whisk them really well.
2. Transfer the mix to a ramekin, place it in your air fryer's basket and cook at 360°F for 6 minutes

NUTRITION: Calories: 180; Fat: 7g; Fiber: 1g; Carbs: 5g; Protein: 7g

639. Crustless Pizza

Preparation Time: 10 minutes

Servings: 1

INGREDIENTS

- 2 slices sugar-free bacon; cooked and crumbled
- 7 slices pepperoni
- ½ cup shredded mozzarella cheese
- ¼ cup cooked ground sausage
- 2 tbsp. low-carb, sugar-free pizza sauce, for dipping
- 1 tbsp. grated Parmesan cheese

DIRECTIONS

1. Cover the bottom of a 6-inch cake pan with mozzarella. Place pepperoni, sausage and bacon on top of cheese and sprinkle with Parmesan
2. Place pan into the air fryer basket. Adjust the temperature to 400 Degrees F and set the timer for 5 minutes.
3. Remove when cheese is bubbling and golden. Serve warm with pizza sauce for dipping.

NUTRITION: Calories: 466; Protein: 28.1g; Fiber: 0.5g; Fat: 34.0g; Carbs: 5.2g

640. Olives and Zucchini Cakes

Preparation Time: 17 minutes

Servings: 6

INGREDIENTS

- 3spring onions; chopped.
- ½ cup kalamata olives, pitted and minced
- 3zucchinis; grated
- ½ cup parsley; chopped.
- ½ cup almond flour
- 1egg
- Cooking spray
- Salt and black pepper to taste.

DIRECTIONS

1. Take a bowl and mix all the ingredients except the cooking spray, stir well and shape medium cakes out of this mixture
2. Place the cakes in your air fryer's basket, grease them with cooking spray and cook at 380°F for 6 minutes on each side. Serve as an appetizer.

NUTRITION: Calories: 165; Fat: 5g; Fiber: 2g; Carbs: 3g; Protein: 7g

641. Tomato Bites

Preparation Time: 25 minutes

Servings: 6

INGREDIENTS

- 6tomatoes; halved
- 2oz. watercress
- 3oz. cheddar cheese; grated
- 1tbsp. olive oil
- 3tsp. sugar-free apricot jam
- 2tsp. oregano; dried
- A pinch of salt and black pepper

DIRECTIONS

1. Spread the jam on each tomato half, sprinkle oregano, salt and pepper and drizzle the oil all over them
2. Introduce them in the fryer's basket, sprinkle the cheese on top and cook at 360°F for 20 minutes
3. Arrange the tomatoes on a platter, top each half with some watercress and serve as an appetizer.

NUTRITION: Calories: 131; Fat: 7g; Fiber: 2g; Carbs: 4g; Protein: 7g

642. Spinach Rolls

Preparation Time: 26 minutes

Servings: 6

INGREDIENTS:

- 3cups mozzarella; shredded
- 6oz. spinach; chopped.
- 4oz. cream cheese, soft
- ½ cup almond flour
- 2eggs; whisked
- ¼ cup parmesan; grated
- 2tbsp. ghee; melted
- 4tbsp. coconut flour

- A pinch of salt and black pepper

DIRECTIONS

1. Take a bowl and mix the mozzarella with coconut and almond flour, eggs, salt and pepper, stir well until you obtain a dough and roll it well on a parchment paper
2. Cut into triangles and leave them aside for now
3. Take a bowl and mix the spinach with parmesan, cream cheese, salt and pepper and stir really well.
4. Divide this into the center of each dough triangle, roll and seal the edges
5. Brush the rolls with the ghee, place them in your air fryer's basket and cook at 360°F for 20 minutes
6. Servings as an appetizer.

NUTRITION: Calories: 210; Fat: 8g; Fiber: 1g; Carbs: 3g; Protein: 8g

643. Ranch Roasted Almonds

Preparation Time: 11 minutes

Servings: 2 cups

INGREDIENTS

- ½ (1-oz. ranch) dressing mix packet
- 2cups raw almonds.
- 2tbsp. unsalted butter; melted.

DIRECTIONS

1. Take a large bowl, toss almonds in butter to evenly coat. Sprinkle ranch mix over almonds and toss. Place almonds into the air fryer basket
2. Adjust the temperature to 320 Degrees F and set the timer for 6 minutes. Shake the basket two- or three-times during cooking
3. Let cool at least 20 minutes. Almonds will be soft but become crunchier during cooling. Store in an airtight container up to 3 days.

NUTRITION: Calories: 190; Protein: 6.0g; Fiber: 3.0g; Fat: 16.7g; Carbs: 7.0g

644. Pickled Snack

Preparation Time: 25 minutes

Servings: 4

INGREDIENTS

- 4dill pickle spears; sliced in half and quartered
- 1cup avocado mayonnaise
- 8bacon slices; halved

DIRECTIONS:

1. Wrap each pickle spear in a bacon slice, put them in your air fryer's basket and cook at 400°F for 20 minutes.
2. Serve as a snack with the mayonnaise

NUTRITION: Calories: 100; Fat: 4g; Fiber: 2g; Carbs: 3g; Protein: 4g

645. Avocado Bites

Preparation Time: 13 minutes

Servings: 4

INGREDIENTS

- 4avocados, peeled, pitted and cut into wedges
- 1½ cups almond meal
- 1egg; whisked
- A pinch of salt and black pepper
- Cooking spray

DIRECTIONS

1. Put the egg in a bowl and the almond meal in another.

2. Season avocado wedges with salt and pepper, coat them in egg and then in meal almond
3. Arrange the avocado bites in your air fryer's basket, grease them with cooking spray and cook at 400°F for 8 minutes Servings as a snack right away

NUTRITION: Calories: 200; Fat: 12g; Fiber: 3g; Carbs: 5g; Protein: 16g

646. Asparagus Wraps

Preparation Time: 20 minutes

Servings: 8

INGREDIENTS

- 16asparagus spears; trimmed
- 16bacon strips
- 1tbsp. lemon juice
- 2tbsp. olive oil
- 1tsp. oregano; chopped.
- 1tsp. thyme; chopped.
- A pinch of salt and black pepper

DIRECTIONS

1. Take a bowl and mix the oil with lemon juice, the herbs, salt and pepper and whisk well.
2. Brush the asparagus spears with this mix and wrap each in a bacon strip
3. Arrange the asparagus wraps in your air fryer's basket and cook at 390°F for 15 minutes.

NUTRITION: Calories: 173; Fat: 4g; Fiber: 2g; Carbs: 3g; Protein: 6g

647. Warm Tomato Salsa

Preparation Time: 13 minutes

Servings: 4

INGREDIENTS

- 2spring onions; chopped.
- 1garlic clove; minced
- 4tomatoes; cubed
- 3chili peppers; minced
- 2tbsp. lime juice
- 2tsp. parsley; chopped.
- 2tsp. cilantro; chopped.
- Cooking spray

DIRECTIONS

1. Grease a pan that fits your air fryer with the cooking spray and mix all the ingredients inside.
2. Introduce the pan in the machine and cook at 360°F for 8 minutes. Divide into bowls and serve

NUTRITION: Calories: 148; Fat: 1g; Fiber: 2g; Carbs: 3g; Protein: 5g

648. Zucchini Chips

Preparation Time: 20 minutes

Servings: 6

INGREDIENTS

- 3zucchinis, thinly sliced
- 1cup almond flour
- 2eggs; whisked
- Salt and black pepper to taste.

DIRECTIONS

1. Take a bowl and mix the eggs with salt and pepper. Put the flour in a second bowl.
2. Dredge the zucchinis in flour and then in eggs
3. Arrange the chips in your air fryer's basket, cook at 350°F for 15 minutes and serve as a snack.

NUTRITION: Calories: 120; Fat: 4g; Fiber: 2g; Carbs: 3g; Protein: 5g

649. Parsley Meatballs

Preparation Time: 25 minutes

Servings: 6

INGREDIENTS

- 1lb. beef meat, ground
- 2tbsp. parsley; chopped.
- 1tsp. onion powder
- 1tsp. garlic powder
- Cooking spray
- A pinch of salt and black pepper

DIRECTIONS

1. Take a bowl and mix all the ingredients except the cooking spray, stir well and shape medium meatballs out of this mix
2. Pace them in your lined air fryer's basket, grease with cooking spray and cook at 360°F for 20 minutes

NUTRITION: Calories: 180; Fat: 5g; Fiber: 2g; Carbs: 5g; Protein: 7g

650. Cheese Chips

Preparation Time: 7 minutes

Servings: 4

INGREDIENTS

- 8oz. cheddar cheese; shredded
- 1tsp. sweet paprika

DIRECTIONS:

1. Divide the cheese in small heaps in a pan that fits the air fryer, sprinkle the paprika on top, introduce the pan in the machine and cook at 400°F for 5 minutes
2. Cool down the chips and serve them.

NUTRITION: Calories: 150; Fat: 4g; Fiber: 3g; Carbs: 4g; Protein: 6g

651. Sweet Pepper Poppers

Preparation Time: 23 minutes

Servings: 16 halves

INGREDIENTS

- 8mini sweet peppers
- 4slices sugar-free bacon; cooked and crumbled
- ¼ cup shredded pepper jack cheese
- 4oz. full-fat cream cheese; softened.

DIRECTIONS:

1. Remove the tops from the peppers and slice each one in half lengthwise. Use a small knife to remove seeds and membranes
2. In a small bowl, mix cream cheese, bacon and pepper jack
3. Place 3 tsp. of the mixture into each sweet pepper and press down smooth. Place into the fryer basket. Adjust the temperature to 400 Degrees F and set the timer for 8 minutes
4. Servings warm.

NUTRITION: Calories: 176; Protein: 7.4g; Fiber: 0.9g; Fat: 13.4g; Carbs: 3.6g

652. Bacon Wrapped Onion Rings.

Preparation Time: 15 minutes

Servings: 4

INGREDIENTS

- 1large onion; peeled.
- 8slices sugar-free bacon.
- 1tbsp. sriracha

DIRECTIONS

1. Slice onion into ¼-inch-thick slices. Brush sriracha over the onion slices. Take two slices of onion and wrap bacon around the rings. Repeat with remaining onion and bacon
2. Place into the air fryer basket. Adjust the temperature to 350 Degrees F and set the timer for 10 minutes.
3. Use tongs to flip the onion rings halfway through the cooking time. When fully cooked, bacon will be crispy. Serve warm

NUTRITION: Calories: 105; Protein: 7.5g; Fiber: 0.6g; Fat: 5.9g; Carbs: 4.3g

653. Zucchini Salsa

Preparation Time: 20 minutes

Servings: 6

INGREDIENTS

- 1½ lb. zucchinis, roughly cubed
- 2 tomatoes; cubed
- 2 spring onions; chopped.
- 1 tbsp. balsamic vinegar
- Salt and black pepper to taste.

DIRECTIONS

1. In a pan that fits your air fryer, mix all the ingredients, toss, introduce the pan in the fryer and cook at 360°F for 15 minutes
2. Divide the salsa into cups and serve cold.

NUTRITION: Calories: 164; Fat: 6g; Fiber: 2g; Carbs: 3g; Protein: 8g

654. Mushroom Platter

Preparation Time: 17 minutes

Servings: 4

INGREDIENTS

- 12oz. Portobello mushrooms; sliced
- 2 tbsp. olive oil
- 2 tbsp. balsamic vinegar
- ½ tsp. rosemary; dried
- ½ tsp. thyme; dried
- ½ tsp. basil; dried
- ½ tsp. tarragon; dried
- A pinch of salt and black pepper

DIRECTIONS

1. Take a bowl and mix all the ingredients and toss well.
2. Arrange the mushroom slices in your air fryer's basket and cook at 380°F for 12 minutes. Arrange the mushroom slices on a platter and serve

NUTRITION: Calories: 147; Fat: 8g; Fiber: 2g; Carbs: 3g; Protein: 3g

655. Crab Balls

Preparation Time: 25 minutes

Servings: 8

INGREDIENTS

- 16oz. lump crabmeat; chopped.
- 2/3 cup almond meal
- ½ cup coconut cream
- 1 egg; whisked
- 2 tbsp. chives, mined
- 1 tsp. lemon juice
- 1 tsp. mustard
- A pinch of salt and black pepper
- Cooking spray

DIRECTIONS

1. Take a bowl and mix all the ingredients except the cooking spray and stir well.

2. Shape medium balls out of this mix, place them in the fryer and cook at 390°F for 20 minutes

NUTRITION: Calories: 141; Fat: 7g; Fiber: 2g; Carbs: 4g; Protein: 9g

656. Bacon Wrapped Brie

Preparation Time: 15 minutes

Servings: 8

INGREDIENTS

- 1(8-oz. round Brie
- 4 slices sugar-free bacon.

DIRECTIONS

1. Place two slices of bacon to form an X. Place the third slice of bacon horizontally across the center of the X. Place the fourth slice of bacon vertically across the X. It should look like a plus sign (+on top of an X. Place the Brie in the center of the bacon
2. Wrap the bacon around the Brie, securing with a few toothpicks. Cut a piece of parchment to fit your air fryer basket and place the bacon-wrapped Brie on top. Place inside the air fryer basket.
3. Adjust the temperature to 400 Degrees F and set the timer for 10 minutes. When 3 minutes remain on the timer, carefully flip Brie
4. When cooked, bacon will be crispy and cheese will be soft and melty. To serve; cut into eight slices.

NUTRITION: Calories: 116; Protein: 7.7g; Fiber: 0.0g; Fat: 8.9g; Carbs: 0.2g

657. Shrimp Balls

Preparation Time: 20 minutes

Servings: 4

INGREDIENTS

- 1lb. shrimp, peeled, deveined and minced
- 1 egg; whisked
- ½ cup coconut flour
- 1tbsp. avocado oil
- 3tbsp. coconut; shredded
- 1tbsp. cilantro; chopped.

DIRECTIONS

1. Take a bowl and mix all the ingredients, stir well and shape medium balls out of this mix.
2. Place the balls in your lined air fryer's basket, cook at 350°F for 15 minutes and serve

NUTRITION: Calories: 184; Fat: 5g; Fiber: 2g; Carbs: 4g; Protein: 7g

DESSERTS

658. Awesome Chinese Doughnuts

Preparation Time: 10 minutes

Cooking Time: 8 minutes

Servings: 8

NUTRITION: Calories: 259 Fat: 15.9 g Carbs: 27 g Protein: 3.8 g

INGREDIENTS

- 1tbsp. baking powder
- 6tbsps. coconut oil
- ¾ cup of coconut milk
- 2tsps. sugar
- 2cup all-purpose flour
- ½ tsp. sea salt

DIRECTIONS

1. Preheat the air fryer to 3500F.
2. Mix baking powder, flour, sugar, and salt in a bowl.
3. Add coconut oil and mix well. Add coconut milk and mix until well combined.
4. Knead dough for 3-4 minutes.
5. Roll dough half inch thick and using cookie cutter cut doughnuts.
6. Place doughnuts in cake pan and brush with oil. Place cake pan in air fryer basket and air fry doughnuts for 5 minutes. Turn doughnuts to other side and air fry for 3 minutes more.
7. Serve and enjoy.

659. Crispy Bananas

Preparation Time: 10 minutes

Cooking Time: 10 minutes

Servings: 4

NUTRITION: Calories: 282 Fat: 9 g Carbs: 46 g Protein: 5 g

INGREDIENTS

- 4sliced ripe bananas
- 1egg
- ½ cup breadcrumbs
- 1½ tbsps. cinnamon sugar
- 1tbsp. almond meal
- 1½ tbsps. coconut oil
- 1tbsp. crushed cashew
- ¼ cup corn flour

DIRECTIONS

1. Set the pan on fire to heat the coconut oil over medium heat and add breadcrumbs in the pan and stir for 3-4 minutes.
2. Remove pan from heat and transfer breadcrumbs in a bowl.
3. Add almond meal and crush cashew in breadcrumbs and mix well.
4. Dip banana half in corn flour then in egg and finally coat with breadcrumbs.
5. Place coated banana in air fryer basket. Sprinkle with Cinnamon Sugar.
6. Air fry at 350 F/ 176 C for 10 minutes.
7. Serve and enjoy.

660. Air-Fried Banana and Walnuts Muffins

Preparation Time: 10 minutes

Cooking Time: 10 minutes

Servings: 2

NUTRITION: Calories: 192 Fat: 12.3 g Carbs: 19.4 g Protein: 1.9 g

Desserts

INGREDIENTS

- ¼ cup flour
- ½ tsp. baking powder
- ¼ cup mashed banana
- ¼ cup butter
- 1tbsp. chopped walnuts
- ¼ cup oats

DIRECTIONS

1. Spray four muffin molds with cooking spray and set aside.
2. In a bowl, mix together mashed bananas, walnuts, sugar, and butter.
3. In another bowl, mix oat flour, and baking powder.
4. Combine the flour mixture to the banana mixture.
5. Pour batter into prepared muffin mold.
6. Place in air fryer basket and cook at 320 F/ 160 C for 10 minutes.
7. Remove muffins from air fryer and allow to cool completely.
8. Serve and enjoy.

661. Air-Fryer Blueberry Muffins

Preparation Time: 10 minutes

Cooking Time: 14 minutes

Servings: 2

NUTRITION: Calories: 435 Fat: 20.9 g Carbs: 55 g Protein: 9 g

INGREDIENTS

- 1/3 cup milk
- 2tbsps. sugar
- 2/3 cup flour
- ¾ cup blueberries
- 3tbsps. melted butter
- 1egg
- 1tsp. baking powder

DIRECTIONS

1. Spray four silicone muffin cups with cooking spray and set aside.
2. In a bowl, mix together all ingredients until well combined.
3. Pour batter into prepared muffin cups.
4. Place muffin cups in air fryer basket and cook at 320 F/ 160 C for 14 minutes.
5. Serve and enjoy.

662. Nutty Mix

Preparation Time: 5 minutes

Cooking Time: 4 minutes

Servings: 6

NUTRITION:

- Calories: 316
- Fat: 29 g
- Carbs: 11.3 g
- Protein: 7.6 g
- Ingredients:
- 2cup mix nuts
- 1tsp. ground cumin
- 1tsp. chili powder
- 1tbsp. melted butter
- 1tsp. salt
- 1tsp. pepper

DIRECTIONS

1. Set all ingredients in a large bowl and toss until well coated.
2. Preheat the air fryer at 3500F for 5 minutes.
3. Add mix nuts in air fryer basket and air fry for 4 minutes. Shake basket halfway through.
4. Serve and enjoy.

663. Vanilla Spiced Soufflé

Preparation Time: 20 minutes

Cooking Time: 32 minutes

Servings: 6

NUTRITION: Calories: 215 Fat: 12.2g Carbs: 18.98g Protein: 6.66g

INGREDIENTS

- ¼ cup all-purpose flour
- 1 cup whole milk
- 2 tsps. vanilla extract
- 1 tsp. cream of tartar
- 1 vanilla bean
- 4 egg yolks
- 1-oz. sugar
- ¼ cup softened butter
- ¼ cup sugar
- 5 egg whites

DIRECTIONS

1. Combine flour and butter in a bowl until the mixture becomes a smooth paste.
2. Set the pan over medium flame to heat the milk. Add sugar and stir until dissolved.
3. Mix in the vanilla bean and bring to a boil.
4. Beat the mixture using a wire whisk as you add the butter and flour mixture.
5. Lower the heat to simmer until thick. Discard the vanilla bean. Turn off the heat.
6. Place them on an ice bath and allow to cool for 10 minutes.
7. Grease 6 ramekins with butter. Sprinkle each with a bit of sugar.
8. Beat the egg yolks in a bowl. Add the vanilla extract and milk mixture. Mix until combined.
9. Whisk together the tartar cream, egg whites, and sugar until it forms medium stiff peaks.
10. Gradually fold egg whites into the soufflé base. Transfer the mixture to the ramekins.
11. Put 3 ramekins in the cooking basket at a time. Cook for 16 minutes at 330 degrees. Move to a wire rack for cooling and cook the rest.
12. Sprinkle powdered sugar on top and drizzle with chocolate sauce before serving.

664. Apricot Blackberry Crumble

Preparation Time: 10 minutes

Cooking Time: 20 minutes

Servings: 8

NUTRITION: Calories: 217 Fat: 7.44g Carbs: 36.2g Protein: 2.3g

INGREDIENTS

- 1 cup flour
- 18 oz. fresh apricots
- 5 tbsps. cold butter
- ½ cup sugar
- 5½ oz. fresh blackberries
- Salt
- 2 tbsps. lemon juice

DIRECTIONS

1. Put the apricots and blackberries in a bowl. Add lemon juice and 2 tbsps. of sugar. Mix until combined.
2. Transfer the mixture to a baking dish.
3. Put flour, the rest of the sugar, and a pinch of salt in a bowl. Mix well. Add a tbsp. of cold butter.
4. Combine the mixture until it becomes crumbly. Put this on top of the fruit mixture and press it down lightly.
5. Set the baking tray in the cooking basket.
6. Cook for 20 minutes at 390 degrees.
7. Allow to cool before slicing and serving.

665. Chocolate Cup cakes

Preparation Time: 5 minutes

Cooking Time: 12 minutes

Servings: 6

NUTRITION: Calories: 289 Protein: 8.72 g Fat: 11.5 g Carbs: 38.94 g

INGREDIENTS

- 3eggs
- ¼ cup caster sugar
- ¼ cup cocoa powder
- 1tsp. baking powder
- 1cup milk
- ¼ tsp. vanilla essence
- 2cup all-purpose flour
- 4tbsps. butter

DIRECTIONS

1. Preheat your Air Fryer to a temperature of 400°F (200°C).
2. Beat eggs with sugar in a bowl until creamy.
3. Add butter and beat again for 1-2 minutes.
4. Now add flour, cocoa powder, milk, baking powder, and vanilla essence, mix with a spatula.
5. Fill ¾ of muffin tins with the mixture and place them into Air Fryer basket.
6. Let cook for 12 minutes.
7. Serve!

666. Stuffed Baked Apples

Preparation Time: 3 minutes

Cooking Time: 12 minutes

Servings: 4

NUTRITION: Calories: 324 Protein: 2.8 g Fat: 6.99 g Carbs: 70.31 g

INGREDIENTS

- 4tbsps. honey

Desserts

- ¼ cup brown sugar
- ½ cup raisins
- ½ cup crushed walnuts
- 4large apples

DIRECTIONS:

1. Preheat Air Fryer to a temperature of 350°F (180°C).
2. Cut the apples from the stem and remove the inner using spoon.
3. Now fill each apple with raisins, walnuts, honey, and brown sugar.
4. Transfer apples in a pan and place in Air Fryer basket, cook for 12 minutes.
5. Serve.

667. Roasted Pineapples with Vanilla Zest

Preparation Time: 5 minutes

Cooking Time: 8 minutes

Servings: 4

NUTRITION: Calories: 90 Protein: 0.79 g Fat: 0.17 g Carbs: 23.22 g

INGREDIENTS

- 2anise stars
- ¼ cup orange juice
- 1tsp. lime juice
- 1vanilla pod
- 2tbsps. caster sugar
- ¼ cup pineapple juice
- 1lb. pineapple slices

DIRECTIONS

1. Preheat Air Fryer to a temperature of 350°F (180°C).
2. Take a baking pan that can fit into Air Fryer basket.
3. Now add pineapple juice, sugar, orange juice, anise stars, and vanilla pod into a pan and mix well.

4. Place in pineapple slices evenly and transfer pan into Air Fryer basket.
5. Cook for 8 minutes.
6. Serve!

668. Vanilla Coconut Pie

Preparation Time: 15 minutes

Cooking Time: 12 minutes

Servings: 4

NUTRITION: Calories: 272   Fat: 27 g   Carbs: 7.8 g   Protein: 5.3 g

INGREDIENTS

- Shredded coconut, 1 cup
- Granulated monk fruit, ½ cup
- Vanilla extract, 1 ½ tsps.
- Eggs,
- Almond milk, 1 ½ cup
- Coconut flour, ½ cup
- Butter, ¼ cup

DIRECTIONS

1. Combine all the ingredients in a suitable mixing bowl using a wooden spatula to form a batter.
2. Pour this batter into a 6-inch pie pan then place this pan in the air fryer basket.
3. Return the basket to the air fryer then cook the pie for 12 minutes at 3700 F on Air Fry Mode.
4. Allow it to cool then serve.

669. Cookie Dough Ball

Preparation Time: 15 minutes

Cooking Time: 5 minutes

Servings: 4

NUTRITION: Calories: 179   Fat: 10.7 g   Carbs: 24.2 g   Protein: 6.9 g

INGREDIENTS:

- Vanilla extract, ½ tsp.
- Swerve sugar substitute, 1 tbsp.
- Egg,
- Mini sugar-free chocolate chips, 3 tbsps.
- Coconut flour, ½ cup
- Xanthan gum, ¼ tsp.
- Coconut oil.
- Baking powder, ½ tsp.
- Almond flour, ½ cup
- Trivia sugar substitute, ½ tbsp.
- Melted butter, ½ tbsp.
- Cinnamon, ¼ tsp.

DIRECTIONS

1. In a mixing bowl, incorporate all the ingredients.
2. Whisk in egg, vanilla, and melted butter.
3. Mix well until a smooth dough forms then fold in chocolate chips.
4. Roll the dough into a ball then refrigerate until air fryer is ready.
5. Grease the air fryer basket with coconut oil and preheat the fryer to 375 degrees F.
6. Divide the dough into cookie-sized balls and place them in the basket.
7. Set the basket back to the air fryer and cook them for 5 minutes on Air Fry Mode.
8. Serve.

670. Pumpkin Bread Cake

Preparation Time: 15 minutes

Cooking Time: 25 minutes

Servings: 6

NUTRITION: Calories: 84   Fat: 3.7 g   Carbs: 9.1 g   Protein: 3.6 g

INGREDIENTS

- Pumpkin puree, ¼ cup
- Large brown eggs,
- Pumpkin pie spice mix, 1 tsp.
- Stevia, 2 tsps.
- Vanilla extract, 1 tsp.
- Himalayan pink salt, 1/8 tsp.
- Unsweetened almond milk, 2 tbsps.
- Organic coconut flour, ¼ cup
- Baking powder, 1 tsp.

DIRECTIONS

1. Whisk eggs with almond milk, pumpkin puree, and vanilla in a mixer.
2. Mix in the remaining ingredients to incorporate until smooth.
3. Spread this batter into a 7-inch pan lined with parchment paper.
4. Move the pan to the air fryer basket and return the basket to the fryer.
5. Cook the cake batter for 25 minutes at 3500 F on Air Fry Mode.
6. Slice after cooling to serve

671. Air Fried Beignets

Preparation Time: 15 minutes

Cooking Time: 5 minutes

Servings: 4

NUTRITION: Calories: 114 Fat: 9 g Carbs: 7.1 g Protein: 3.7 g

INGREDIENTS

- Almond flour, 1 ½ cup
- Coconut milk, ½ cup
- Egg,
- Vanilla extract, 1 tbsp.
- Salt, ¼ tsp.
- Swerve sugar substitute, 3 tbsps.
- Cornstarch, ¼ tsp.
- Swerve confectioner sugar substitute
- Butter, 1 tbsp.
- Cooking oil

DIRECTIONS

1. Mix almond flour with salt, and cornstarch in a suitable bowl.
2. Heat milk in the microwave then mix it with Swerve and butter.
3. Once slightly cooled, whisk in vanilla and egg.
4. Combine the flour mixture and milk mixture with a hand blender.
5. Cover this batter and refrigerate it for 30 minutes.
6. Grease the air fryer basket with cooking oil and drop the batter into the basket using an ice cream scoop.
7. Add more scoops with sufficient distance in between, spray these balls with cooking oil.
8. Set the basket back to the air fryer and cook the beignets for 5 minutes at 3300 F on Air Fry Mode.
9. Serve once cooled and garnish with Swerve confectioner's sugar substitute.

672. Chocolate Mayo Cake

Preparation Time: 15 minutes

Cooking Time: 2 minutes

Servings: 2

NUTRITION: Calories: 239 Fat: 17.1 g Carbs: 4.2 g Protein: 6.9 g

INGREDIENTS

- Large egg,
- Water, 2 tbsps.
- Swerve sugar substitute, 3 tbsps.
- Dark cocoa powder, 2 tbsps.
- Mayonnaise, ¼ cup
- Vanilla extract, ½ tsp.
- Cooking oil
- Baking powder, 1 tsp.

- Almond flour, 4 tbsps.
- Coconut flour, 1½ tbsps.

DIRECTIONS

1. Combine the dry ingredients in a 4-cup mixing bowl.
2. Whisk in the remaining ingredients to create a smooth batter.
3. Divide the batter into two 4-ounce ramekins, greased with cooking oil.
4. Place the ramekins in the air fryer basket and return the basket to the air fryer.
5. Cook them for 2 minutes on air fry mode at 3500 F.
6. Garnish with whipped cream.
7. Serve.

673. Homemade French Fries

Preparation time: 30 minutes

Cooking time: 28 minutes

Servings: 4

INGREDIENTS

- 2reddish potatoes, cut into strips of 76 x 25 mm
- 1liter of cold water, to soak the potatoes
- 15ml of oil
- 3g garlic powder
- 2g of paprika
- Salt and pepper to taste
- Tomato sauce or ranch sauce, to serve

DIRECTION:

1. Cut the potatoes into 76 x 25 mm strips and soak them in water for 15 minutes.
2. Drain the potatoes, rinse with cold, dry water with paper towels.
3. Add oil and spices to the potatoes, until they are completely covered.
4. Preheat the air fryer, set it to 195°C.
5. Add the potatoes to the preheated air fryer. Set the timer to 28 minutes.
6. Be sure to shake the baskets in the middle of cooking.
7. Remove the baskets from the air fryer when you have finished cooking and season the fries with salt and pepper.
8. Serve with tomato sauce or ranch sauce.

NUTRITION: Calories: 390 Fat: 36g Carbohydrates: 42g Protein: 5g Sugar: 4g Cholesterol: 0mg

674. Sweet Potato Chips

Preparation time: 5 minutes

Cooking time: 10 minutes

Servings: 4

INGREDIENTS

- 2large sweet potatoes, cut into strips 25 mm thick
- 15ml of oil
- 10g of salt
- 2g black pepper
- 2g of paprika
- 2g garlic powder
- 2g onion powder

DIRECTION:

1. Cut the sweet potatoes into strips 25 mm thick.
2. Preheat the air fryer for a few minutes.
3. Add the cut sweet potatoes in a large bowl and mix with the oil until the potatoes are all evenly coated.
4. Sprinkle salt, black pepper, paprika, garlic powder and onion powder. Mix well.
5. Place the French fries in the preheated baskets and cook for 10 minutes at 205°C. Be sure to shake the baskets halfway through cooking.

NUTRITION: Calories: 130 Fat: 0g Carbohydrates: 29g Protein: 2g Sugar: 9g Cholesterol: 0mg

675. Cajun Style French Fries

Preparation time: 30 minutes

Cooking time: 28 minutes

Servings: 4

INGREDIENTS

- 2 reddish potatoes, peeled and cut into strips of 76 x 25 mm
- 1 liter of cold water
- 15ml of oil
- 7g of Cajun seasoning
- 1g cayenne pepper
- Tomato sauce or ranch sauce, to serve

DIRECTION:

1. Cut the potatoes into 76 x 25 mm strips and soak them in water for 15 minutes.
2. Drain the potatoes, rinse with cold, dry water with paper towels.
3. Preheat the air fryer, set it to 195°C.
4. Add oil and spices to the potatoes, until they are completely covered.
5. Add the potatoes to the preheated air fryer and set the timer to 28 minutes.
6. Be sure to shake the baskets in the middle of cooking
7. Remove the baskets from the air fryer when you have finished cooking and season the fries with salt and pepper.
8. Serve with tomato sauce or ranch sauce.

NUTRITION: Calories: 156 Fat: 8.01g Carbohydrate: 20.33g Protein: 1.98g Sugar: 0.33g Cholesterol: 0mg

676. Fried Zucchini

Preparation time: 10 minutes

Cooking time: 8 minutes

Servings: 4

INGREDIENTS

- 2 medium zucchinis, cut into strips 19 mm thick
- 60g all-purpose flour
- 12g of salt
- 2g black pepper
- 2 beaten eggs
- 15ml of milk
- 84g Italian seasoned breadcrumbs
- 25g grated Parmesan cheese
- Nonstick Spray Oil
- Ranch sauce, to serve

DIRECTION:

1. Cut the zucchini into strips 19 mm thick.
2. Mix with the flour, salt, and pepper on a plate. Mix the eggs and milk in a separate dish. Put breadcrumbs and Parmesan cheese in another dish.
3. Cover each piece of zucchini with flour, then dip them in egg and pass them through the crumbs. Leave aside.
4. Preheat the air fryer, set it to 175°C.
5. Place the covered zucchini in the preheated air fryer and spray with oil spray. Set the timer to 8 minutes and press Start / Pause.
6. Be sure to shake the baskets in the middle of cooking.
7. Serve with tomato sauce or ranch sauce.

NUTRITION: Calories: 67 Fat: 4.1g Carbohydrates: 4.5g Protein: 3.3g : 1.47g Cholesterol: 20.7mg

677. Fried Avocado

Preparation time: 15 minutes

Cooking time: 10 minutes

Servings: 2

INGREDIENTS

- 2 avocados cut into wedges 25 mm thick

- 50g Pan crumbs bread
- 2g garlic powder
- 2g onion powder
- 1g smoked paprika
- 1g cayenne pepper
- Salt and pepper to taste
- 60g all-purpose flour
- 2 eggs, beaten
- Nonstick Spray Oil
- Tomato sauce or ranch sauce, to serve

DIRECTION:

1. Cut the avocados into 25 mm thick pieces.
2. Combine the crumbs, garlic powder, onion powder, smoked paprika, cayenne pepper and salt in a bowl.
3. Separate each wedge of avocado in the flour, then dip the beaten eggs and stir in the breadcrumb mixture.
4. Preheat the air fryer.
5. Place the avocados in the preheated air fryer baskets, spray with oil spray and cook at 205°C for 10 minutes. Turn the fried avocado halfway through cooking and sprinkle with cooking oil.
6. Serve with tomato sauce or ranch sauce.

NUTRITION: Calories: 96 Fat: 8.8g Carbohydrates: 5.12g Protein: 1.2g Sugar: 0.4g Cholesterol: 0mg

678. Vegetables In air Fryer

Preparation time: 20 minutes

Cooking time: 30 minutes

Servings: 2

INGREDIENTS

- 2 potatoes
- 1 zucchini
- 1 onion
- 1 red pepper
- 1 green pepper

DIRECTION:

1. Cut the potatoes into slices.
2. Cut the onion into rings.
3. Cut the zucchini slices
4. Cut the peppers into strips.
5. Put all the ingredients in the bowl and add a little salt, ground pepper and some extra virgin olive oil.
6. Mix well.
7. Pass to the basket of the air fryer.
8. Select 1600C, 30 minutes.
9. Check that the vegetables are to your liking.

NUTRITION: Calories: 135 Fat: 11g Carbohydrates: 8g Protein: 1g Sugar: 2g Cholesterol: 0mg

679. Crispy Rye Bread Snacks with Guacamole and Anchovies

Preparation time: 10 minutes

Cooking time: 10 minutes

Servings: 4

INGREDIENTS

- 4 slices of rye bread
- Guacamole
- Anchovies in oil

DIRECTION:

1. Cut each slice of bread into 3 strips of bread.
2. Place in the basket of the air fryer, without piling up, and we go in batches giving it the touch you want to give it. You can select 1800C, 10 minutes.
3. When you have all the crusty rye bread strips, put a layer of guacamole on top, whether homemade or commercial.

4. In each bread, place 2 anchovies on the guacamole.

NUTRITION: Calories: 180 Fat: 11.6g Carbohydrates: 16g Protein: 6.2g Sugar: 0g Cholesterol: 19.6mg

680. Mushrooms Stuffed with Tomato

Preparation time: 5 minutes

Cooking time: 50 minutes

Servings: 4

INGREDIENTS

- 8large mushrooms
- 250g of minced meat
- 4cloves of garlic
- Extra virgin olive oil
- Salt
- Ground pepper
- Flour, beaten egg and breadcrumbs
- Frying oil
- Fried Tomato Sauce

DIRECTION:

- Remove the stem from the mushrooms and chop it. Peel the garlic and chop. Put some extra virgin olive oil in a pan and add the garlic and mushroom stems.
- Sauté and add the minced meat. Sauté well until the meat is well cooked and season.
- Fill the mushrooms with the minced meat.
- Press well and take the freezer for 30 minutes.
- Pass the mushrooms with flour, beaten egg and breadcrumbs. Beaten egg and breadcrumbs.
- Place the mushrooms in the basket of the air fryer.
- Select 20 minutes, 1800C.
- Distribute the mushrooms once cooked in the dishes.
- Heat the tomato sauce and cover the stuffed mushrooms.

NUTRITION: Calories: 160 Fat: 7.96g Carbohydrates: 19.41g Protein: 7.94g Sugar: 9.19g Cholesterol: 0mg

681. Spiced Potato Wedges

Preparation time: 1

Cooking time: 40 minutes

Servings 4

INGREDIENTS

- 8medium potatoes
- Salt
- Ground pepper
- Garlic powder
- Aromatic herbs, the one we like the most
- 2tbsp extra virgin olive oil
- 4tbsp breadcrumbs or chickpea flour

DIRECTION:

1. Put the unpeeled potatoes in a pot with boiling water and a little salt.
2. Let cook 5 minutes. Drain and let cool. Cut into thick segments, without peeling.
3. Put the potatoes in a bowl and add salt, pepper, garlic powder, the aromatic herb that we have chosen oil and breadcrumbs or chickpea flour.
4. Stir well and leave 15 minutes. Pass to the basket of the air fryer and select 20 minutes, 1800C.
5. From time to time shake the basket so that the potatoes mix and change position. Check that they are tender.

NUTRITION: Calories: 121 Fat: 3g Carbohydrates: 19g Protein: 2g Sugar: 0g Cholesterol: 0mg

682. Egg Stuffed Zucchini Balls

Preparation time: 15 minutes

Cooking time: 45-60 minutes

Servings: 4

INGREDIENTS

- 2zucchinis
- 1onion
- 1egg
- 120g of grated cheese
- 4eggs
- Salt
- Ground pepper
- Flour

DIRECTION:

1. Chop the zucchini and onion in the Thermomix, 10 seconds speed 8, in the Cuisine with the kneader chopper at speed 10 about 15 seconds or we can chop the onion by hand and the zucchini grate. No matter how you do it, the important thing is that the zucchini and onion are as small as possible.
2. Put in a bowl and add the cheese and the egg. Pepper and bind well.
3. Incorporate the flour, until you have a very brown dough with which you can wrap the eggs without problems.
4. Cook the eggs and peel.
5. Cover the eggs with the zucchini dough and pass through the flour.
6. Place the four balls in the basket of the air fryer and paint with oil.
7. Select 1800C and leave for 45 to 60 minutes or until you see that the balls are crispy on the outside.
8. Serve over a layer of mayonnaise or aioli.

NUTRITION: Calories: 23 Fat: 0.5g Carbohydrates: 2g Protein: 1.8g Sugar: 0g Cholesterol: 15mg

683. Vegetables with Provolone

Preparation time: 10 minutes

Cooking time: 30 minutes

Servings: 4

INGREDIENTS

- 1bag of 400g of frozen tempura vegetables
- Extra virgin olive oil
- Salt
- 1slice of provolone cheese

DIRECTION:

1. Put the vegetables in the basket of the air fryer. Add some strands of extra virgin olive oil and close.
2. Select 20 minutes, 2000C.
3. Pass the vegetables to a clay pot and place the provolone cheese on top.
4. Take to the oven, 1800C, about 10 minutes or so or until you see that the cheese has melted to your liking.

NUTRITION: Calories: 104 Fat: 8g Carbohydrates: 0g Protein: 8g Sugar: 0g Cholesterol: 0mg

684. Spicy Potatoes

Preparation time: 10 minutes

Cooking time: 30 minutes

Servings: 4

INGREDIENTS

- 400g potatoes
- 2tbsp spicy paprika
- 1tbsp olive oil
- Catupiry or cottage cheese
- Salt to taste

DIRECTION:

1. Wash the potatoes with a brush. Unpeeled, cut vertically in a crescent shape, about 1 finger thick Place the potatoes in a bowl and cover with water. Let stand for about half an hour.
2. Preheat the air fryer. Set the timer of 5 minutes and the temperature to 2000C.
3. Drain the water from the potatoes and dry with paper towels or a clean cloth. Put them back in the bowl and pour the oil, salt and paprika over them. Mix well with your hands so that all of them are covered evenly with the spice mixture. Pour the spiced potatoes in the basket of the air fryer. Set the timer for 30 minutes and press the power button. Stir the potatoes in half the time.
4. Remove the potatoes from the air fryer, place on a plate.
5. Serve with cheese and sauce.

NUTRITION: Calories: 153 Fat: 4g Carbohydrates: 26 Protein: 3g Sugar: 0g Cholesterol: 5mg

685. Scrambled Eggs with Beans, Zucchini, Potatoes and Onions

Preparation time: 30 minutes

Cooking time: 35 minutes

Servings: 4

INGREDIENTS

- 300g of beans
- 2onions
- 1zucchini
- 4potatoes
- 8eggs
- Extra virgin olive oil
- Salt
- Ground pepper
- A splash of soy sauce

DIRECTION:

1. Put the beans taken from their pod to cook in abundant saltwater. Drain when they are tender and reserve.
2. Peel the potatoes and cut into dice. Season and put some threads of oil. Mix and take to the air fryer. Select 1800C, 15 minutes.
3. After that time, add together with the potatoes, diced zucchini, and onion in julienne, mix and select 1800C, 20 minutes.
4. From time to time mix and stir.
5. Pass the contents of the air fryer together with the beans to a pan.
6. Add a little soy sauce and salt to taste.
7. Sauté and peel the eggs.
8. Do the scrambled.

NUTRITION: Calories: 65 Fat: 0.4g Carbohydrates: 8.6g Proteins: 4.6g Sugar: 0g Cholesterol: 0mg

686. French Toast

Preparation time: 5 minutes

Cooking time: 15 minutes

Servings: 8

INGREDIENTS

For the bread:

- 500g of flour
- 25g of oil
- 300g of water
- 25g of fresh bread yeast
- 12g of salt

For French toast:

- Milk and cinnamon or milk and sweet wine
- Eggs
- Honey

DIRECTION:

1. The first thing is to make bread a day before. Put in the MasterChef Gourmet the ingredients of the bread and knead 1 minute at speed Let the dough rise 1 hour and knead 1 minute at speed 1 again. Remove the dough and divide into 4 portions. Make a ball and spread like a pizza. Roll up to make a small loaf of bread and let rise 1 hour or so.
2. Take to the oven and bake 40 minutes, 2000C. Let the bread cool on a rack and reserve for the next day. Cut the bread into slices and reserve. Prepare the milk to wet the slices of bread. To do so, put the milk to heat, like 500 ml or so with a cinnamon stick or the same milk with a glass of sweet wine, as you like. When the milk has started to boil, remove from heat, and let cool.
3. Beat the eggs. Place a rack on a plate and we dip the slices of bread in the cold milk, then in the beaten egg and pass to the rack with the plate underneath to release the excess liquid. Put the slices of bread in the bucket of the air fryer, in batches, not piled up, and we take the air fryer, 180 degrees, 10 minutes each batch.
4. When you have all the slices passed through the air fryer, put the honey in a casserole, like 500g, next to 1 small glass of water and 4 tablespoons of sugar. When the honey starts to boil, lower the heat, and pass the bread slices through the honey. Place in a fountain and the rest of the honey we put it on top, bathing again the French toast. Ready our French toast, when they cool, they can already be eaten.

NUTRITION: Calories: 224 Fat: 15.2g Carbohydrates: 17.39g Protein: 4.81g Sugar: 5.76g Cholesterol: 84mg

687. Sweet Potato Salt and Pepper

Preparation time: 5 minutes

Cooking time: 20 minutes

Servings: 4

INGREDIENTS

- 1large sweet potato
- Extra virgin olive oil
- Salt
- Ground pepper

DIRECTION:

1. Peel the sweet potato and cut into thin strips, if you have a mandolin it will be easier for you.
2. Wash well and put salt.
3. Add a little oil to impregnate the sweet potato in strips and place in the air fryer basket.
4. Select 1800C, 30 minutes or so. From time to time, shake the basket so that the sweet potato moves.
5. Pass to a tray or plate and sprinkle with fine salt and ground pepper.

NUTRITION: Calories: 107 Fat: 0.6g Carbohydrates: 24.19g Protein: 1.61g Sugar: 5.95g Cholesterol: 0mg

688. Potatoes with Provencal Herbs With Cheese

Preparation time: 5 minutes

Cooking time: 20 minutes

Servings: 4

INGREDIENTS

A. 1kg of potatoes

B. Provencal herbs

C. Extra virgin olive oil

D. Salt

E. Grated cheese

DIRECTION:

1. Peel the potatoes and cut the cane salt and sprinkle with Provencal herbs.
2. Put in the basket and add some strands of extra virgin olive oil.
3. Take the air fryer and select 1800C, 20 minutes.
4. Take out and move on to a large plate.
5. Cover cheese.
6. Gratin in the microwave or in the oven, a few minutes until the cheese is melted.

NUTRITION: Calories: 437 Fat: 25g Carbohydrates: 42g Protein: 9g Sugar: 0g Cholesterol: 0mg

689. Potato Wedges

Preparation time: 3 minutes

Cooking time: 20 minutes

Servings: 4

INGREDIENTS:

- 2 large thick potatoes, rinsed and cut into wedges 102 mm long
- 23ml of olive oil
- 3g garlic powder
- 1g onion powder
- 3g of salt
- 1g black pepper
- 5g grated Parmesan cheese
- Tomato sauce or ranch sauce, for server

DIRECTION:

1. Cut the potatoes into 102 mm long pieces.
2. Preheat the air fryer for 5 minutes. Set it to 195°C.
3. Cover the potatoes with olive oil and mix the condiments and Parmesan cheese until they are well covered.
4. Add the potatoes to the preheated fryer. Set the time to 20 minutes.
5. Be sure to shake the baskets in the middle of cooking.
6. Serve with tomato sauce or ranch sauce.

NUTRITION: Calories: 156 Fat: 8.01g Carbohydrate: 20.33g Protein: 1.98g Sugar: 0.33g Cholesterol: 0mg

690. Onion Rings

Preparation time: 10 minutes

Cooking time: 20 minutes

Servings: 2

INGREDIENTS

- 1 small white onion, cut into rounds 13 mm thick and separated into rings
- 84g crusty bread
- 2g smoked paprika
- 5g of salt
- 2 eggs
- 224 ml whey
- 60g all-purpose flour
- Nonstick Spray Oil

DIRECTION:

1. Cut a sliced onion 13 mm thick and separate the layers into rings.
2. Combine breadcrumbs, paprika and salt in a bowl. Leave aside.
3. Beat eggs and buttermilk until completely mixed.
4. Dip each onion ring in the flour, then in the beaten eggs and finally in the breadcrumb mixture.
5. Preheat the air fryer, set it to 190°C.
6. Sprinkle the onion rings with cooking oil.
7. Place the onion rings in a single layer in the baskets of the preheated air fryer and cook in batches at 190°C for 10 minutes until golden brown. Be sure to use oil

spray in the middle of cooking to cook evenly.
8. Serve with your favorite sauce.

NUTRITION: Calories: 276 Fat: 15.51g Carbohydrates: 31.32g Protein: 3.7g Sugar: 0g Cholesterol: 14mg

691. Onion Flower

Preparation time: 15 minutes

Cooking time: 25 minutes

Servings: 3

INGREDIENTS

- 1 large onion
- 120g all-purpose flour
- 7g of paprika
- 12g of salt
- 7g garlic powder
- 3g chili powder
- 1g black pepper
- 1g dried oregano
- 295 ml of water
- 56g Italian breadcrumbs
- Nonstick Spray Oil

DIRECTION:

1. Peel the onion and cut the top. Place it on a cutting board. Cut down, from the center out on the cutting board. Repeat to create 8 evenly separated cuts around the onion. Make sure your cut goes through all the layers, but leave the onion connected in the center. Leave aside.
2. Cover the onion in cold water for at least 2 hours and then dry it. Put the flour, paprika, salt, garlic powder, chili powder, black pepper, oregano, and water until a mixture forms.
3. Preheat the air fryer for 5 minutes at 1800C.
4. Cover the onion with the mixture, spreading it over the layers and making sure they are all covered. Then, sprinkle the top and bottom of the onion with the crumbs. Spray the bottom of the air fryer with cooking oil spray and place the onion inside cut up. Spray the top of the onion generously with oil spray.
5. Cook the onion at 205 ° C for 10 minutes, then cook for another 15 minutes at 175°C.

NUTRITION: Calories: 120 Fat: 9.02g Carbohydrate: 8.67g Protein: 1.72g Sugar: 3.76g Cholesterol: 16mg

692. Hasselback Potatoes

Preparation time: 3 minutes

Cooking time: 40 minutes

Servings: 2

INGREDIENTS

- 4 medium reddish potatoes washed and drained
- 30ml of olive oil
- 12g of salt
- 1g black pepper
- 1g garlic powder
- 28g melted butter
- 8g parsley, freshly chopped, to decorate

DIRECTION:

1. Wash and scrub potatoes. Let them dry with a paper towel.
2. Cut the slits, 6 mm away, on the potatoes, stopping before you cut them completely, so that all the slices are connected approximately 13 mm at the bottom of the potato.
3. Preheat the air fryer for 6 minutes, set it to 175°C.
4. Cover the potatoes with olive oil and season evenly with salt, black pepper, and garlic powder.

5. Add the potatoes in the air fryer and cook for 30 minutes at 175°C.
6. Brush the melted butter over the potatoes and cook for another 10 minutes at 175 °C.
7. Garnish with freshly chopped parsley.

NUTRITION: Calories: 415 Fat: 42g Carbohydrate: 9g Protein: 1g

693. Roasted Potatoes

Preparation time: 3 minutes

Cooking time: 20 minutes

Servings: 4

INGREDIENTS:

- 227g of small fresh potatoes, cleaned and halved
- 30 ml of olive oil
- 3g of salt
- 1g black pepper
- 2g garlic powder
- 1g dried thyme
- 1g dried rosemary

DIRECTION:

1. Preheat the air fryer for a few minutes. Set it to 195°C.
2. Cover the potatoes in half with olive oil and mix the seasonings.
3. Place the potatoes in the preheated air fryer. Set the time to 20 minutes. Be sure to shake the baskets in the middle of cooking.

NUTRITION: Calories: 93 Fat: 0.13g Carbohydrates: 21.04g Protein: 2.49g Sugar: 1.g Cholesterol: mg

694. Honey Roasted Carrots

Preparation time: 5 minutes

Cooking time: 12 minutes

Servings: 2-4

INGREDIENTS

- 454g of rainbow carrots, peeled and washed
- 15ml of olive oil
- 30ml honey
- 2sprigs of fresh thyme
- Salt and pepper to taste

DIRECTION:

1. Wash the carrots and dry them with a paper towel. Leave aside.
2. Preheat the air fryer for a few minutes a 1800C.
3. Place the carrots in a bowl with olive oil, honey, thyme, salt, and pepper. Place the carrots in the air fryer at 1800C for 12 minutes. Be sure to shake the baskets in the middle of cooking.
4. Serve hot.

NUTRITION: Calories: 125 Fat: 7g Carbohydrates: 15.6g Protein: 1.2g Sugar: 8.6g Cholesterol: 0mg

695. Roasted Broccoli with Garlic

Preparation time: 3 minutes

Cooking time: 10 minutes

Servings 3

INGREDIENTS

- 1large broccoli cut 5
- 15ml of olive oil
- 3g garlic powder
- 3g of salt
- 1g black pepper

DIRECTION:

1. Preheat the air fryer for 5 minutes. Set it to 150°C.
2. Sprinkle the broccoli pieces with olive oil and mix them until they are well covered.
3. Mix broccoli with seasonings.
4. Add the broccoli to the preheated air fryer at 1500C for 5 minutes.

NUTRITION: Calories: 278 Fat: 5.1g Carbohydrates: 6.58g Proteins: 1.9g

696. Roasted Cauliflower

Preparation time: 2 minutes

Cooking time: 10 minutes

Servings: 2-3

INGREDIENTS

- 284g cauliflower
- 10ml of olive oil
- 3g of salt
- 1g black pepper

DIRECTION:

1. Preheat the air fryer, set it to 150°C.
2. Place the cauliflower florets in a container, sprinkle with olive oil and season with salt and pepper, covering the florets evenly.
3. Add the cauliflower to the preheated air fryer at 1500C for 5 minutes.

NUTRITION: Calories: 94 Fat: 3.1g Carbohydrates: 15.4g Proteins: 4.5g Sugar: 0g Cholesterol: 0.0mg

697. Roasted Corn

Preparation time: 2 minutes

Cooking time: 10 minutes

Servings: 2

INGREDIENTS

- 1ear of corn, with husks and silks removed, and cut in half
- 14g melted butter
- 2g of salt

DIRECTION:

1. Preheat the air fryer for 3 minutes at 1800C.
2. Pass the melted butter over the corn and season with salt.
3. Place the corn in the preheated air fryer at 1800C for 7 minutes.
4. Be sure to shake the baskets in the middle of cooking.

NUTRITION: Calories: 86 Fat: 1.2g Carbohydrates: 19g Proteins: 3.2g

698. Roasted Pumpkin

Preparation time: 10 minutes

Cooking time: 12 minutes

Servings: 2-4

INGREDIENTS

- 1pumpkin, peeled, seeded, and cut into 25 mm cubes
- 15ml of olive oil, plus a little more to spray
- 1g of thyme leaves
- 6g of salt
- 1g black pepper

DIRECTION:

1. Preheat the air fryer for a few minutes at 1800C.
2. Cover the pumpkin cubes seasoned with olive oil and season with thyme, salt, and pepper.

3. Add seasoned squash to the preheated air fryer at 1800C for 10 minutes.
4. Be sure to shake the baskets in the middle of cooking.
5. Sprinkle with olive oil when you finish cooking and serve.

NUTRITION: Calories: 50.0 Total Fat: 0.62g Carbohydrates: 10.81g Proteins: 2.48g

699. Roasted Eggplant

Preparation time: 5 minutes

Cooking time: 10 minutes

Servings: 1-2

INGREDIENTS

- 1 Japanese eggplant, sliced 13 mm thick
- 30ml of olive oil
- 3g of salt
- 2g garlic powder
- 1g black pepper
- 1g onion powder
- 1g ground cumin

DIRECTION:

1. Preheat the air fryer for 5 minutes at 1800C.
2. Cut the peeled eggplant into 13 mm thick slices.
3. Combine the oil and seasonings in a large bowl until well combined and mix the eggplant until all the pieces are well covered.
4. Place the eggplant in the preheated air fryer and cook at 205°C for 10 minutes.

NUTRITION: Calories: 325 Carbohydrates: 6.8g Fat: 4.2g Proteins: 1.9g Sugar: 3.5g Cholesterol: 0mg

700. Corn And Cheese Cakes

Preparation time: 8 minutes

Cooking time: 15 minutes

Servings: 6

INGREDIENTS

- 60g all-purpose flour
- 79g cornmeal
- 38g white sugar
- 6g of salt
- 7g baking powder
- 118ml of milk
- 45g melted butter
- 1 egg
- 165g of corn
- 3 scallions, chopped
- 120g grated cheddar cheese
- Nonstick Spray Oil

DIRECTION:

1. Put flour, cornmeal, sugar, salt, and baking powder in a bowl and mix everything.
2. Beat the milk, butter, and egg until well joined.
3. Mix the dry ingredients with the wet ingredients. Fold the corn, chives, and cheddar cheese.
4. Preheat the air fryer for 5 minutes. Set it to 160°C.
5. Grease the muffin molds with oil spray and place the mixture in the molds until they are a.
6. Add the muffins to the preheated air fryer at 1800C. Set the time to 15 minutes.
7. Serve the muffins with butter or enjoy them alone.

NUTRITION: Calories: 35 Fat: 0.2g Carbohydrates: 7.5g Protein: 0.7g Sugar: 2.1g Cholesterol: 0mg

701. Olives, Bacon and Green beans

Preparation Time: 20 minutes

Servings: 4

INGREDIENTS

- ½ lb. green beans, trimmed and halved
- ¼ cup tomato sauce
- ¼ cup bacon, cooked and crumbled
- 1cup black olives, pitted and halved
- 1tbsp. olive oil

DIRECTIONS

1. In a pan that fits the air fryer, combine all the ingredients, toss, put the pan in the air fryer and cook at 380°F for 15 minutes
2. Divide between plates and serve.

NUTRITION: Calories: 160; Fat: 4g; Fiber: 3g; Carbs: 5g; Protein: 4g

702. Endives and Walnuts

Preparation Time: 20 minutes

Servings: 4

INGREDIENTS

- 4endives, trimmed
- ½ cup walnuts; chopped.
- 3tbsp. olive oil
- 2tbsp. white vinegar
- 1tsp. mustard
- A pinch of salt and black pepper

DIRECTIONS

1. Take a bowl and mix the oil with salt, pepper, mustard and vinegar and whisk really well.
2. Add the endives, toss and transfer them to your air fryer's basket. Cook at 350°F for 15 minutes, divide between plates and serve with walnuts sprinkled on top

NUTRITION: Calories: 154; Fat: 4g; Fiber: 3g; Carbs: 6g; Protein: 7g

703. Asparagus and Yogurt Sauce

Preparation Time: 14 minutes

Servings: 4

INGREDIENTS

- 1lb. asparagus, trimmed
- 2garlic cloves; minced
- ¼ cup chives; chopped
- ¼ cup lemon juice
- 1cup Greek yogurt
- 1cup basil; chopped
- ½ cup parsley; chopped
- 2tbsp. olive oil
- 1tsp. garlic powder
- 1tsp. oregano; dried
- A pinch of salt and black pepper

DIRECTIONS

1. Take a bowl and mix the asparagus with the oil, salt, pepper, oregano and garlic powder and toss.
2. Put the asparagus in the air fryer's basket and cook at 400°F for 10 minutes
3. Meanwhile, in a blender, mix the yogurt with basil, chives, parsley, lemon juice and garlic cloves and pulse well
4. Divide the asparagus between plates, drizzle the sauce all over and serve.

NUTRITION: Calories: 194; Fat: 6g; Fiber: 2g; Carbs: 4g; Protein: 8g

704. Vinegar Broccoli

Preparation Time: 30 minutes

Servings: 4

INGREDIENTS

- 6bacon slices, cooked and crumbled
- 1broccoli head, florets separated
- ½ cup cranberries

- ½ cup almonds; chopped
- 2 shallots; chopped
- 3 tbsp. balsamic vinegar
- A pinch of salt and black pepper

DIRECTIONS

1. In a pan that fits the air fryer, combine the broccoli with the rest of the ingredients and toss.
2. Put the pan in the air fryer and cook at 380°F for 25 minutes
3. Divide between plates and serve.

NUTRITION: Calories: 173; Fat: 7g; Fiber: 2g; Carbs: 4g; Protein: 8g

705. Veggie Quesadilla

Preparation Time: 15 minutes

Servings: 2

INGREDIENTS

- 4 flatbread dough tortillas
- ⅔ cup shredded pepper jack cheese
- ½ medium avocado; peeled, pitted and mashed
- ½ medium green bell pepper; seeded and chopped
- ¼ cup diced red onion
- ¼ cup chopped white mushrooms
- ¼ cup full-fat sour cream.
- ¼ cup mild salsa
- 1 tbsp. coconut oil

DIRECTIONS

1. In a medium skillet over medium heat, warm coconut oil. Add pepper, onion and mushrooms to skillet and sauté until peppers begin to soften, 3–5 minutes
2. Place two tortillas on a work surface and sprinkle each with half of cheese. Top with sautéed veggies, sprinkle with remaining cheese and place remaining two tortillas on top
3. Place quesadillas carefully into the air fryer basket.
4. Adjust the temperature to 400 Degrees F and set the timer for 5 minutes.
5. Flip the quesadillas halfway through the cooking time. Serve warm with avocado, sour cream and salsa.

NUTRITION: Calories: 795; Protein: 34.5g; Fiber: 6.5g; Fat: 61.3g; Carbs: 19.4g

706. Cajun Olives and Peppers

Preparation Time: 16 minutes

Servings: 4

INGREDIENTS

- ½ lb. mixed bell peppers; sliced
- 1 cup black olives, pitted and halved
- ½ tbsp. Cajun seasoning
- 1 tbsp. olive oil

DIRECTIONS:

1. In a pan that fits the air fryer, combine all the ingredients.
2. Put the pan it in your air fryer and cook at 390°F for 12 minutes. Divide the mix between plates and serve

NUTRITION: Calories: 151; Fat: 3g; Fiber: 2g; Carbs: 4g; Protein: 5g

707. Chili Broccoli

Preparation Time: 20 minutes

Servings: 4

INGREDIENTS:

- 1 lb. broccoli florets
- Juice of 1 lime
- 2 tbsp. chili sauce

- 2 tbsp. olive oil
- A pinch of salt and black pepper

DIRECTIONS

1. Take a bowl and mix the broccoli with the other ingredients and toss well.
2. Put the broccoli in your air fryer's basket and cook at 400°F for 15 minutes
3. Divide between plates and serve.

NUTRITION: Calories: 173; Fat: 6g; Fiber: 2g; Carbs: 6g; Protein: 8g

708. Balsamic Kale

Preparation Time: 14 minutes

Servings: 6

INGREDIENTS

- 2½ lb. kale leaves
- 3 garlic cloves; minced
- 2 tbsp. olive oil
- 2 tbsp. balsamic vinegar
- Salt and black pepper to taste.

DIRECTIONS

1. In a pan that fits the air fryer, combine all the ingredients and toss.
2. Put the pan in your air fryer and cook at 300°F for 12 minutes. Divide between plates and serve

NUTRITION: Calories: 122; Fat: 4g; Fiber: 3g; Carbs: 4g; Protein: 5g

709. Mustard Greens and Green Beans

Preparation Time: 22 minutes

Servings: 4

INGREDIENTS

- 1 lb. green beans; halved
- ¼ cup tomato puree
- 3 garlic cloves; minced
- 1 bunch mustard greens, trimmed
- 2 tbsp. olive oil
- 1 tbsp. balsamic vinegar
- Salt and black pepper to taste.

DIRECTIONS

1. In a pan that fits your air fryer, mix the mustard greens with the rest of the ingredients, toss, put the pan in the fryer and cook at 350°F for 12 minutes
2. Divide everything between plates and serve.

NUTRITION: Calories: 163; Fat: 4g; Fiber: 3g; Carbs: 4g; Protein: 7g

710. Olives and Cilantro Vinaigrette

Preparation Time: 17 minutes

Servings: 4

INGREDIENTS

- 1 cup baby spinach
- 2 cups black olives, pitted
- 1 tbsp. olive oil
- 2 tbsp. balsamic vinegar
- A bunch of cilantro; chopped.
- Salt and black pepper to taste.

DIRECTIONS

1. In a pan that fits the air fryer, combine all the ingredients and toss.
2. Put the pan in the air fryer and cook at 370°F for 12 minutes
3. Transfer to bowls and serve.

NUTRITION: Calories: 132; Fat: 4g; Fiber: 2g; Carbs: 4g; Protein: 4g

711. Broccoli and Tomatoes

Preparation Time: 20 minutes

Servings: 4

INGREDIENTS

- 1 broccoli head, florets separated
- 2 cups cherry tomatoes, quartered
- 1 tbsp. cilantro; chopped.
- Juice of 1 lime
- A drizzle of olive oil
- A pinch of salt and black pepper

DIRECTIONS

1. In a pan that fits the air fryer, combine the broccoli with tomatoes and the rest of the ingredients except the cilantro, toss, put the pan in the air fryer and cook at 380°F for 15 minutes
2. Divide between plates and serve with cilantro sprinkled on top.

NUTRITION: Calories: 141; Fat: 3g; Fiber: 2g; Carbs: 4g; Protein: 5g

712. Kale and Mushrooms

Preparation Time: 20 minutes

Servings: 4

INGREDIENTS

- 1 lb. brown mushrooms; sliced
- 1 lb. kale, torn
- 14 oz. coconut milk
- 2 tbsp. olive oil
- Salt and black pepper to taste.

DIRECTIONS

1. In a pan that fits your air fryer, mix the kale with the rest of the ingredients and toss
2. Put the pan in the fryer, cook at 380°F for 15 minutes, divide between plates and serve

NUTRITION: Calories: 162; Fat: 4g; Fiber: 1g; Carbs: 3g; Protein: 5g

713. Spicy Olives and Avocado

Preparation Time: 20 minutes

Servings: 4

INGREDIENTS

- 2 small avocados, pitted; peeled and sliced
- ¼ cup cherry tomatoes; halved
- 2 cups kalamata olives, pitted
- 1 tbsp. coconut oil; melted
- juice of 1 lime

DIRECTIONS:

1. In a pan that fits the air fryer, combine the olives with the other ingredients, toss.
2. Put the pan in your air fryer and cook at 370°F for 15 minutes
3. Divide the mix between plates and serve.

NUTRITION: Calories: 153; Fat: 3g; Fiber: 3g; Carbs: 4g; Protein: 6g

714. Lemon Endives

Preparation Time: 20 minutes

Servings: 4

INGREDIENTS

- 12 endives, trimmed
- 3 tbsp. ghee; melted
- 1 tbsp. lemon juice
- A pinch of salt and black pepper

DIRECTIONS

1. take a bowl and mix the endives with the ghee, salt, pepper and lemon juice and toss.

2. put the endives in the fryer's basket and cook at 350°f for 15 minutes
3. divide between plates and serve.

NUTRITION: Calories: 163; Fat: 4g; Fiber: 3g; Carbs: 5g; Protein: 6g

715. Roasted Lemon Cauliflower

Preparation Time: 20 minutes

Servings: 4

INGREDIENTS

- 1 medium head cauliflower
- 1 medium lemon.
- 2 tbsp. salted butter; melted.
- 1 tsp. dried parsley.
- ½ tsp. garlic powder.

DIRECTIONS

1. Remove the leaves from the head of cauliflower and brush it with melted butter. Cut the lemon in half and zest one half onto the cauliflower. Squeeze the juice of the zested lemon half and pour it over the cauliflower.
2. Sprinkle with garlic powder and parsley. Place cauliflower head into the air fryer basket. Adjust the temperature to 350 Degrees F and set the timer for 15 minutes
3. Check cauliflower every 5 minutes to avoid overcooking. It should be fork tender.
4. To serve, squeeze juice from other lemon half over cauliflower. Serve immediately.

NUTRITION: Calories: 91; Protein: 3.0g; Fiber: 3.2g; Fat: 5.7g; Carbs: 8.4g

716. Creamy Kale

Preparation Time: 20 minutes

Servings: 4

INGREDIENTS

- 2 lb. kale, torn
- 2 garlic cloves; minced
- ½ cup parmesan, grated
- 1½ cups coconut cream
- 2 tbsp. olive oil
- ½ tsp. nutmeg, ground
- A pinch of salt and black pepper

DIRECTIONS

1. In a pan that fits your air fryer, mix the kale with the rest of the ingredients, toss, introduce the pan in the fryer and cook at 400°F for 15 minutes. Divide between plates and serve

NUTRITION: Calories: 135; Fat: 3g; Fiber: 2g; Carbs: 4g; Protein: 6g

717. Mustard Asparagus

Preparation Time: 17 minutes

Servings: 4

INGREDIENTS

- 1 lb. asparagus, trimmed
- ½ cup parmesan, grated
- ¼ cup mustard
- 3 garlic cloves; minced
- 2 tbsp. olive oil

DIRECTIONS

1. Take a bowl and mix the asparagus with the oil, garlic and mustard and toss really well.
2. Put the asparagus spears in your air fryer's basket and cook at 400°F for 12 minutes
3. Divide between plates, sprinkle the parmesan on top and serve.

NUTRITION: Calories: 162; Fat: 4g; Fiber: 4g; Carbs: 6g; Protein: 9g

718. Kale and Brussels Sprouts

Preparation Time: 20 minutes

Servings: 8

INGREDIENTS

- 1lb. Brussels sprouts, trimmed
- 3oz. mozzarella, shredded
- 2cups kale, torn
- 1tbsp. olive oil
- Salt and black pepper to taste.

DIRECTIONS

1. In a pan that fits the air fryer, combine all the ingredients except the mozzarella and toss.
2. Put the pan in the air fryer and cook at 380°F for 15 minutes.
3. Divide between plates, sprinkle the cheese on top and serve.

NUTRITION: Calories: 170; Fat: 5g; Fiber: 3g; Carbs: 4g; Protein: 7g

719. Butter Broccoli

Preparation Time: 20 minutes

Servings: 4

INGREDIENTS

- 1lb. broccoli florets
- ½ tbsp. butter; melted
- 1tsp. sweet paprika
- a pinch of salt and black pepper

DIRECTIONS

1. Take a bowl and mix the broccoli with the rest of the ingredients and toss.
2. Put the broccoli in your air fryer's basket, cook at 350°F for 15 minutes, divide between plates and serve

NUTRITION: Calories: 130; Fat: 3g; Fiber: 3g; Carbs: 4g; Protein: 8g

720. Oregano Kale

Preparation Time: 15 minutes

Servings: 4

INGREDIENTS

- 1lb. kale, torn
- 2tbsp. oregano; chopped
- 1tbsp. olive oil
- A pinch of salt and black pepper

DIRECTIONS

1. In a pan that fits the air fryer, combine all the ingredients and toss.
2. Put the pan in the air fryer and cook at 380°F for 10 minutes. Divide between plates and serve

NUTRITION: Calories: 140; Fat: 3g; Fiber: 2g; Carbs: 3g; Protein: 5g

721. Savoy Cabbage

Preparation Time: 20 minutes

Servings: 4

INGREDIENTS

- 1Savoy cabbage head, shredded
- 1tbsp. dill; chopped.
- 1½ tbsp. ghee; melted
- ¼ cup coconut cream
- Salt and black pepper to taste.

DIRECTIONS

1. In a pan that fits the air fryer, combine all the ingredients except the coconut cream, toss, put the pan in the air fryer and cook at 390°F for 10 minutes

2. Add the cream, toss, cook for 5 minutes more, divide between plates and serve

NUTRITION: Calories: 173; Fat: 5g; Fiber: 3g; Carbs: 5g; Protein: 8g

722. Broccoli and Tomato Sauce

Preparation Time: 20 minutes

Servings: 4

INGREDIENTS

- 1 broccoli head, florets separated
- ¼ cup scallions; chopped
- ½ cup tomato sauce
- 1 tbsp. olive oil
- 1 tbsp. sweet paprika
- Salt and black pepper to taste.

DIRECTIONS

1. In a pan that fits the air fryer, combine the broccoli with the rest of the ingredients, toss.
2. Put the pan in the fryer and cook at 380°F for 15 minutes
3. Divide between plates and serve.

NUTRITION: Calories: 163; Fat: 5g; Fiber: 2g; Carbs: 4g; Protein: 8g

723. Italian Olives

Preparation Time: 20 minutes

Servings: 4

INGREDIENTS

- 12 oz. tomatoes; chopped.
- 2 cups black olives, pitted and halved
- 4 garlic cloves; minced
- 2 rosemary springs; chopped.
- 2 red bell peppers; sliced
- A handful basil; chopped.
- 2 tbsp. olive oil

DIRECTIONS

1. In a pan that fits the air fryer, combine the olives with the rest of the ingredients, toss.
2. Put the pan in the fryer and cook at 380°F for 15 minutes
3. Divide between plates and serve.

NUTRITION: Calories: 173; Fat: 6g; Fiber: 2g; Carbs: 4g; Protein: 5g

724. Kale and Olives

Preparation Time: 20 minutes

Servings: 4

INGREDIENTS

- 1 an ½ lb. kale, torn
- 1 tbsp. hot paprika
- 2 tbsp. olive oil
- 2 tbsp. black olives, pitted and sliced
- Salt and black pepper to taste.

DIRECTIONS

1. In a pan that fits the air fryer, combine all the ingredients and toss.
2. Put the pan in your air fryer, cook at 370°F for 15 minutes, divide between plates and serve

NUTRITION: Calories: 154; Fat: 3g; Fiber: 2g; Carbs: 4g; Protein: 6g

725. Broccoli Casserole

Preparation Time: 35 minutes

Servings: 4

INGREDIENTS

- 1 lb. broccoli florets
- 15 oz. coconut cream
- 2 eggs, whisked

- 2 cups cheddar, grated
- 1 cup parmesan, grated
- 1 tbsp. parsley; chopped
- 3 tbsp. ghee; melted
- 1 tbsp. mustard
- A pinch of salt and black pepper

DIRECTIONS

1. Grease a baking pan that fits the air fryer with the ghee and arrange the broccoli on the bottom.
2. Add the cream, mustard, salt, pepper and the eggs and toss
3. Sprinkle the cheese on top, put the pan in the air fryer and cook at 380°F for 30 minutes
4. Divide between plates and serve.

NUTRITION: Calories: 244; Fat: 12g; Fiber: 3g; Carbs: 5g; Protein: 12g

726. Cheesy Zoodle Bake

Preparation Time: 18 minutes

Servings: 4

INGREDIENTS

- ½ cup heavy whipping cream.
- 2 oz. full-fat cream cheese.
- 1 cup shredded sharp Cheddar cheese.
- 2 medium zucchini, spiralized
- ¼ cup diced white onion
- 2 tbsp. salted butter
- ½ tsp. minced garlic

DIRECTIONS

1. In a large saucepan over medium heat, melt butter. Add onion and sauté until it begins to soften, 1–3 minutes. Add garlic and sauté 30 seconds, then pour in cream and add cream cheese
2. Remove the pan from heat and stir in Cheddar. Add the zucchini and toss in the sauce, then put into a 4-cup round baking dish.
3. Cover the dish with foil and place into the air fryer basket. Adjust the temperature to 370 Degrees F and set the timer for 8 minutes
4. After 6 minutes remove the foil and let the top brown for remaining cooking time. Stir and serve.

NUTRITION: Calories: 337; Protein: 9.6g; Fiber: 1.2g; Fat: 28.4g; Carbs: 5.9g

727. Fennel and Collard Greens Sauté

Preparation Time: 17 minutes

Servings: 4

INGREDIENTS

- 1 lb. collard greens, trimmed
- ½ cup tomato sauce
- 2 fennel bulbs, trimmed and quartered
- 2 tbsp. olive oil
- Salt and black pepper to taste.

DIRECTIONS

1. In a pan that fits your air fryer, mix the collard greens with the fennel and the rest of the ingredients, toss, put the pan in the fryer and cook at 350°F for 12 minutes
2. Divide everything between plates and serve.

NUTRITION: Calories: 163; Fat: 4g; Fiber: 3g; Carbs: 5g; Protein: 6g

728. Tomato and Kale Salad

Preparation Time: 20 minutes

Servings: 4

INGREDIENTS

- ½ lb. kale leaves, torn
- ¼ cup veggie stock
- 10 cherry tomatoes; halved
- 2 tbsp. tomato sauce
- Salt and black pepper to taste.

DIRECTIONS

1. In a pan that fits your air fryer, mix tomatoes with the remaining ingredients, toss.
2. Put the pan in the fryer and cook at 360°F for 15 minutes
3. Divide between plates and serve right away.

NUTRITION: Calories: 161; Fat: 2g; Fiber: 2g; Carbs: 4g; Protein: 6g

729. Beef Stuffed Bell Peppers

Preparation Time: 50 minutes

Servings: 4

INGREDIENTS

- Ground beef – 1 pound
- Ground coriander – 1 tsp
- Medium white onion, peeled and chopped – 1
- Minced garlic – 1 ½ tsp
- Turmeric powder – 1/2 tsp
- Hot curry powder – 1 tbsp
- Olive oil – 2 tbsps
- Grated ginger – 1 tbsp
- Ground cumin – 1/2 tsp
- Salt – 1/2 tsp
- Ground black pepper – 1/2 tsp
- Egg – 1
- Medium green bell peppers; halves and cored – 4
- Raisins – 1/3 cup
- Chopped walnuts – 1/3 cup

DIRECTIONS

1. Place a medium skillet pan over medium-high heat, add oil and when hot, add onion and cook for 4 to 5 minutes or until softened, stirring frequently.
2. Then add garlic and beef, stir well and continue cooking for 10 minutes.
3. Add remaining ingredients except for bell pepper, stir well until combined and remove the pan from heat.
4. Plug in the air fryer, insert fryer basket greased with oil, shut with lid and preheat at 320 0F for 10 minutes.
5. In the meantime, stuff pepper halves with prepared beef mixture.
6. Place stuffed peppers into heated air fryer in a single layer, spray with oil and cook for 20 minutes.
7. Serve straightaway.

NUTRITION: Calories: 170; Fat: 4; Fiber: 3; Carbs: 7; Protein: 12

730. Crispy Leeks with Lemon

Preparation Time: 12 minutes

Servings: 4

INGREDIENTS

- Medium leeks; washed, ends cut off and halved – 4
- Unsalted butter; melted – 1 tbsp
- Salt – ½ tsp
- Ground black pepper – ½ tsp
- Lemon juice – 1 tbsp

DIRECTIONS

1. Plug in the air fryer, insert fryer basket greased with oil, shut with lid and preheat at 350 0F for 5 minutes.
2. Meanwhile, rub melted butter all over leeks and then season with salt and black pepper.

3. Place leeks into the air fryer and cook for 7 minutes or until done.
4. When done, transfer leeks onto a serving plate, drizzle with lemon juice and serve.

NUTRITION: Calories: 100; Fat: 4; Fiber: 2; Carbs: 6; Protein: 2

731. Okra Salad with Tomato and Corn

Preparation Time: 22 minutes

Servings: 6

INGREDIENTS

- Okra; trimmed – 1 pound
- Scallions; chopped – 6
- Tomatoes; chopped – 28 ounce
- Medium green bell peppers; chopped – 3
- Salt – ½ tsp
- Ground black pepper – ¼ tsp
- Olive oil – 2 tbsps
- Sugar – 1 tsp
- Corn – 1 cup

DIRECTIONS

1. Plug in the air fryer, insert fryer basket, shut with lid and preheat at 360 0F for 10 minutes.
2. In the meantime, place a pan that fits into air fryer over medium heat, add oil and when hot, add scallions and bell pepper and cook for 5 minutes.
3. Then add okra, tomatoes and corn, season with salt and black pepper and stir until mixed.
4. Insert pan into the air fryer and cook for 7 minutes or until done.
5. Serve immediately.

NUTRITION: Calories: 152; Fat: 4; Fiber: 3; Carbs: 18; Protein: 4

732. Cheesy Fennel

Preparation Time: 18 minutes

Servings: 4

INGREDIENTS

- Fennel bulbs; cut into quarters – 2
- Olive oil – 3 tbsps
- Lemon, juiced – 1/2
- Salt – ½ tsp
- Ground black pepper – ¼ tsp
- Minced garlic – ½ tsp
- Red chili pepper; chopped – 1
- Vegetable stock – 3/4 cup
- White wine – 1/4 cup
- Grated parmesan cheese – 1/4 cup

DIRECTIONS

1. Plug in the air fryer, insert fryer basket, shut with lid and preheat at 350 0F for 10 minutes.
2. In the meantime, place a pan that fits into air fryer over medium-high heat, add oil and when hot, add chili peppers and garlic and cook for 2 minutes.
3. Add fennel and parmesan cheese, pour in lemon juice, wine and stock, season with salt and black pepper and stir until mixed.
4. Insert pan into the air fryer and cook for 6 minutes or until done/
5. Serve straightaway.

NUTRITION: Calories: 100; Fat: 4; Fiber: 8; Carbs: 4; Protein: 4

733. Parmesan Swiss Chard with Sausage

Preparation Time: 30 minutes

Servings: 8

INGREDIENTS

- Swiss chard; chopped – 8 cups
- White onion; chopped – 1/2 cup
- Grated parmesan cheese – 1/4 cup
- Sausage; chopped – 1 pound
- Olive oil – 1 tbsp

- Minced garlic – ½ tsp
- Salt – ½ tsp
- Ground black pepper – ¼ tsp
- Eggs – 3
- Ricotta cheese – 2 cups
- Shredded mozzarella cheese – 1 cup
- Ground nutmeg – 1/8 tsp

DIRECTIONS

1. Plug in the air fryer, insert fryer basket, shut with lid and preheat at 320 0F for 10 minutes.
2. In the meantime, place a pan that fits into air fryer over medium heat, add oil and when hot, add Swiss chard, onion, and garlic, season with salt, black pepper and nutmeg and stir until mixed.
3. Cook Swiss chard for 2 minutes, then remove the pan from heat and set aside.
4. Crack eggs in a bowl, add cheeses, whisk until combined, then pour the mixture over Swiss chard's and toss until mixed.
5. Insert pan into the air fryer and cook for 17 minutes or until done.
6. Serve straightaway.

NUTRITION: Calories: 332; Fat: 13; Fiber: 3; Carbs: 14; Protein: 23

734. Beet, Red Onion and Tomato Mix with Goat Cheese

Preparation Time: 44 minutes

Servings: 8

INGREDIENTS

- Small beets; trimmed, peeled and halved – 8
- Medium red onion; peeled and sliced – 1
- Sugar – 2 tbsps
- Mixed cherry tomatoes; halved – 1 pint
- Pecans – 2 ounce
- Olive oil – 2 tbsps
- Goat cheese; crumbled – 4 ounce
- Balsamic vinegar – 1 tbsp
- Salt – ½ tsp
- Ground black pepper – ½ tsp

DIRECTIONS

1. Plug in the air fryer, insert fryer basket greased with oil, shut with lid and preheat at 350 0F for 5 minutes.
2. Then add beets into the air fryer, season with salt and black pepper and cook for 14 minutes or until done.
3. When done, transfer beets into a salad bowl, then add onion, tomatoes, and pecans and toss until mixed.
4. Whisk together sugar, oil, and vinegar into a small bowl until sugar dissolves completely and then drizzle this mixture over salad.
5. Add cheese, toss until mixed and serve.

NUTRITION: Calories: 124; Fat: 7; Fiber: 5; Carbs: 12; Protein: 6

735. Brussels Sprouts with Cherry Tomatoes and Green Onions

Preparation Time: 15 minutes

Servings: 4

INGREDIENTS

- Brussels sprouts; trimmed – 1 pound
- Cherry tomatoes; halved – 6
- Green onions; chopped – 1/4 cup
- Olive oil – 1 tbsp
- Salt – ¾ tsp
- Ground black pepper – ¼ tsp

DIRECTIONS

1. Plug in the air fryer, insert fryer basket greased with oil, shut with lid and preheat at 350 0F for 5 minutes.
2. Add sprouts, season with salt and black pepper and cook for 10 minutes or until done.

3. When done, transfer sprouts into a bowl, add tomatoes, onion, and olive oil and toss until mixed.
4. Serve straightaway.

NUTRITION: Calories: 121; Fat: 4; Fiber: 4; Carbs: 11; Protein: 4

736. Cheesy Radish Hash Browns

Preparation Time: 17 minutes

Servings: 4

INGREDIENTS

- Onion powder – 1/2 tsp
- Grated parmesan cheese – 1/3 cup
- Eggs – 4
- Radishes; sliced – 1 pound
- Garlic powder – 1/2 tsp
- Salt – ½ tsp
- Ground black pepper – ¼ tsp

DIRECTIONS

1. Plug in the air fryer, insert fryer basket, shut with lid and preheat at 350 0F for 5 minutes.
2. Meanwhile, place radish in a bowl, add eggs, onion powder, garlic powder, cheese, then season with salt, black pepper and stir well until combined.
3. Spoon radish into a pan that fits into the air fryer, then insert it into the fryer and cook for 7 minutes or until done.
4. Divide hash evenly and serve.

NUTRITION: Calories: 80; Fat: 5; Fiber: 2; Carbs: 5; Protein: 7

737. Spinach Stuffed Spinach Pie

Preparation Time: 45 minutes

Servings: 4

INGREDIENTS

- Flour – 7 ounce
- Unsalted butter – 2 tbsps
- Spinach – 7 ounce
- Olive oil – 1 tbsp
- Medium white onion; peeled and chopped – 1
- Eggs – 2
- Milk – 2 tbsps
- Cottage cheese – 3 ounce
- Salt – 1 ½ tsp
- Ground black pepper – 1 tsp

DIRECTIONS

1. Place flour in a bowl, season with ¾ tsp salt and ¼ tsp black pepper, add butter, 1 egg and milk and blend using an immersion blender until well combined.
2. Knead the mixture for 5 minutes and then let rest for 10 minutes at room temperature.
3. Then place a skillet pan over medium-high heat, add oil and when hot, add onion and spinach and cook for 2 minutes.
4. Season with remaining salt and black pepper, add cottage cheese and remaining eggs, stir well and remove the pan from heat.
5. Plug in the air fryer, insert fryer basket greased with oil, shut with lid and preheat at 360 0F for 5 minutes.
6. Divide dough evenly into four portions, then roll each dough and place on the bottom of the ramekin and stuff with spinach filling.
7. Place ramekins into the air fryer and cook for 15 minutes until done.
8. Serve straightaway.

NUTRITION: Calories: 250; Fat: 12; Fiber: 2; Carbs: 23; Protein: 12

738. Shrimp Stuffed Peppers

Preparation Time: 16 minutes

Servings: 4

INGREDIENTS:

- Baby bell peppers; cut into halves lengthwise – 12
- Shrimp; cooked, peeled and de-veined – 1 pound
- Red pepper flakes; crushed – 1/4 tsps
- Basil pesto – 6 tbsps
- Lemon juice – 1 tbsp
- Olive oil – 1 tbsp
- Salt – ¾ tsp
- Ground black pepper – ½ tsp
- Chopped parsley – 2 tbsps

DIRECTIONS

1. Plug in the air fryer, insert fryer basket greased with oil, shut with lid and preheat at 320 0F for 5 minutes.
2. Meanwhile, place shrimps in a bowl, add parsley, pesto, lemon juice and oil, season with salt, black pepper, and red pepper flakes and whisk until well combined.
3. Stuff the shrimp mixture into peppers and then place into the fryer, spraying with oil and cook for 6 minutes or until done.
4. Serve straightaway.

NUTRITION: Calories: 130; Fat: 2; Fiber: 1; Carbs: 3; Protein: 15

739. Balsamic Cherry Tomatoes Salad

Preparation Time: 47 minutes

Servings: 4

INGREDIENTS

- Balsamic vinegar – 3 tbsps
- Minced garlic – 1 ½ tsp
- Chopped thyme – 1 tbsp
- Cherry tomatoes – 24
- Olive oil – 2 tbsp
- Salt – 1 tsp
- Ground black pepper – ½ tsp
- For the dressing:
- Balsamic vinegar – 2 tbsps
- Salt – 1/8 tsp
- Ground black pepper – 1/8 tsp
- Olive oil – 4 tbsps

DIRECTIONS

1. Place minced garlic, thyme, oil and vinegar in a bowl, season with salt and black pepper and whisk until well mixed.
2. Then add tomatoes, toss until evenly coated and set aside for 30 minutes.
3. When ready to cook, plug in the air fryer, insert fryer basket greased with oil, shut with lid and preheat at 360 0F for 5 minutes.
4. In the meantime, thread marinated tomatoes onto skewers.
5. Place tomatoes into the air fryer and cook for 6 minutes.
6. In the meantime, whisk together ingredients for the dressing until combined.
7. When tomatoes are cooked, divide them evenly on a plate, then drizzle with dressing and serve.

NUTRITION: Calories: 140; Fat: 1; Fiber: 1; Carbs: 2; Protein: 7

740. Chinese Broccoli Salad

Preparation Time: 18 minutes

Servings: 4

INGREDIENTS

- Broccoli head; cut into florets – 1
- Chinese rice wine vinegar – 1 tbsp
- Peanut oil – 1 tbsp

- Minced garlic – 3 tsps
- Salt – 1 tsp
- Ground black pepper – ½ tsp

DIRECTIONS

1. Plug in the air fryer, insert fryer basket greased with oil, shut with lid and preheat at 350 0F for 5 minutes.
2. Meanwhile, place broccoli florets in a bowl, add half of the oil, season with salt and black pepper and toss until mixed.
3. Add seasoned broccoli into the air fryer and cook for 8 minutes, shaking halfway through.
4. When done, transfer broccoli to a salad bowl, add remaining ingredients and toss until mixed.
5. Serve straightaway.

NUTRITION: Calories: 121; Fat: 3; Fiber: 4; Carbs: 4; Protein: 4

741. Beet Salad with Parsley Dressing

Preparation Time: 40 minutes

Servings: 4

INGREDIENTS

- Medium beets – 4
- Balsamic vinegar – 2 tbsps
- Bunch of parsley; chopped – 1
- Olive oil – 1 tbsp
- Minced garlic – ½ tsp
- Capers – 2 tbsps
- Salt – ¾ tsp
- Ground black pepper – ½ tsp

DIRECTIONS

1. Plug in the air fryer, insert fryer basket greased with oil, shut with lid and preheat at 360 0F for 5 minutes.
2. Then place beets in a single layer and cook for 14 minutes.
3. In the meantime, stir together garlic, parsley, capers, salt, black pepper, and oil until combined.
4. When beets are done, transfer them onto a cutting board, then let cool for 15 minutes and peel.
5. Cut beets into slices, then place them into a salad bowl, season with capers mixture and drizzle with vinegar.
6. Toss until beets are evenly coated and serve.

NUTRITION: Calories: 70; Fat: 2; Fiber: 1; Carbs: 6; Protein: 4

742. Eggplant and Garlic Sauce Recipe

Preparation Time: 20 minutes

Servings: 4

INGREDIENTS

- Olive oil – 2 tbsps
- Minced garlic – 1 tsp
- Grated ginger – ½ tsp
- Soy sauce – 1 tbsp
- Eggplants; halved and sliced – 3
- Red chili pepper; chopped – 1
- Green onion stalk; chopped – 1
- Balsamic vinegar – 1 tbsp

DIRECTIONS

1. Plug in the air fryer, insert fryer basket greased with oil, shut with lid and preheat at 320 0F for 5 minutes.
2. Meanwhile, take a pan that fits into the air fryer, place it over medium-high heat, then add oil and when hot, add eggplant and cook for 2 minutes per side.
3. Add remaining ingredients, stir well and insert pan into the air fryer.
4. Cook eggplant for 7 minutes or until done and serve.

NUTRITION: Calories: 130; Fat: 2; Fiber: 4; Carbs: 7; Protein: 9

743. Cherry Tomatoes with Basil and Parmesan

Preparation Time: 20 minutes

Servings: 8

INGREDIENTS

- Jalapeno pepper; chopped – 1
- Minced garlic – 2 tsps
- Dried oregano – 1/2 tsp
- Chopped basil – 1/4 cup
- Cherry tomatoes; halved – 2 pounds
- Salt – 1 tsp
- Ground black pepper – ½ tsp
- Olive oil – 1/4 cup
- Grated parmesan cheese – 1/2 cup

DIRECTIONS

1. Plug in the air fryer, insert fryer basket greased with oil, shut with lid and preheat at 380 0F for 5 minutes.
2. Meanwhile, place tomatoes and peppers in a bowl, add garlic and oil, season with salt, black pepper, and oregano and toss until evenly coated.
3. Then place tomatoes into the air fryer and cook for 15 minutes until done.
4. When ready, transfer tomatoes into a salad bowl, add basil and parmesan, toss until coated and serve.

NUTRITION: Calories: 140; Fat: 2; Fiber: 2; Carbs: 6; Protein: 8

744. Lemony Eggplant and Zucchini Mix

Preparation Time: 18 minutes

Servings: 4

INGREDIENTS

- Medium eggplant; roughly cubed – 1
- Medium zucchinis; roughly cubed – 3
- Lemon juice – 2 tbsps
- Dried thyme – 1 tsp
- Salt – 1 tsp
- Ground black – ½ tsp
- Dried oregano – 1 tsp
- Olive oil – 3 tbsps

DIRECTIONS

1. Plug in the air fryer, insert fryer basket, shut with lid and preheat at 360 0F for 5 minutes.
2. Take a pan that fits into an air fryer, place eggplant in the bottom, then add zucchini, drizzle with lemon juice and season with salt, black pepper, thyme, and oregano.
3. Toss until well mixed, then place the pan into the air fryer and cook for 8 minutes until done.
4. When ready, divide evenly between plates and serve.

NUTRITION: Calories: 152; Fat: 5; Fiber: 7; Carbs: 19; Protein: 5

745. Mexican Style Stuffed Bell Peppers

Preparation Time: 35 minutes

Servings: 4

INGREDIENTS:

- Medium green bell peppers; tops cut off and seeds removed – 4
- Tomato juice – 1/2 cup
- Medium white onion; chopped – 1/4 cup
- Green peppers; chopped – /4 cup
- Tomato sauce – 2 cups
- Jalapeno peppers; chopped – 2 tbsps
- Chicken breasts – 4
- Tomatoes; chopped – 1 cup
- Salt – 1 tsp
- Ground black pepper – ½ tsp
- Onion powder – 2 tsps
- Red pepper; crushed – 1/2 tsp

- Red chili powder – 1 tsp
- Garlic powder – 1/2 tsp
- Ground cumin – 1 tsp

DIRECTIONS

1. Plug in the air fryer, insert fryer basket greased with oil, shut with lid and preheat at 350 0F for 5 minutes.
2. Take a pan that fits into air fryer, place chicken in it along with remaining ingredients except for bell peppers and stir until mixed.
3. Insert the pan into the air fryer and cook for 15 minutes or until done.
4. Then shred chicken using two forks, stir well and stuff into bell peppers.
5. Place stuffed bell peppers into the air fryer and cook for 10 minutes at 320 0F.
6. Serve straightaway.

NUTRITION: Calories: 180; Fat: 4; Fiber: 3; Carbs: 7; Protein: 14

746. **Balsamic Artichokes with Oregano**

Preparation Time: 15 minutes

Servings: 4

INGREDIENTS

- Large artichokes; trimmed – 4
- Lemon juice – 2 tbsps
- Balsamic vinegar – 2 tsps
- Dried oregano – 1 tsp
- Olive oil – 1/4 cup
- Minced garlic – 1 tsp
- Salt – 1 ½ tsp
- Ground black pepper – 1 tsp

DIRECTIONS

1. Plug in the air fryer, insert fryer basket greased with oil, shut with lid and preheat at 360 0F for 5 minutes.
2. Meanwhile, place artichokes in a bowl, season with 1 tsp salt and ½ tsp black pepper, drizzle with half of the lemon juice and oil and toss until evenly coated.
3. Place artichokes into the air fryer and cook for 7 minutes or until done.
4. In the mean time prepare vinaigrette and for this, whisk together remaining oil, lemon juice, salt, and black pepper, add garlic and oregano and stir well until combined.
5. When artichokes are ready, place them on a serving plate, drizzle with prepared vinaigrette and toss until coated.
6. Serve straightaway.

NUTRITION: Calories: 200; Fat: 3; Fiber: 6; Carbs: 12; Protein: 4

747. **Artichokes with Anchovy Sauce**

Preparation Time: 15 minutes

Servings: 2

INGREDIENTS

- Medium artichokes; trimmed – 2
- Minced garlic – 1 tsp
- Olive oil – ½ tsp
- Lemon juice – 1 tbsp
- For the sauce:
- Anchovy fillets – 3
- Coconut oil – 1/4 cup
- Olive oil – 1/4 cup
- Minced garlic – 1 ½ tsp

DIRECTIONS

1. Plug in the air fryer, insert fryer basket greased with oil, shut with lid and preheat at 360 0F for 5 minutes.
2. Meanwhile, place artichokes in a bowl, add minced garlic, lemon juice, and oil and toss until evenly coated.
3. Place artichokes into the air fryer and cook for 6 minutes or until done.
4. In the meantime prepare sauce and for this, blend all the ingredients for the

sauce in a blender for 2 minutes or until smooth.
5. When artichokes are ready, divide evenly between plates, then drizzle with anchovy sauce and serve.

NUTRITION: Calories: 261; Fat: 4; Fiber: 7; Carbs: 20; Protein: 12

748. Beets and Arugula Salad with Cider Dressing

Preparation Time: 20 minutes

Servings: 4

INGREDIENTS

- Beets; peeled and quartered – 1 ½ pound
- Brown sugar – 2 tbsps
- Scallions; chopped – 2
- Mustard – 2 tsps
- Olive oil – 1/8 tsp
- Orange zest; grated – 2 tsps
- Apple cider vinegar – 2 tbsps
- Orange juice – 1/2 cup
- Arugula – 2 cups

DIRECTIONS

1. Plug in the air fryer, insert fryer basket greased with oil, shut with lid and preheat at 360 0F for 5 minutes.
2. Meanwhile, rub each beet with orange juice and oil.
3. Place beets into the air fryer and cook for 10 minutes until done.
4. Then transfer beets into a bowl, add scallion and arugula, sprinkle with orange zest and toss until mixed.
5. Whisk together sugar, vinegar, and mustard until well combined, then drizzle this over beets and toss until evenly coated.
6. Serve straightaway.

NUTRITION: Calories: 121; Fat: 2; Fiber: 3; Carbs: 11; Protein: 4

749. Cheesy Artichokes

Preparation Time: 15 minutes

Servings: 6

INGREDIENTS:

- Artichoke hearts – 14 ounce
- Cream cheese – 8 ounce
- Shredded mozzarella cheese – 8 ounce
- Sour cream – 1/2 cup
- Minced garlic – 1 ½ tsp
- Grated parmesan cheese – 16 ounce
- Spinach – 10 ounce
- Chicken stock – 1/2 cup
- Mayonnaise – 1/2 cup
- Onion powder – 1 tsp

DIRECTIONS

1. Plug in the air fryer, insert fryer basket, shut with lid and preheat at 360 0F for 5 minutes.
2. Meanwhile, take a pan that fits into air fryer, place artichokes in it, add remaining ingredients except for cheeses and stir until mixed.
3. Insert the pan into the air fryer and cook for 6 minutes or until done.
4. When ready, add cheese into artichokes, toss until mixed and serve.

NUTRITION: Calories: 261; Fat: 12; Fiber: 2; Carbs: 12; Protein: 15

750. Parmesan Brussels Sprouts

Preparation Time: 18 minutes

Servings: 4

INGREDIENTS

- Brussels sprouts; washed – 1 pound
- Lemon, juiced – 1
- Unsalted butter – 2 tbsps

- Grated parmesan cheese – 3 tbsps
- Salt – 1 tsp
- Ground black pepper – ½ tsp

DIRECTIONS

1. Plug in the air fryer, insert fryer basket greased with oil, shut with lid and preheat at 350 0F for 5 minutes.
2. Then add Brussels sprouts and cook for 8 minutes until done.
3. Meanwhile, place a skillet pan over medium heat, add butter and when it melts, add salt, black pepper, and lemon juice and whisk well until smooth, remove the pan from heat and set aside.
4. When sprouts are ready, transfer them into a bowl, top with butter sauce and set aside.

NUTRITION: Calories: 152; Fat: 6; Fiber: 6; Carbs: 8; Protein: 12

751. Simple and Sweet Baby Carrots

Preparation Time: 15 minutes

Servings: 4

INGREDIENTS

- Baby carrots – 2 cups
- Salt – 1/8 tsp
- Ground black pepper – 1/8 tsp
- Brown sugar – 1 tbsp
- Butter; melted – 1/2 tbsp

DIRECTIONS

1. Plug in the air fryer, insert fryer basket, shut with lid and preheat at 350 0F for 5 minutes.
2. Meanwhile, take a pan that fits into the air fryer, add carrots in it along with butter, then sprinkle with salt, black pepper and sugar and toss until mixed.
3. Insert pan into the air fryer and cook for 10 minutes or until done.
4. Serve straightaway.

NUTRITION: Calories: 100; Fat: 2; Fiber: 3; Carbs: 7; Protein: 4

SNACKS

752. Jackfruit Air-Fryer Fries

Cooking Time: 20 minutes

Servings: 4

INGREDIENTS

- 1cup Jackfruit, seeded
- 1teaspoon olive oil
- 1teaspoon turmeric
- 1teaspoon liquid stevia
- 2teaspoons sugar-free syrup
- 1teaspoon salt

DIRECTIONS:

1. In a mixing bowl, add syrup, olive oil, stevia, turmeric, and salt. Add mixture to strips of jackfruit. Toss ingredients and allow to stand for 30-minutes. Preheat your air fryer to 370°Fahrenheit for 2-minutes. Place the jackfruit into air fryer and cook for 20-minutes. Shake basket a few times through the cook time.

NUTRITION: Calories: 155, Total Fat: 0.5g, Carbs: 39.2g, Protein: 2.43g

753. Sweet & Sour Air-Fried Yam

Cooking Time: 20 minutes

Servings: 4

INGREDIENTS

- 1teaspoon olive oil
- 2tablespoons chives, minced
- Salt and pepper to taste
- 1teaspoon lemon zest
- 1tablespoon liquid stevia
- 1tablespoon tamarind paste
- 2cups Yam, cut into strips

DIRECTIONS

1. Wash the veggies and peel the skin from yams. Cut the yams into strips and put in a mixing bowl. Add stevia and tamarind paste into a bowl. Add minced chives into a bowl. Season with salt and pepper. Sprinkle with lemon zest. Marinate yams for 30-minutes. Preheat your air-fryer to 380°Fahrenheit. Add yams to the air-fryer basket and spray teaspoon of olive oil on jicama. Cook for 20-minutes until crispy. Shake the basket a few times during cook time. Serve warm.

NUTRITION: Calories: 49, Total Fat: 0.12g, Carbs: 11.47g, Proteins: 0.94g

754. Air-Fried Sesame Tofu with Broccoli & Bell Pepper Salad

Cooking Time: 20 minutes

Servings: 5

INGREDIENTS

- ¾ cups red bell pepper, sliced
- 1cup broccoli
- 1teaspoon sesame oil
- 1teaspoon olive oil
- 1tablespoon lemon zest
- 1tablespoon Shaoxing wine
- Salt and pepper to taste
- 1tablespoon sriracha sauce
- 1tablespoon sugar-free syrup
- ½ cup sesame seeds
- 1cup of tofu

DIRECTIONS

1. Prepare broccoli and red bell pepper. Soak the broccoli in warm water

and rinse in cold water. Cut it into florets and set aside. Slice the red pepper into cubes. In a bowl, mix vegetables. Add Shaoxing wine, olive oil, lemon zest into bowl, season with salt and pepper and toss to combine. Rinse and drain a cup of tofu. Cut tofu into small cubes. Place tofu in mixing bowl, add sesame seeds to the bowl. Season with sriracha sauce and syrup. Mix well. Preheat your air-fryer to 370°Fahrenheit for 2-minutes. Place tofu mixture into air-fryer and spray it with sesame oil. Cook the tofu mixture for 20-minutes. Shake the basket a few times through cook time. Add the tofu to the bowl of veggies and toss. Serve right away

NUTRITION: Calories: 340, Total Fat: 18g, Carbs: 18g, Protein: 22g

755. Coconut Pumpkin Curry

Cooking Time: 25 minutes

Servings: 4

INGREDIENTS

- 2cups pumpkin, cubed
- 1tablespoon sesame seeds
- 2-inches ginger, minced
- 1tablespoon parsley, chopped
- 2teaspoons curry powder
- 1teaspoon black pepper
- ¼ cup coconut cream
- 1tablespoon shredded coconut
- 1red chili for garnish
- 1red chili, minced
- ¼ cup water

DIRECTIONS

1. Place the cubed pumpkin into the pan with minced ginger. Add ¼ cup water and ¼ cup coconut cream into the pan. Cook for 15-minutes at 300°Fahrenheit. Slightly mash pumpkin cubes. Add the minced chili, curry powder, pepper, and stir. Cook for another 10-minutes. Transfer to a large bowl. Garnish with chopped parsley and red chili. Serve warm.

NUTRITION: Calories: 115, Total Fat: 4.38g, Carbs: 19.85, Protein: 2.7g

756. Tomato Vegetable Curry

Cooking Time: 25 minutes

Servings: 4

INGREDIENTS

- 1teaspoon oregano
- 1tablespoon basil leaves, chopped
- 1tablespoon cilantro leaves, chopped
- 2teaspoons curry powder
- 2cloves garlic, minced
- 1large onion, diced
- ¼ cup chickpeas
- ½ cup water
- ½ cup coconut milk
- ¼ cup potatoes, diced
- ½ cup tomatoes, chopped

DIRECTIONS

1. Cut washed veggies into small cubes. Chop the herbs into small pieces and save for later use. Soak and rinse chickpeas with water. Drain and set aside. Add ½ cup coconut milk and ½ cup water to your air-fryer. Add the garlic, onions and cubed vegetables. Season with curry powder, pepper, and oregano. Cook for 20-minutes. Add the basil and cilantro leaves. Cook for another 5-minutes until the soup thickens. Serve warm with Jasmine rice.

NUTRITION: Calories: 53,Total Fat: 0.82g, Carbs: 9.7g, Protein: 1.9g

757. Crispy Air-Fried Gourd

Cooking Time: 15 minutes

Servings: 6

INGREDIENTS

- 2medium size bitter gourd (sliced
- 1tablespoon rice vinegar
- 1teaspoon salt
- 1teaspoon turmeric powder
- 1teaspoon sugar-free maple syrup
- 2teaspoons liquid stevia
- 2tablespoons cornstarch
- 2teaspoons of coconut oil cooking spray

DIRECTIONS

1. Remove the pit from a bitter gourd, cut in half length-wise. Place the sliced bitter gourd into a mixing bowl. Add stevia, maple syrup, rice vinegar, turmeric powder to the bowl. Season with salt and stir with wooden spoon. Let the bitter gourd soak in the mixture for about an hour before cooking. In another bowl, add cornstarch. Coat the marinated bitter gourd with cornstarch and set aside. Preheat your air-fryer to 380°Fahrenheit for 2-minutes. Place the bitter gourd into the air-fryer basket and spray it with coconut oil spray. Cook for 15-minutes or until crispy, shake the basket every 5-minutes during cook time.

NUTRITION: Calories: 34, Total Fat: 0.2g, Carbs: 7g, Protein: 3.6g

758. Air-Fried Vegan Noodles

Cooking Time: 11 minutes

Servings: 4

INGREDIENTS

- 1large green bell pepper
- 4cups of rice noodles
- 1large red bell pepper
- 1tablespoon white sesame seeds
- 2teaspoons sesame oil
- 1tablespoon basil leaves, minced
- 2teaspoons rice vinegar
- 1teaspoon vegan oyster sauce
- 1teaspoon pepper
- 2teaspoons ketchup
- ½ teaspoon chili powder

DIRECTIONS

1. Allow noodles to soak in a pot of hot water for 3-minutes and then allow them to dry. Preheat your air-fryer to 400°Fahrenheit for 2-minutes. Place noodles into the air-fryer basket and drizzle them with sesame oil, toss to coat. Cook noodles for 8-minutes, toss after 4-minutes of cooking. Once noodles are cooked transfer them to a bowl and set aside. Cut bell peppers into strips, mince spring onions and basil leaves. Place veggies in a mixing bowl. Add soy sauce, vegan oyster sauce, rice vinegar, and ketchup. Add cooked noodles into bowl with veggies and toss to combine. Sprinkle with pepper and chili powder and garnish with sesame seeds. Serve warm.

NUTRITION: Calories: 235, Total Fat: 10.9, Carbs: 34.7g, Protein: 13.9g

759. Sweet & Spicy Tofu with Steamed Spinach

Cooking Time: 24 minutes

Servings: 6

INGREDIENTS

- 6cups of spinach, chopped
- 2teaspoons rice vinegar
- 1teaspoon agave syrup

- 1 teaspoon salt
- 2-inches ginger, minced
- 1 teaspoon sesame oil
- 1 tablespoon vegan oyster sauce
- 1 teaspoon red pepper flakes
- 1 lb. tofu cubed

DIRECTIONS

1. Rinse and drain the tofu. Make sure to press the tofu to remove excess water. Cut tofu into small cubes and place them in a mixing bowl. Add minced ginger to bowl with tofu. Add agave syrup, season with salt, red pepper flakes and stir. Let mixture stand for 30-minutes before frying.
2. Prepare spinach by steaming for 4-minutes, then transfer spinach to bowl. Add vegan oyster sauce and rice vinegar and toss and save for later use. Preheat air-fryer to 370°Fahrenheit. Add the marinated tofu and spray with a teaspoon of sesame oil. Cook for 20-minutes and shake the air-fryer basket every 5-minutes during cook time. Once cooked, transfer the tofu to bowl with steamed spinach mix. Toss all ingredients and serve warm.

NUTRITION: Calories: 169, Total Fat: 10.8g, Carbs: 6.8g, Protein: 15.2g

760. Air-Fried Walnuts & Green Beans

Cooking Time: 20 minutes

Servings: 5

INGREDIENTS

- ½ teaspoon chili powder
- 4 cups green beans, cut into 3-inch long pieces
- ¼ cup walnuts, roasted
- 4 garlic cloves, chopped
- 1 tablespoon light soy sauce
- 1 teaspoon sugar-free maple syrup
- 1 teaspoon sesame oil
- Salt and pepper to taste

DIRECTIONS

1. After washing and chopping vegetable place into a bowl. Prepare by using a mortar and pestle, pound walnuts lightly and then transfer to a bowl of vegetables. Add remaining ingredients to a bowl, except sesame oil. Preheat your air-fryer to 390°Fahrenheit. Add marinated beans and walnuts to air-fryer and spray them with sesame oil. Cook for 20-minutes and shake the basket a couple of times during the cook time. Serve warm.

NUTRITION: Calories: 155, Total Fat: 12.41g, Carbs: 9.18g, Protein: 4.68g

761. Air-Fried Avocado & Yellow Pepper Salad

Cooking Time: 10 minutes

Servings: 6

INGREDIENTS

- 2 tablespoons potato starch
- 3 large avocados, diced
- ½ cup sweet corn kernels
- 6 lettuce leaves
- 3 large tomatoes, cut into wedges
- 3 yellow pepper, seeded and sliced into small pieces
- 2 teaspoons lemon zest
- 2 tablespoons basil leaves, chopped
- Salt and pepper to taste
- 1 tablespoon vinegar
- 2 tablespoons flaxseed mixed with 3 tablespoons water
- 1 tablespoon olive oil

DIRECTIONS

1. Cut avocado in half and remove seed. Scoop the avocado flesh and cut into cubes. Chop tomatoes, yellow peppers, and basil into small pieces and set aside. Slice yellow peppers into thin slices. In blender ad flax seed and water and blend until fluffy. Transfer to a bowl and mix with potato starch. Season with salt and pepper. Mix all the ingredients and coat cubed avocado. In another mixing bowl, combine lettuce leaves with sweet corn kernels, and chopped tomatoes, yellow peppers, and basil leaves. Add vinegar and lemon zest. Whisk all ingredients and save for later.
2. Preheat your air-fryer to 390°Fahrenheit. Spray olive oil over the avocados. Place avocados into air-fryer and cook for 10-minutes. Shake basket halfway through cook time. Once cooked transfer avocados to bowl with lettuce salad and toss with two large salad spoons. Serve right away.

762. **Onion Strings**

Cooking Time: 7 minutes

Serving: 6

INGREDIENTS

- 8large onions, shredded
- 2tablespoons cornstarch
- ½ teaspoon cayenne powder
- 1teaspoon pepper
- 1teaspoon apple cider vinegar
- 1teaspoon olive oil
- 1teaspoon baking soda

DIRECTIONS

1. Remove outer skin from onions, using a vegetable shredder, cut onions into thin strips and set aside. Add baking soda, apple cider vinegar and blend until it becomes fluffy. Transfer mixture to a bowl. Add salt and pepper. Season with cayenne pepper. Add shredded onions into a bowl and toss to combine. In another bowl, add cornstarch. Mix the marinated onions in the bowl of cornstarch, coating them well. Preheat your air-fryer to 390°Fahrenheit. Add onions to the air-fryer basket and spray with olive oil. Cook for 7-minutes, shake halfway through cook time. Once cooked, transfer to plate. Serve warm.

NUTRITION: Calories: 22, Total Fat: 1.3g, Carbs: 5.6g, Protein: 1.2g

763. **Air-Fried Banana Turmeric Chips**

Cooking Time: 8 minutes

Servings: 4

INGREDIENTS

- 1teaspoon of sesame oil
- ½ teaspoon pepper
- 1teaspoon turmeric
- 4large bananas, sliced
- ½ teaspoon salt
- 2teaspoons agave syrup

DIRECTIONS

1. In a bowl, mix agave syrup, and turmeric. Season with salt and pepper. Add sliced bananas and toss to combine. Set aside. Preheat your air-fryer to 370°Fahrenheit. Spray sesame oil over sliced bananas and place into the air-fryer basket. Cook bananas for 8-minutes, shake basket halfway through cook time. Serve warm.

NUTRITION: Calories: 176, Total Fat: 9.9g, Carbs: 23.4g, Protein: 1.13g

764. Spicy Air-Fried Eggplant

Cooking Time: 20 minutes

Servings: 4

INGREDIENTS

- 2 garlic cloves, minced
- 2 large eggplants, sliced
- 2 red chili peppers, chopped
- 2 green chili peppers, minced
- 1 teaspoon sesame oil
- 1 tablespoon light soy sauce
- Pepper and salt to taste

DIRECTIONS

1. Cut eggplants and set aside. Chop chilies and mince garlic and save for later use. In a bowl, mix garlic, green and red chili peppers. Add soy sauce and sprinkle with pepper, add eggplant slices, toss and set aside. Preheat your air-fryer to 350°Fahrenheit. Add eggplant slices and spray with sesame oil. Cook for 20-minutes, shake basket every 5-minutes during cook time. Once cooked garnish eggplant slices with chili peppers and garlic. Serve warm.

NUTRITION: Calories: 223, Total Fat: 6.4g, Carbs: 11.8g, Protein: 3.2g

765. Air-Fried Carrots with Lemon

Cooking Time: 18 minutes

Servings: 4

INGREDIENTS

- 2 cups carrots (julienned
- 1 tablespoon parsley, chopped
- 1 teaspoon paprika
- 2 teaspoon lemon juice
- ½ teaspoon pepper
- 1 teaspoon salt
- 2 teaspoons olive oil
- 1 tablespoon lemon zest

DIRECTIONS

1. In a bowl, combine lemon zest, lemon juice, paprika, salt, pepper, olive oil, carrots, and toss. Combine ingredients and allow to stand for 30-minutes before air-frying.
2. Preheat air-fryer to 390°Fahrenheit. Add carrots to the air-fryer basket and cook for 18-minutes. Give the basket a shake a couple of times during the cook time. Serve warm.

NUTRITION: Calories: 201, Total Fat: 11.48g, Carbs: 25.3g, Protein: 1.08

766. Air-Fried Radish Cake

Cooking Time: 15 minutes

Servings: 4

INGREDIENTS

- 2 cups radish, cut into big strips
- ¼ cup potato flour
- 1 tablespoon Sriracha sauce
- 1 teaspoon black pepper
- ½ teaspoon salt
- 1 teaspoon olive oil
- 1 tablespoon flax seed combined with 3 tablespoons water

DIRECTIONS

1. In a blender add the flax seed and water and blend until smooth. In a mixing bowl, add Sriracha sauce, salt, and pepper. Stir, add strips of radish. Add flax seed mix to the bowl and mix well. Add the potato flour to another bowl. Coat the radish sticks with flour and set aside.
2. Preheat your air-fryer to 350°Fahrenheit. Add coated radish to air-

fryer and spray with olive oil. Cook for 15-minutes, shake a couple of times during cook time. Serve warm.

NUTRITION: Calories: 78, Total Fat: 6.07g, Carbs: 7.14g, Protein: 1.3g

767. Air-Fried Roasted Potatoes with Rosemary

Cooking Time: 30 minutes

Servings: 4

INGREDIENTS

- 2cups potatoes, diced
- 2teaspoons rosemary, dried
- 1teaspoon sesame oil
- 1teaspoon black pepper

DIRECTIONS

1. Preheat your air-fryer to 370°Fahrenheit. Add potatoes and spray them with sesame oil. Heat for 30-minutes and shake air-fryer basket a couple of times during cook time. Garnish with rosemary and serve warm.

NUTRITION: Calories: 203, Total Fat: 9.53g, Carbs: 27.28g, Protein: 3.11g

768. Potato Fries with Bean Sprouts & Peanut Herb Salad

Cooking Time: 20 minutes

Servings: 4

INGREDIENTS

- 2cups potato (cut into strips
- ¾ cup bean sprouts
- 2tablespoons parsley leaves, chopped
- 2tablespoons basil leaves, chopped
- 1teaspoon, pepper
- 1teaspoon salt
- 1tablespoon Sriracha sauce
- ½ cup roasted peanuts
- 1tablespoon rice vinegar
- 2teaspoons olive oil

DIRECTIONS

2. Preheat your air-fryer to 390°Fahrenheit and then place potato fries into the air-fryer basket. Spray a teaspoon of olive oil and season with salt. Cook for 15-minutes and shake basket a few times during cook time. After potato fries are cooked, save them for later use.
3. Prepare half a cup of peanuts. Preheat your air-fryer to 400°Fahrenheit and put half a cup of peanuts in the basket. Spray a teaspoon of olive oil and cook for 5-minutes. Once roasted, set aside.
4. Now, get a large mixing bowl, combine bean sprouts, chopped parsley, basil leaves in a bowl. Add the potato fries and roasted into a bowl. Season with Sriracha sauce and rice vinegar. Sprinkle with pepper. Toss and serve right away.

NUTRITION: Calories: 163, Total Fat: 0.7g, Carbs: 34.2g, Protein: 5.03g

769. Tuna with Roast Yams

Cooking Time: 30 minutes

Servings: 2

INGREDIENTS

- 2large yams
- 1green onion, finely sliced into rings
- 1can tuna, in oil, drained
- 2tablespoons greek plain yogurt
- ½ tablespoon olive oil
- 1teaspoon chili powder
- 1tablespoon capers
- 2tablespoons red onion diced for garnish

DIRECTIONS

1. Preheat your air-fryer to 300°Fahrenheit and brush the yams with olive oil and place them into the air-fryer basket. Cook yams for 20-minutes. Finely mash the tuna in a bowl, add yogurt, chili powder, and half of the green onions. Add salt and pepper to taste.
2. Place the yams on plates and cut them lengthwise. Place the fish blend onto the open yams. Sprinkle filling with capers and leftover green onion. Serve topped with diced red onion and with a crisp salad of your choice.

NUTRITION: Calories: 214, Total Fat: 3.2g, Carbs: 36.4g, Protein: 3.4

770. Air-Fried Ratatouille

Cooking Time: 15 minutes

Servings: 4

INGREDIENTS

- 1onion, peeled, cubed
- 1clove garlic, crushed
- 1tablespoon olive oil
- 2tomatoes, chopped
- Fresh ground pepper
- 2teaspoons Provencal herbs
- 1large zucchini, sliced
- 1yellow bell pepper, chopped

DIRECTIONS

1. Preheat your air-fryer to 300°Fahrenheit. In an oven-proof bowl, add vegetables, salt, pepper and olive oil and mix well. Put the bowl in the basket in air fryer. Cook for 15-minutes, stirring halfway through cook time. Serve with fricasseed meat.

Nutritional Values per serving: Calories: 154, Total Fat: 12.05g, Carbs: 11.94g, Protein: 1.69g

771. Toad in the Hole

Cooking Time: 30 minutes

Servings: 4

INGREDIENTS

- 1cup milk
- ½ cup cold water
- 1tablespoon basil, fresh sprigs
- 1red onion, finely sliced
- 1½ cups almond flour
- 8small sausages
- 1tablespoon olive oil
- 1clove of garlic, pressed

DIRECTIONS

1. Use an ovenproof dish that fits in your air-fryer and coat with oil. Sift the flour in a medium-sized bowl and beat the eggs into it. Gradually include the milk, water, the hacked onion and garlic and season to taste with salt and pepper. Combine everything. Pierce and stick the sprigs of basil into sausages and place into a dish. Pour the batter over sausages. Preheat your air-fryer to 300°Fahrenheit and cook for 30-minutes.

772. Glass Noodle & Tiger Shrimp Salad

Cooking Time: 8 minutes

Servings: 4

INGREDIENTS

- 12tiger shrimps, butterflied
- Zest of one lemon
- Zest of one lime
- ¼ cup olive oil
- 2tablespoons mixed spice

- 2 tablespoons olive oil
- A handful of basil, fried for garnish
- For the salad:
- 4 baby yellow bell peppers, sliced
- 4 baby red bell peppers, sliced
- 2 scallions, bias cut
- 2 cups green papaya, peeled, seeded, julienned
- ½ cup mint leaves
- ½ cup cilantro leaves
- 16-ounces of glass noodles, cooked and chilled
- 1 English cucumber, peeled, seeded, sliced
- 1 carrot, peeled and julienned
- 2 tablespoons basil leaves, julienned
- For dressing:
- 4-ounces of honey
- 2 cups grapeseed oil
- 1 cup soy sauce
- 4-ounces ginger, peeled and grated
- 1 bunch scallions, sliced
- 2 tablespoons of sweet chili sauce

DIRECTIONS

1. Preheat your air-fryer to 390°Fahrenheit for 10-minutes. Mix olive oil and mixed spice and brush mixture over shrimp. Sprinkle the lemon and lime juice over the shrimps. Season with salt and pepper. Place the shrimp in the basket and cook for 4-minutes. Chill shrimps on a plate and repeat cooking process with remaining shrimp. Whisk lemon juice, soy sauce, honey, ginger, scallion and sweet chili sauce in a bowl. Whisk in oil. Add mixture to blend and mix to get a puree consistency. Season to taste. In a bowl, toss mixed greens and salad dressing mix, along with noodles, then divide it between serving plates. Top each plate of salad with 3 shrimps. Garnish with cilantro and basil.

NUTRITION: Calories: 258, Total Fat: 15.89g, Carbs: 4.41g, Protein: 23.59g

773. Air-Fried Fingerling Potatoes

Cooking Time: 30 minutes

Servings: 4

INGREDIENTS

- 2 lbs. Fingerling potatoes, peeled, cubed
- 2 tablespoons chives, minced
- 2 tablespoons parsley leaves, minced
- 2 garlic cloves, smashed
- 2 tablespoons butter, melted
- 1 shallot, quartered

DIRECTIONS

1. Add cubed potatoes to an oven-proof dish. Brush potatoes with melted butter. Sprinkle with cubed potatoes the rest of ingredients. Set your air-fryer for 320°Fahrenheit and cook for 30-minutes. Stir a few times during cook time. Serve warm.

NUTRITION: Calories: 213, Total Fat: 5.2g, Carbs: 32.1g, Protein: 4.68g

774. Parmesan Chicken Meatballs

Cooking Time: 10 minutes

Servings: 4

INGREDIENTS

- ½ cup whole-wheat breadcrumbs
- Pepper and salt to taste
- ½ lime, zested
- 1/3 cup parmesan cheese, grated
- ½ teaspoon paprika
- 1 teaspoon basil, dried
- 3 garlic cloves, minced
- ½ lb. ground chicken
- 1/3 teaspoon mustard seeds
- 1½ tablespoons melted butter
- 2 eggs, beaten

DIRECTIONS

1. In a non-stick skillet that is preheated over medium heat, place ground chicken, garlic and cook until chicken is no longer pink, about 5-minutes.
2. Throw the remaining ingredients into skillet. Remove from heat. Allow to cool down and roll into balls. Roll each ball into beaten eggs, then roll them in breadcrumbs and transfer them into the air-fryer basket. Cook for 8-minutes at 385°Fahrenheit.

NUTRITION: Calories: 52, Total Fat: 2.46g, Carbs: 2.94g, Protein: 7.8g

775. Meatballs with Mediterranean Dipping Sauce

Cooking Time: 15 minutes

Servings: 4

INGREDIENTS

- For the meatballs:
- 1½ tablespoons melted butter
- 2 eggs
- ½ tablespoon red pepper flakes, crushed
- 2 tablespoons fresh mint leaves, finely chopped
- 4 garlic cloves, finely minced
- ½ lb. ground pork
- 2 tablespoons capers
- For the Mediterranean dipping sauce:
- 1/3 cup black olives, pitted, chopped finely
- 2 tablespoons fresh rosemary
- ½ teaspoon dill, dried
- 1/3 cup Greek yogurt
- ½ teaspoon lemon zest
- 2 tablespoons parsley

DIRECTIONS

1. Start the preheating of your air-fryer at 395°Fahrenheit. In a large bowl, add meatball ingredients and combine well. Shape into golf ball size balls. Cook the meatballs for about 9-minutes. Meanwhile, prepare your dipping sauce, by whisking all the ingredients. Serve meatballs warm with Mediterranean sauce.

NUTRITION: Calories: 52, Total Fat: 2.32g, Carbs: 3.04g, Protein: 7.45g

776. Mayo-Cheddar Jacket Potatoes

Cooking Time: 10 minutes

Servings: 8

INGREDIENTS

- 1/3 cup cheddar cheese, grated
- 3 tablespoons mayonnaise
- Sea salt, ground black pepper and cayenne pepper to taste
- 2 tablespoons chives, chopped
- 1½ tablespoons olive oil
- 8 Russet potatoes
- ½ cup soft cheese, softened

DIRECTIONS

1. Stab potatoes with a fork. Preheat your air-fryer to 360°Fahrenheit. Bake the potatoes for 10-minutes in the air-fryer basket. Meanwhile, prepare your filling by mixing the rest of the above ingredients. Stuff potatoes with the prepared filling. Serve immediately!

NUTRITION: Calories: 327, Total Fat: 7g, Carbs: 59g, Protein: 9.4g

777. Pork & Brie Meatballs

Cooking Time: 17 minutes

Servings: 8

INGREDIENTS

- 1 teaspoon cayenne pepper
- 2 teaspoons mustard
- Sea salt and black pepper to taste
- 1½ lbs. ground pork
- 2 small yellow onions, chopped
- 5 garlic cloves, minced
- 2 tablespoons Brie cheese, grated

DIRECTIONS

1. Mix all the above ingredients until all is well combined. Form into golf ball size balls. Cook at 375°Fahrenheit for 17-minutes.

NUTRITION Values per serving: Calories: 275, Total Fat: 18.6g, Carbs: 2.7g, Protein: 22.9g

778. Potato Chips & Tangy Dipping Sauce

Cooking Time: 18 minutes

Servings: 6

INGREDIENTS

- 1/3 teaspoon marjoram, dried
- 2 tablespoons garlic paste
- 1/3 cup sour cream
- 5 Russet potatoes, cut into fries
- 2½ tablespoons olive oil
- 1 teaspoon seasoned salt
- 1½ tablespoons mayonnaise
- 1/3 teaspoon red pepper flakes, crushed

DIRECTIONS

1. Soak the potatoes in water for 35-minutes; change the water a few times to remove the starch. Preheat your air-fryer to 325°Fahrenheit and cook fries for 18-minutes. Meanwhile, combine remaining ingredients to make a dipping sauce and enjoy it on the side!

NUTRITION: Calories: 326, Total Fat: 8.4g, Carbs: 57.5g, Protein: 7.5g

779. Beef Meatballs in Blueberry Chipotle Sauce

Cooking Time: 20 minutes

Servings: 4

INGREDIENTS

- 2 tablespoons Dijon mustard
- Salt and black pepper to taste
- 1 tablespoon herb vinegar
- ½ teaspoon cumin
- 1 teaspoon liquid stevia
- 1½ teaspoons garlic, minced
- ½ lb. ground beef
- 1/3 cup blueberry chipotle ketchup
- 2 tablespoons scallions, minced
- 1½ Worcestershire sauce

DIRECTIONS

1. In a large dish mix meat, cumin, scallions, salt, pepper, combine well. Form meatballs and cook them in your air-fryer at 375°Fahrenheit for 15-minutes. Meanwhile, add the other ingredients into a pan over medium heat and cook for 5-minutes. Add the meatballs to pan and stir, cook for an additional 5-minutes.

NUTRITION: Calories: 112, Total Fat: 8.28g, Carbs: 2.4g, Protein: 9.75g

780. Lemon Pepper Broccoli Crunch

Preparation time: 5 minutes

Cooking time: 6 Hours

Servings: 4

INGREDIENTS

- 4cups broccoli florets, chopped into bite sized pieces
- 1Tbsp olive oil
- 1tsp sea salt
- 1tsp lemon pepper seasoning

DIRECTIONS:

1. Preheat your air fryer to 135 degrees F.
2. Wash and drain the broccoli florets.
3. Place the broccoli in a large bowl and toss with the olive oil and sea salt.
4. Add the broccoli to the basket of your air fryer or spread them in a flat layer on the tray of your air fryer (either option will work!).
5. Cook in the air fryer for about 6 hours, tossing the broccoli every hour or so to cook evenly. Essentially, you will be dehydrating the broccoli.
6. Once the broccoli is fully dried, remove it from the air fryer, toss with the lemon pepper seasoning, and then let cool. It will keep crisping as it cools.
7. Enjoy fresh or store in an airtight container for up to a month.

NUTRITION: Calories 53, Total Fat 3g, Saturated Fat 0g, Total Carbs 3g, Net Carbs 1g, Protein 2g, Sugar 0g, Fiber 2g, Sodium 629mg, Potassium 0g

781. Sweet Broccoli Crunch

Preparation time: 5 minutes

Cooking time: 6 Hours

Servings: 4

INGREDIENTS

- 4cups broccoli florets, chopped into bite sized pieces
- 1Tbsp olive oil
- 1tsp sea salt
- 1tsp granulated erythritol

DIRECTIONS:

1. Preheat your air fryer to 135 degrees F.
2. Wash and drain the broccoli florets.
3. Place the broccoli in a large bowl and toss with the olive oil, erythritol, and sea salt.
4. Add the broccoli to the basket of your air fryer or spread them in a flat layer on the tray of your air fryer (either option will work!).
5. Cook in the air fryer for about 6 hours, tossing the broccoli every hour or so to cook evenly. Essentially, you will be dehydrating the broccoli.
6. Once the broccoli is fully dried, remove it from the air fryer and then let cool. It will keep crisping as it cools.
7. Enjoy fresh or store in an airtight container for up to a month.

NUTRITION: Calories 62, Total Fat 3g, Saturated Fat 0g, Total Carbs 5g, Net Carbs 2g, Protein 2g, Sugar 0g, Fiber 3g, Sodium 610mg, Potassium 0g

782. Maple Broccoli Crunch

Preparation time: 5 minutes

Cooking time: 6 Hours

Servings: 4

INGREDIENTS

- 4cups broccoli florets, chopped into bite sized pieces
- 1Tbsp olive oil
- 1tsp sea salt
- 1½ tsp maple extract

DIRECTIONS:

1. Preheat your air fryer to 135 degrees F.
2. Wash and drain the broccoli florets.
3. Place the broccoli in a large bowl and toss with the olive oil, maple extract, and sea salt.

4. Add the broccoli to the basket of your air fryer or spread them in a flat layer on the tray of your air fryer (either option will work!).
5. Cook in the air fryer for about 6 hours, tossing the broccoli every hour or so to cook evenly. Essentially, you will be dehydrating the broccoli.
6. Once the broccoli is fully dried, remove it from the air fryer and then let cool. It will keep crisping as it cools.
7. Enjoy fresh or store in an airtight container for up to a month.

NUTRITION: Calories 54, Total Fat 3g, Saturated Fat 0g, Total Carbs 3g, Net Carbs 1g, Protein 2g, Sugar 1g, Fiber 2g, Sodium 610mg, Potassium 0g

783. Veggie Crunch

Preparation time: 5 minutes

Cooking time: 6 Hours

Servings: 4

INGREDIENTS

- 2cups broccoli florets, chopped into bite sized pieces
- 2cups cauliflower florets, chopped into bite sized pieces
- 1Tbsp olive oil
- 1tsp sea salt

DIRECTIONS:

1. Preheat your air fryer to 135 degrees F.
2. Wash and drain the florets.
3. Place the florets in a large bowl and toss with the olive oil and sea salt.
4. Add the florets to the basket of your air fryer or spread them in a flat layer on the tray of your air fryer (either option will work!).
5. Cook in the air fryer for about 6 hours, tossing the florets every hour or so to cook evenly. Essentially, you will be dehydrating the veggies.
6. Once the florets is fully dried, remove it from the air fryer and then let cool. It will keep crisping as it cools.
7. Enjoy fresh or store in an airtight container for up to a month.

NUTRITION: Calories 53, Total Fat 3g, Saturated Fat 0g, Total Carbs 3g, Net Carbs 1g, Protein 2g, Sugar 0g, Fiber 2g, Sodium 610mg, Potassium 0g

784. Chili Lime Broccoli Crunch

Preparation time: 5 minutes

Cooking time: 6 Hours

Servings: 4

INGREDIENTS

- 4cups broccoli florets, chopped into bite sized pieces
- 1Tbsp olive oil
- 1tsp sea salt
- 1tsp lime zest
- 1Tbsp lime juice
- 1tsp chili powder

DIRECTIONS:

1. Preheat your air fryer to 135 degrees F.
2. Wash and drain the broccoli florets.
3. Place the broccoli in a large bowl and toss with the olive oil, lime juice, lime zest and sea salt.
4. Add the broccoli to the basket of your air fryer or spread them in a flat layer on the tray of your air fryer (either option will work!).
5. Cook in the air fryer for about 6 hours, tossing the broccoli every hour or so to cook evenly. Essentially, you will be dehydrating the broccoli.
6. Once the broccoli is fully dried, remove it from the air fryer, toss with the chili

powder, and then let cool. It will keep crisping as it cools.

7. Enjoy fresh or store in an airtight container for up to a month.

NUTRITION: Calories 62, Total Fat 3g, Saturated Fat 0g, Total Carbs 3g, Net Carbs 1g, Protein 2g, Sugar 1g, Fiber 2g, Sodium 647mg, Potassium 0g

785. Zucchini Chips

Preparation time: 15 minutes

Cooking time: 4 Hours

Servings: 8

INGREDIENTS

- 4cups very thin zucchini slices
- 2Tbsp olive oil
- 2tsp sea salt

DIRECTIONS:

1. Preheat your air fryer to 135 degrees F.
2. Toss the thin zucchini slices with the oil and sea salt.
3. Place the zucchini on the air fryer tray or in the air fryer basket.
4. Cook for 4 hours, tossing the zucchini occasionally to allow it to dehydrate evenly.
5. Once crisp, remove the zucchini from the air fryer and enjoy!

NUTRITION: Calories 40, Total Fat 4g, Saturated Fat 0g, Total Carbs 3g, Net Carbs 2g, Protein 1g, Sugar 2g, Fiber 1g, Sodium 570mg, Potassium 0g

786. Cayenne Zucchini Chips

Preparation time: 15 minutes

Cooking time: 4 Hours

Servings: 8

INGREDIENTS

- 4cups very thin zucchini slices
- 2Tbsp olive oil
- 2tsp sea salt
- 1tsp cayenne pepper

DIRECTIONS:

1. Preheat your air fryer to 135 degrees F.
2. Toss the thin zucchini slices with the oil, cayenne and sea salt.
3. Place the zucchini on the air fryer tray or in the air fryer basket.
4. Cook for 4 hours, tossing the zucchini occasionally to allow it to dehydrate evenly.
5. Once crisp, remove the zucchini from the air fryer and enjoy!

NUTRITION: Calories 42, Total Fat 4g, Saturated Fat 0g, Total Carbs 3g, Net Carbs 2g, Protein 1g, Sugar 2g, Fiber 1g, Sodium 575mg, Potassium 0g

787. Salt and Vinegar Zucchini Chips

Preparation time: 15 minutes

Cooking time: 4 Hours

Servings: 8

INGREDIENTS

- 4cups very thin zucchini slices
- 2Tbsp olive oil
- 2tsp sea salt
- 1Tbsp white balsamic vinegar

DIRECTIONS:

1. Preheat your air fryer to 135 degrees F.
2. Toss the thin zucchini slices with the oil, vinegar and sea salt.
3. Place the zucchini on the air fryer tray or in the air fryer basket.

4. Cook for 4 hours, tossing the zucchini occasionally to allow it to dehydrate evenly.
5. Once crisp, remove the zucchini from the air fryer and enjoy!

NUTRITION: Calories 42, Total Fat 4g, Saturated Fat 0g, Total Carbs 3g, Net Carbs 2g, Protein 1g, Sugar 2g, Fiber 1g, Sodium 570mg, Potassium 0g

788. Smoked Zucchini Chips

Preparation time: 15 minutes

Cooking time: 4 Hours

Servings: 8

INGREDIENTS

- 4cups very thin zucchini slices
- 2Tbsp olive oil
- 2tsp smoked sea salt

DIRECTIONS:

1. Preheat your air fryer to 135 degrees F.
2. Toss the thin zucchini slices with the oil and smoked sea salt.
3. Place the zucchini on the air fryer tray or in the air fryer basket.
4. Cook for 4 hours, tossing the zucchini occasionally to allow it to dehydrate evenly.
5. Once crisp, remove the zucchini from the air fryer and enjoy!

NUTRITION: Calories 40, Total Fat 4g, Saturated Fat 0g, Total Carbs 3g, Net Carbs 2g, Protein 1g, Sugar 2g, Fiber 1g, Sodium 570mg, Potassium 0g

789. Yellow Zucchini Chips

Preparation time: 15 minutes

Cooking time: 4 Hours

Servings: 8

INGREDIENTS

- 4cups very thin yellow zucchini slices
- 2Tbsp olive oil
- 2tsp sea salt

DIRECTIONS:

1. Preheat your air fryer to 135 degrees F.
2. Toss the thin zucchini slices with the oil and sea salt.
3. Place the zucchini on the air fryer tray or in the air fryer basket.
4. Cook for 4 hours, tossing the zucchini occasionally to allow it to dehydrate evenly.
5. Once crisp, remove the zucchini from the air fryer and enjoy!

NUTRITION: Calories 45, Total Fat 4g, Saturated Fat 0g, Total Carbs 3g, Net Carbs 2g, Protein 1g, Sugar 2g, Fiber 1g, Sodium 570mg, Potassium 0g

790. Soft Pretzels

Preparation time: 15 minutes

Cooking time: 14 minutes

Servings: 6

INGREDIENTS

- 2cups almond flour
- 1Tbsp baking powder
- 1tsp garlic powder
- 1tsp onion powder
- 3eggs
- 5tbsp softened cream cheese
- 3cups mozzarella cheese, grated
- 1tsp sea salt

DIRECTIONS:

1. Preheat your air fryer to 400 degrees F and prepare the air fryer tray with parchment paper.

2. Place the almond flour, onion powder, baking powder and garlic powder in a large bowl and stir well.
3. Combine the cream cheese and mozzarella in a separate bowl and melt in the microwave, heating slowly and stirring several times to ensure the cheese melts and does not burn.
4. Add two eggs to the almond flour mix along with the melted cheese. Stir well until a dough forms.
5. Divide the dough into six equal pieces and roll into your desired pretzel shape.
6. Place the pretzels on the prepared sheet tray.
7. Whisk the remaining eggs and brush over the pretzels then sprinkle them all with the sea salt.
8. Bake in the air fryer for 12 minutes or until the pretzels are golden brown.
9. Remove from the air fryer and enjoy while warm!

NUTRITION: Calories 449, Total Fat 36g, Saturated Fat 7g, Total Carbs 10g, Net Carbs 6g, Protein 28, Sugar 3g, Fiber 4g, Sodium 234mg, Potassium 48g

791. Soft Garlic Parmesan Pretzels

Preparation time: 15 minutes

Cooking time: 14 minutes

Servings: 6

INGREDIENTS

- 2cups almond flour
- 1Tbsp baking powder
- 1tsp garlic powder
- 1tsp onion powder
- 3eggs
- 5Tbsp softened cream cheese
- 3cups mozzarella cheese, grated
- 1tsp sea salt
- ½ tsp garlic powder
- ¼ cup parmesan cheese

DIRECTIONS:

1. Preheat your air fryer to 400 degrees F and prepare the air fryer tray with parchment paper.
2. Place the almond flour, onion powder, baking powder and 1 tsp garlic powder in a large bowl and stir well.
3. Combine the cream cheese and mozzarella in a separate bowl and melt in the microwave, heating slowly and stirring several times to ensure the cheese melts and does not burn.
4. Add two eggs to the almond flour mix along with the melted cheese. Stir well until a dough forms.
5. Divide the dough into six equal pieces and roll into your desired pretzel shape.
6. Place the pretzels on the prepared sheet tray.
7. Whisk the remaining eggs and brush over the pretzels then sprinkle them all with the sea salt, parmesan, and ½ tsp garlic powder.
8. Bake in the air fryer for 12 minutes or until the pretzels are golden brown.
9. Remove from the air fryer and enjoy while warm!

NUTRITION: Calories 493, Total Fat 39g, Saturated Fat 8g, Total Carbs 10g, Net Carbs 6g, Protein 28, Sugar 3g, Fiber 4g, Sodium 234mg, Potassium 48g

792. Soft Cinnamon Pretzels

Preparation time: 15 minutes

Cooking time: 14 minutes

Servings: 6

INGREDIENTS

- 2cups almond flour
- 1Tbsp baking powder

- 1 tsp salt
- 3 eggs
- 5 Tbsp softened cream cheese
- 3 cups mozzarella cheese, grated
- ½ tsp ground cinnamon

DIRECTIONS:

1. Preheat your air fryer to 400 degrees F and prepare the air fryer tray with parchment paper.
2. Place the almond flour, baking powder and salt in a large bowl and stir well.
3. Combine the cream cheese and mozzarella in a separate bowl and melt in the microwave, heating slowly and stirring several times to ensure the cheese melts and does not burn.
4. Add two eggs to the almond flour mix along with the melted cheese. Stir well until a dough forms.
5. Divide the dough into six equal pieces and roll into your desired pretzel shape.
6. Place the pretzels on the prepared sheet tray.
7. Whisk the remaining eggs and brush over the pretzels then sprinkle them all with the cinnamon.
8. Bake in the air fryer for 12 minutes or until the pretzels are golden brown.
9. Remove from the air fryer and enjoy while warm!

NUTRITION: Calories 432, Total Fat 34g, Saturated Fat 7g, Total Carbs 10g, Net Carbs 6g, Protein 28, Sugar 3g, Fiber 4g, Sodium 212mg, Potassium 48g

793. Soft Pecan Pretzels

Preparation time: 15 minutes

Cooking time: 14 minutes

Servings: 6

INGREDIENTS

- 2 cups almond flour
- 1 Tbsp baking powder
- 1 tsp garlic powder
- 1 tsp onion powder
- 3 eggs
- 5 Tbsp softened cream cheese
- 3 cups mozzarella cheese, grated
- 1 tsp sea salt
- ¼ cup chopped pecans

DIRECTIONS:

1. Preheat your air fryer to 400 degrees F and prepare the air fryer tray with parchment paper.
2. Place the almond flour, onion powder, baking powder and garlic powder in a large bowl and stir well.
3. Combine the cream cheese and mozzarella in a separate bowl and melt in the microwave, heating slowly and stirring several times to ensure the cheese melts and does not burn.
4. Add two eggs to the almond flour mix along with the melted cheese. Stir well until a dough forms.
5. Divide the dough into six equal pieces and roll into your desired pretzel shape.
6. Place the pretzels on the prepared sheet tray.
7. Whisk the remaining eggs and brush over the pretzels then sprinkle them all with the sea salt and chopped pecans
8. Bake in the air fryer for 12 minutes or until the pretzels are golden brown.
9. Remove from the air fryer and enjoy while warm!

NUTRITION: Calories 512, Total Fat 41g, Saturated Fat 10g, Total Carbs 10g, Net Carbs 6g, Protein 31g, Sugar 3g, Fiber 4g, Sodium 234mg, Potassium 48g

794. Soft Cheesy Pretzels

Preparation time: 15 minutes

Cooking time: 14 minutes

Servings: 6

INGREDIENTS

- 2cups almond flour
- 1Tbsp baking powder
- 1Tbsp grated parmesan cheese
- 1tsp garlic powder
- 3eggs
- 5Tbsp softened cream cheese
- 3cups mozzarella cheese, grated
- 1tsp sea salt
- ½ grated cheddar cheese

DIRECTIONS:

1. Preheat your air fryer to 400 degrees F and prepare the air fryer tray with parchment paper.
2. Place the almond flour, parmesan, baking powder and garlic powder in a large bowl and stir well.
3. Combine the cream cheese and mozzarella in a separate bowl and melt in the microwave, heating slowly and stirring several times to ensure the cheese melts and does not burn.
4. Add two eggs to the almond flour mix along with the melted cheese. Stir well until a dough forms.
5. Divide the dough into six equal pieces and roll into your desired pretzel shape.
6. Place the pretzels on the prepared sheet tray.
7. Whisk the remaining eggs and brush over the pretzels then sprinkle them all with the sea salt and the grated cheddar cheese.
8. Bake in the air fryer for 12 minutes or until the pretzels are golden brown.
9. Remove from the air fryer and enjoy while warm!

Snack

NUTRITION: Calories 513, Total Fat 40g, Saturated Fat 10g, Total Carbs 10g, Net Carbs 6g, Protein 28, Sugar 3g, Fiber 4g, Sodium 234mg, Potassium 48g

795. Sweet Zucchini Chips

Preparation time: 15 minutes

Cooking time: 4 Hours

Servings: 8

INGREDIENTS

- 4cups very thin zucchini slices
- 2Tbsp olive oil
- 2tsp sea salt
- 1Tbsp granulated erythritol

DIRECTIONS:

1. Preheat your air fryer to 135 degrees F.
2. Toss the thin zucchini slices with the oil, erythritol and sea salt.
3. Place the zucchini on the air fryer tray or in the air fryer basket.
4. Cook for 4 hours, tossing the zucchini occasionally to allow it to dehydrate evenly.
5. Once crisp, remove the zucchini from the air fryer and enjoy!

NUTRITION: Calories 40, Total Fat 4g, Saturated Fat 0g, Total Carbs 6g, Net Carbs 5g, Protein 1g, Sugar 4g, Fiber 1g, Sodium 570mg, Potassium 0g

796. Cucumber Chips

Preparation time: 15 minutes

Cooking time: 3 Hours

Servings: 4

INGREDIENTS

- 4cups very thin cucumber slices
- 2Tbsp apple cider vinegar
- 2tsp sea salt

DIRECTIONS:

1. Preheat your air fryer to 200 degrees F.
2. Place the cucumber slices on a paper towel and layer another paper towel on top to absorb the moisture in the cucumbers.
3. Place the dried slices in a large bowl and toss with the vinegar and salt.
4. Place the cucumber slices on a tray lined with parchment and then bake in the air fryer for 3 hours. The cucumbers will begin to curl and brown slightly.
5. Turn off the air fryer and let the cucumber slices cool inside the fryer (this will help them dry a little more).
6. Enjoy right away or store in an airtight container.

NUTRITION: Calories 15, Total Fat 0g, Saturated Fat 0g, Total Carbs 4g, Net Carbs 3g, Protein 1g, Sugar 2g, Fiber 1g, Sodium 34mg, Potassium 0g

797. Dill and Onion Cucumber Chips

Preparation time: 15 minutes

Cooking time: 3 Hours

Servings: 4

INGREDIENTS

- 4cups very thin cucumber slices
- 2Tbsp apple cider vinegar
- 2tsp sea salt
- 1tsp dried dill
- 1tsp ground onion powder

DIRECTIONS:

1. Preheat your air fryer to 200 degrees F.
2. Place the cucumber slices on a paper towel and layer another paper towel on top to absorb the moisture in the cucumbers.
3. Place the dried slices in a large bowl and toss with the vinegar, dried dill, onion powder and salt.
4. Place the cucumber slices on a tray lined with parchment and then bake in the air fryer for 3 hours. The cucumbers will begin to curl and brown slightly.
5. Turn off the air fryer and let the cucumber slices cool inside the fryer (this will help them dry a little more).
6. Enjoy right away or store in an airtight container.

NUTRITION: Calories 17, Total Fat 0g, Saturated Fat 0g, Total Carbs 4g, Net Carbs 3g, Protein 1g, Sugar 2g, Fiber 1g, Sodium 34mg, Potassium 0g

798. Smokey Cucumber Chips

Preparation time: 15 minutes

Cooking time: 3 Hours

Servings: 4

INGREDIENTS

- 4cups very thin cucumber slices
- 2Tbsp apple cider vinegar
- 2tsp smoked sea salt

DIRECTIONS:

1. Preheat your air fryer to 200 degrees F.
2. Place the cucumber slices on a paper towel and layer another paper towel on top to absorb the moisture in the cucumbers.
3. Place the dried slices in a large bowl and toss with the vinegar and salt.
4. Place the cucumber slices on a tray lined with parchment and then bake in the air fryer for 3 hours. The cucumbers will begin to curl and brown slightly.

5. Turn off the air fryer and let the cucumber slices cool inside the fryer (this will help them dry a little more).
6. Enjoy right away or store in an airtight container.

NUTRITION: Calories 18, Total Fat 0g, Saturated Fat 0g, Total Carbs 4g, Net Carbs 3g, Protein 1g, Sugar 2g, Fiber 1g, Sodium 34mg, Potassium 0g

799. Garlic Parmesan Cucumber Chips

Preparation time: 15 minutes

Cooking time: 3 Hours

Servings: 4

INGREDIENTS

- 4cups very thin cucumber slices
- 2Tbsp apple cider vinegar
- 2tsp sea salt
- 1tsp garlic powder
- ¼ cup parmesan cheese

DIRECTIONS:

1. Preheat your air fryer to 200 degrees F.
2. Place the cucumber slices on a paper towel and layer another paper towel on top to absorb the moisture in the cucumbers.
3. Place the dried slices in a large bowl and toss with the vinegar, garlic powder, parmesan, and salt.
4. Place the cucumber slices on a tray lined with parchment and then bake in the air fryer for 3 hours. The cucumbers will begin to curl and brown slightly.
5. Turn off the air fryer and let the cucumber slices cool inside the fryer (this will help them dry a little more).
6. Enjoy right away or store in an airtight container.

Snack

NUTRITION: Calories 34, Total Fat 1g, Saturated Fat 0g, Total Carbs 5g, Net Carbs 4g, Protein 1g, Sugar 3g, Fiber 1g, Sodium 34mg, Potassium 0g

800. Sea Salt and Black Pepper Cucumber Chips

Preparation time: 15 minutes

Cooking time: 3 Hours

Servings: 4

INGREDIENTS

- 4cups very thin cucumber slices
- 2Tbsp apple cider vinegar
- 2tsp sea salt
- 1Tsp ground black pepper

DIRECTIONS:

1. Preheat your air fryer to 200 degrees F.
2. Place the cucumber slices on a paper towel and layer another paper towel on top to absorb the moisture in the cucumbers.
3. Place the dried slices in a large bowl and toss with the vinegar, ground black pepper, and salt.
4. Place the cucumber slices on a tray lined with parchment and then bake in the air fryer for 3 hours. The cucumbers will begin to curl and brown slightly.
5. Turn off the air fryer and let the cucumber slices cool inside the fryer (this will help them dry a little more).
6. Enjoy right away or store in an airtight container.

NUTRITION: Calories 16, Total Fat 0g, Saturated Fat 0g, Total Carbs 4g, Net Carbs 3g, Protein 1g, Sugar 2g, Fiber 1g, Sodium 34mg, Potassium 0g

801. Taco Cucumber Chips

Preparation time: 15 minutes

Cooking time: 3 Hours

Servings: 4

INGREDIENTS

- 4cups very thin cucumber slices
- 2Tbsp apple cider vinegar
- 2tsp sea salt
- 2tsp taco seasoning

DIRECTIONS:

1. Preheat your air fryer to 200 degrees F.
2. Place the cucumber slices on a paper towel and layer another paper towel on top to absorb the moisture in the cucumbers.
3. Place the dried slices in a large bowl and toss with the vinegar, taco seasoning, and salt.
4. Place the cucumber slices on a tray lined with parchment and then bake in the air fryer for 3 hours. The cucumbers will begin to curl and brown slightly.
5. Turn off the air fryer and let the cucumber slices cool inside the fryer (this will help them dry a little more).
6. Enjoy right away or store in an airtight container.

NUTRITION: Calories 23, Total Fat 0g, Saturated Fat 0g, Total Carbs 4g, Net Carbs 3g, Protein 1g, Sugar 2g, Fiber 1g, Sodium 38mg, Potassium 0g

802. **Dilly Almonds**

Preparation time: 5 minutes

Cooking time: 10 minutes

Servings: 6

INGREDIENTS

- 1egg white
- 3cups whole almonds
- 2tsp salt
- 2tsp dried dill
- ½ tsp ground black pepper

DIRECTIONS:

1. Preheat your air fryer to 325 degrees F and prepare the air fryer tray with parchment paper.
2. Place the egg whites in a large bowl and whip until stiff peaks form.
3. Add the almonds and toss to coat.
4. Sprinkle with the seasonings and then place the almonds on the tray, laying them out as evenly as possible on the tray.
5. Bake in the air fryer for 10 minutes. The almonds should be golden brown.
6. Remove from the air fryer and let cool.

NUTRITION: Calories 414, Total Fat 34g, Saturated Fat 8g, Total Carbs 14g, Net Carbs 7g, Protein 14, Sugar 2g, Fiber 8g, Sodium 210mg, Potassium 0g

803. **Garlic Almonds**

Preparation time: 5 minutes

Cooking time: 10 minutes

Servings: 6

INGREDIENTS

- 1egg white
- 3cups whole almonds
- 2tsp salt
- 2tsp garlic powder
- ½ tsp ground black pepper

DIRECTIONS:

1. Preheat your air fryer to 325 degrees F and prepare the air fryer tray with parchment paper.
2. Place the egg whites in a large bowl and whip until stiff peaks form.
3. Add the almonds and toss to coat.

4. Sprinkle with the seasonings and then place the almonds on the tray, laying them out as evenly as possible on the tray.
5. Bake in the air fryer for 10 minutes. The almonds should be golden brown.
6. Remove from the air fryer and let cool.

NUTRITION: Calories 412, Total Fat 34g, Saturated Fat 8g, Total Carbs 14g, Net Carbs 7g, Protein 14, Sugar 2g, Fiber 8g, Sodium 212mg, Potassium 0g

804. Sweet and Salty Almonds

Preparation time: 5 minutes

Cooking time: 10 minutes

Servings: 6

INGREDIENTS

- 1 egg white
- 3 cups whole almonds
- 2 tsp salt
- 1 Tbsp swerve sweetener
- ½ tsp ground black pepper

DIRECTIONS:

1. Preheat your air fryer to 325 degrees F and prepare the air fryer tray with parchment paper.
2. Place the egg whites in a large bowl and whip until stiff peaks form.
3. Add the almonds and toss to coat.
4. Sprinkle with the salt, swerve and ground black pepper, and then place the almonds on the tray, laying them out as evenly as possible on the tray.
5. Bake in the air fryer for 10 minutes. The almonds should be golden brown.
6. Remove from the air fryer and let cool.

NUTRITION: Calories 409, Total Fat 34g, Saturated Fat 8g, Total Carbs 14g, Net Carbs 7g, Protein 14, Sugar 2g, Fiber 8g, Sodium 201mg, Potassium 0g

805. Cayenne Almonds

Preparation time: 5 minutes

Cooking time: 10 minutes

Servings: 6

INGREDIENTS

- 1 egg white
- 3 cups whole almonds
- 2 tsp salt
- 2 tsp cayenne pepper
- ½ tsp ground black pepper

DIRECTIONS:

1. Preheat your air fryer to 325 degrees F and prepare the air fryer tray with parchment paper.
2. Place the egg whites in a large bowl and whip until stiff peaks form.
3. Add the almonds and toss to coat.
4. Sprinkle with the seasonings and then place the almonds on the tray, laying them out as evenly as possible on the tray.
5. Bake in the air fryer for 10 minutes. The almonds should be golden brown.
6. Remove from the air fryer and let cool.

NUTRITION: Calories 414, Total Fat 34g, Saturated Fat 8g, Total Carbs 14g, Net Carbs 7g, Protein 14, Sugar 2g, Fiber 8g, Sodium 210mg, Potassium 0g

806. Black Pepper Almonds

Preparation time: 5 minutes

Cooking time: 10 minutes

Servings: 6

INGREDIENTS

- 1 egg white
- 3 cups whole almonds
- 2 tsp salt
- 1 tsp ground black pepper

DIRECTIONS:

1. Preheat your air fryer to 325 degrees F and prepare the air fryer tray with parchment paper.
2. Place the egg whites in a large bowl and whip until stiff peaks form.
3. Add the almonds and toss to coat.
4. Sprinkle with the salt and pepper and then place the almonds on the tray, laying them out as evenly as possible on the tray.
5. Bake in the air fryer for 10 minutes. The almonds should be golden brown.
6. Remove from the air fryer and let cool.

NUTRITION: Calories 414, Total Fat 34g, Saturated Fat 8g, Total Carbs 14g, Net Carbs 7g, Protein 14, Sugar 2g, Fiber 8g, Sodium 210mg, Potassium 0g

807. Sweet Candied Pecans

Preparation time: 5 minutes

Cooking time: 10 minutes

Servings: 6

INGREDIENTS

- 1 egg white
- 3 cups whole pecans
- 2 tsp salt
- 1 Tbsp swerve

DIRECTIONS:

1. Preheat your air fryer to 325 degrees F and prepare the air fryer tray with parchment paper.
2. Place the egg whites in a large bowl and whip until stiff peaks form.
3. Add the almonds and toss to coat.
4. Sprinkle with the swerve and salt and then place the almonds on the tray, laying them out as evenly as possible on the tray.
5. Bake in the air fryer for 10 minutes. The almonds should be golden brown.
6. Remove from the air fryer and let cool.

NUTRITION: Calories 409, Total Fat 34g, Saturated Fat 8g, Total Carbs 14g, Net Carbs 7g, Protein 14, Sugar 2g, Fiber 8g, Sodium 201mg, Potassium 0g

808. Garlicky Cauliflower Crunch

Preparation time: 5 minutes

Cooking time: 6 Hours

Servings: 4

INGREDIENTS

- 4 cups cauliflower florets, chopped into bite sized pieces
- 1 Tbsp olive oil
- 1 tsp sea salt
- 1 tsp garlic powder

DIRECTIONS:

1. Preheat your air fryer to 135 degrees F.
2. Wash and drain the cauliflower florets.
3. Place the cauliflower in a large bowl and toss with the olive oil and sea salt.
4. Add the cauliflower to the basket of your air fryer or spread them in a flat layer on the tray of your air fryer (either option will work!).
5. Cook in the air fryer for about 6 hours, tossing the cauliflower every hour or so to cook evenly. Essentially, you will be dehydrating the cauliflower.
6. Once the cauliflower is fully dried, remove it from the air fryer, toss it with

the garlic powder, and then let cool. It will keep crisping as it cools.
7. Enjoy fresh or store in an airtight container for up to a month.

NUTRITION: Calories 57, Total Fat 3g, Saturated Fat 0g, Total Carbs 4g, Net Carbs 3g, Protein 1g, Sugar 2g, Fiber 1g, Sodium 619mg, Potassium 320g

809. Cajun Cauliflower Crunch

Preparation time: 5 minutes

Cooking time: 6 Hours

Servings: 4

INGREDIENTS

- 4cups cauliflower florets, chopped into bite sized pieces
- 1Tbsp olive oil
- 1tsp sea salt
- 1tsp Cajun seasoning

DIRECTIONS:

1. Preheat your air fryer to 135 degrees F.
2. Wash and drain the cauliflower florets.
3. Place the cauliflower in a large bowl and toss with the olive oil and sea salt.
4. Add the cauliflower to the basket of your air fryer or spread them in a flat layer on the tray of your air fryer (either option will work!).
5. Cook in the air fryer for about 6 hours, tossing the cauliflower every hour or so to cook evenly. Essentially, you will be dehydrating the cauliflower.
6. Once the cauliflower is fully dried, remove it from the air fryer, toss with the Cajun seasoning, and then let cool. It will keep crisping as it cools.
7. Enjoy fresh or store in an airtight container for up to a month.

NUTRITION: Calories 59, Total Fat 3g, Saturated Fat 0g, Total Carbs 4g, Net Carbs 3g, Protein 1g, Sugar 2g, Fiber 1g, Sodium 621mg, Potassium 320g

810. Air Fried Red Cabbage, Garlic-flavored

Preparation Time: 25 Minutes

Servings: 4

INGREDIENTS

A. Seasoning- Salt and black pepper to the taste
B. Apple cider vinegar-1 tbsps
C. Chopped red cabbage-6 cups
D. Veggie stock-1 cup
E. Applesauce-1 cup
F. Olive oil-1 tbsps Chopped Yellow onion-½ cup
G. 4Minced garlic cloves

DIRECTIONS

1. Combine and mix cabbage with onion, garlic, oil, stock, vinegar, applesauce in a heatproof dish that fits into your 2. air fryer, seasoned with salt and pepper; toss well.
3. Transfer dish into your air fryer's basket and cook for 15minutes at a temperature of 380°F.
4. Share between plates and serve.

811. Healthy Italian Parmesan Mushrooms

Preparation Time: 25 Minutes

Servings: 3

INGREDIENTS

- Italian seasoning-1 tsp
- Melted butter-1 tbsps
- 1egg white
- Mushroom caps-9 button
- 3Crumbled cream cracker slices
- Grated Parmesan -2 tbsps
- Seasoning-A pinch of salt and black pepper

DIRECTIONS

1. Combine and mix crackers with egg white, parmesan, Italian seasoning, butter in a bowl, season with salt and pepper; stir well and stuff mushrooms with this mix
2. Place mushrooms in your air fryer's basket in an orderly manner, cook for 15minutes at a temperature of 360°F.
3. Share among plates and serve.

812. Sweet Tomatoes, Garlic-Herbed Dish

Preparation Time: 25 Minutes

Servings: 4

INGREDIENTS

- 4big tomatoes halved and insides scooped out
- 2minced garlic cloves
- Chopped thyme-½ tsp
- Olive oil-1 tbsps
- Seasoning- Salt and black pepper to the taste

DIRECTIONS

1. Combine and mix tomatoes with salt, pepper, oil, garlic, and thyme in your air fryer; toss well
2. At a temperature of 390°F, cook for 15 minutes. Share among plates and serve.

813. Sweet Potato Chips

Preparation Time: 60 Minutes

Servings: 4

INGREDIENTS

- Olive oil-1 tbsps
- Salt to taste
- 4potatoes scrubbed, peeled into thin chips, soaked in water for 30 minutes, drained and pat dried
- Chopped rosemary-2 tsp

DIRECTIONS

1. Combine and mix potato chips with salt and oil in a bowl toss to coat.
2. Transfer into your air fryer's basket and cook for 30minutes at a temperature of 330°F.
3. Share among plates; drizzle rosemary all over and serve.

814. Herbed Roasted Carrots

Preparation Time: 30 Minutes

Servings: 4

INGREDIENTS

- Orange juice-4 tbsps
- Baby carrots-1-lbs
- Olive oil-2 tsp
- Herbs de Provence-1 tsp

DIRECTIONS

1. Combine and mix carrots with herbs de Provence, oil and orange juice in your air fryer's basket, then toss well.
2. Cook for 20 minutes at a temperature of 320°F.
3. Share among plates and serve.

815. Awesome Barley Risotto Recipe

Preparation Time: 40 Minutes

Servings: 8

INGREDIENTS

- Veggie stock-5 cups
- Olive oil-3 tbsps
- 2Chopped yellow onions

Snack

- 2 Minced garlic cloves
- Chopped and peeled Sweet potato-2-lbss
- Barley-3/4-lbs
- Sliced mushrooms-3-ounce
- skim milk-2-ounces
- Seasoning -Salt and black pepper to the taste
- Dried Thyme-1 tsp
- Dried Tarragon-1 tsp

DIRECTIONS

1. Add stock in a pot, put barley, stir well, with medium temperature bring to a boil and cook for 15 minutes.
2. Heat up your air fryer at a temperature of 350°F, add oil and heat it up
3. Put the following ingredients: barley, onions, garlic, mushrooms, milk, salt, pepper, tarragon, and sweet potato, stir and cook for another 15 minutes.
4. Share among plates and serve.

816. Healthy Cauliflower and Broccoli

Preparation Time: 17 Minutes

Servings: 4

INGREDIENTS:

- 2 cauliflower heads florets separated and steamed
- 1 broccoli head florets separated and steamed
- Chopped capers-1 tbsps
- Juice from 1 orange
- A pinch of hot pepper flakes
- Seasoning -Salt and black pepper to the taste
- Olive oil-4 tbsps
- 4 anchovies
- Zest from 1 orange grated

DIRECTIONS

1. Combine and mix the orange zest with orange juice, pepper flakes, anchovies, capers salt, pepper and olive oil in a bowl, whisk well.
2. Put broccoli and cauliflower ensure it is tossed well.
3. Transfer into your air fryer's basket and cook for 7 minutes at a temperature of 400°F.
4. Share among plates, drizzle all over with some orange vinaigrette and serve.

817. Garlic-Herbed Mayonnaise Brussels Sprouts Dish

Preparation Time: 25 Minutes

Servings: 4

INGREDIENTS

- Mayonnaise-½ cup
- Brussels sprouts trimmed and halved -1-lbs
- Olive oil-6 tsp
- Chopped Thyme-½ tsp
- Seasoning-Salt and black pepper to the taste
- Crushed Roasted garlic -2 tbsps

DIRECTIONS

1. Combine and mix Brussels sprouts with salt, pepper, and oil in a clean bowl, toss well, cook for 15 minutes at a temperature of 390°F.
2. In a separate bowl, mix thyme with mayo and garlic and ensure it is well whisked.
3. Share Brussels sprouts between plates, sprinkle garlic sauce on top and serve.

818. Unusual Risotto Recipe

Preparation Time: 40 Minutes

Servings: 4

INGREDIENTS

- Dried Basil-1 tsp
- Dried oregano-1 tsp
- Rice-1 ½ Cups
- Olive oil-2 tbsps
- 2Chopped yellow onions.
- Beer-2 cups
- Chicken stock-2 cups
- Butter-1 tbsps
- Sliced mushrooms-1 cup
- Grated parmesan-½ cup

DIRECTIONS

1. Combine and mix oil with onions, mushrooms, basil and oregano in a dish that fits your air fryer and stirs well.
2. Add rice, beer, butter, stock, and butter; stir carefully again.
3. Transfer in your air fryer's basket and cook for 30minutes at a temperature of 350°F.
4. Share among plates, add grated parmesan on top and serve.

819. Lip-smacking Buttermilk-Biscuits

Preparation Time: 30 Minutes

Servings: 8

INGREDIENTS

- Buttermilk-1 ⅓ cup
- ½ cup butter+ 1 tbsps melted
- Self-rising flour-2 ⅓ cup
- Grated Cheddar cheese-½ cup
- Flour-1 cup
- Sugar-2 tbsps

DIRECTIONS

1. Combine and mix self-rising flour with ½ cup butter, sugar, cheddar cheese and buttermilk in a bowl, stir well until you obtain a dough

2. Prepare a clean working surface and spread 1 cup of flour on it, roll dough, flatten it, cut 8 circles with a cookie cutter and coat them with flour.
3. Line your air fryer's basket with tin foil, put biscuits, brush them with melted butter and cook for 20 minutes at a temperature of 380°F.
4. Share between plates and serve as a side dish.

820. Spicy Eggplant Dish

Preparation Time: 20 Minutes

Servings: 4

INGREDIENTS

- Tomato paste-1 tbsps
- 1green bell pepper chopped
- Chopped coriander-1 bunch
- Chopped Tomato- 1quantity
- A pinch of dried oregano
- 8baby eggplants; scooped in the center and pulp reserved
- Seasoning- Salt and black pepper to the taste
- Garlic powder-½ tsp
- Olive oil-1 tbsps
- Chopped yellow onion- 1 quantity

DIRECTIONS

1. With medium temperature, heat the oil in a pan, add onion; stir well and cook for 1 minute.
2. Seasoned with salt and pepper, add eggplant pulp, oregano, green bell pepper, tomato paste, garlic powder, coriander, and tomato; stir carefully, and cook for another 2 minutes more, put off heat and cool down.
3. Eggplants should be stuffed with this mix, transfer them in your air fryer's basket and cook for 8 minutes at a temperature of 360°F.

4. Share eggplants between plates and serve.

821. Lip-smacking Mushroom Recipe

Preparation Time: 20 Minutes

Servings: 6

INGREDIENTS

- Seasoning-Salt and black pepper to the taste
- 1green bell pepper chopped
- Mushrooms with stems removed – 24 quantity
- 1Grated carrot
- 2Chopped bacon strips
- 1yellow onion chopped
- Grated Cheddar cheese - 1 cup
- Sour cream-½ cup

DIRECTIONS

1. With medium-high temperature, heat up a pan add bacon, onion, bell pepper, and carrot; stir well and cook for 1 minute.
2. Put salt, pepper, and sour cream, stir well and cook for a minute more put off heat and cool down.
3. Mushrooms should be stuffed with this mix, drizzle cheese on top and cook for 8minutes at a temperature 360°F.
4. Share between plates and serve.

822. Simple Creamy Fried Potato Dish

Preparation Time: 1 hour and 30 Minutes

Servings: 2

INGREDIENTS

- Seasoning-Salt and black pepper to the taste
- 2bacon strips cooked and chopped
- Olive oil-1 tsp
- Big potato- 1 quantity
- Shredded cheddar cheese- 1/3 cup
- Butter-1 tbsps
- Chopped Green onions-1 tbsps
- Heavy cream-2 tbsps

DIRECTIONS

1. Polish potato with oil, season with salt and pepper, transfer in a preheated air fryer and cook for 30 minutes at a temperature of 400°F.
2. Flip potato on both sides, cook for another 30 minutes, transfer to a clean cutting board, cool it down then slice in half lengthwise and scoop pulp in a bowl
3. Put bacon, cheese, butter, heavy cream, green onions, then seasoned with salt and pepper, stir well and stuff potato skins with this mix.
4. Put potatoes back to your air fryer and cook for 20minutes at a temperature of 400°F.
5. Share between plates and serve.

823. Nice Veggie Fries Dish

Preparation Time: 40 Minutes

Servings: 4

INGREDIENTS

- Parsnips cut into medium sticks- 4 quantity
- 2sweet potatoes cut into medium sticks
- Chopped rosemary-2 tbsps
- Olive oil-2 tbsps
- Seasoning-Salt and black pepper to the taste
- 4mixed carrots cut into medium sticks
- Flour-1 tbsps
- Garlic powder-½ tsp

DIRECTIONS

1. In a bowl put veggie fries, add oil, garlic powder, seasoned with salts and pepper, add flour and rosemary, toss well to coat
2. In your preheated air fryer put sweet potatoes, cook them for 10 minutes at a temperature of 350°F and transfer into a platter.
3. Also, in your air fryer put parsnip, and cook for 5 minutes then transfer over potato fries.
4. More also, put carrot fries in your air fryer, cook for 15 minutes at a temperature of 350°F and transfer to the platter with the other fries.
5. Share veggie fries on plates and serve.

824. Enjoyable Green Beans Dish

Preparation Time: 35 Minutes

Servings: 4

INGREDIENTS

- 1½-lbs Green beans trimmed and steamed for 2 minutes
- Olive oil-2 tbsps
- Chopped Shallots-½-lbs
- Toasted Almonds-1/4 cup
- Seasoning-Salt and black pepper to the taste

DIRECTIONS

1. Mix green beans with salt, pepper, shallots, almonds, and oil in your air fryer's basket; toss well and cook for 25 minutes at a temperature of 400°F.
2. Share between plates and serve.

825. Healthy Cinnamon Roasted Pumpkin

Preparation Time: 22 Minutes

Servings: 4

INGREDIENTS

- A pinch of nutmeg ground
- Pumpkin de seeded, sliced and roughly chopped-1½ lbs
- 3garlic cloves; minced
- A pinch of brown sugar
- A pinch of sea salt
- Olive oil-1 tbsps
- A pinch of cinnamon powder

DIRECTIONS

1. Combine and mix, pumpkin with garlic, oil, salt, brown sugar, cinnamon and nutmeg in your air fryer's basket, toss well, cover and cook for 12minutes at a temperature of 370°F.
2. Share between plates and serve.

826. Cinnamon-Mayonnaise-Potato Fries

Preparation Time: 30 Minutes

Servings: 2

INGREDIENTS

- 2sweet potatoes peeled and cut into medium fries
- Mayonnaise -2 tbsps
- Ketchup-1/4 cup
- Olive oil-2 tbsps
- A pinch of ginger powder
- Cumin ground-½ tsp
- A pinch of cinnamon powder
- Curry powder-½ tsp
- Coriander ground-1/4 tsp
- Seasoning-Salt and black pepper to the taste

DIRECTIONS

1. Combine and mix sweet potato fries with salt, pepper, coriander, curry powder and oil in your air fryer's basket, toss well and

cook for 20minutes at a temperature of 370°F, flip potatoes once.
2. Meanwhile, in a separate bowl, mix ketchup with mayo, cumin, ginger, and cinnamon then whisk well.
3. Share fries on plates, sprinkle ketchup mix on top and serve.

827. Delicious Cauliflower Cakes

Preparation Time: 20 Minutes

Servings: 6

INGREDIENTS

- Parmesan; grated-½ cup
- 2eggs
- White flour-1/4 cup
- Cauliflower rice-3 ½ cups
- Seasoning-Salt and black pepper to the taste
- Cooking spray

DIRECTIONS

1. Mix cauliflower rice with salt and pepper in a bowl, stir well and squeeze excess water.
2. Put cauliflower into another bowl, put eggs, salt, and pepper, flour, and parmesan stir really well and shape your cakes.
3. Polish your air fryer with cooking spray, heat it up to a temperature of 400°F, put cauliflower cakes and cook for 10 minutes, flipping them halfway.
4. Share cakes on plates and serve.

828. Tasty Button Mushroom Dish Recipe

Preparation Time: 18 Minutes

Servings: 4

INGREDIENTS

- 10button mushrooms; stems removed
- Italian seasoning -1 tbsps
- Grated Cheddar cheese-2 tbsps
- Olive oil-1 tbsps
- Seasoning-Salt and black pepper to the taste
- Grated Mozzarella-2 tbsps
- Chopped dill-1 tbsps

DIRECTIONS

1. Combine and Mix mushrooms with Italian seasoning, seasoned with salt and pepper, oil and dill in a bowl and rub well.
2. Place mushrooms in your air fryer's basket in an orderly manner; sprinkle mozzarella and cheddar in each.
3. Cook them for 8minutes at a temperature of 360°F.
4. Share between plates and serve.

829. Sweet Buttermilk-Tomatoes

Preparation Time: 15 Minutes

Servings: 4

INGREDIENTS

- Creole seasoning-½ tbsps
- Flour -½ cup
- 2green tomatoes; sliced
- Seasoning-Salt and black pepper to the taste
- Cooking spray
- Buttermilk-1 cup
- Panko bread crumbs-1 cup

DIRECTIONS:

1. Tomato slices should be seasoned with salt and pepper.

2. In three separate bowl, Put flour in one; buttermilk in second and panko crumbs and Creole seasoning in a third one.
3. Tomato slices should be dredged in flour, then in buttermilk and panko bread crumbs.
4. Transfer into your air fryer's basket polished with cooking spray and cook for 5minutes at a temperature of 400°F.
5. Share among plates and serve.

830. Delicious Garlic Potatoes

Preparation Time: 30 Minutes

Servings: 6

INGREDIENTS

- Dried basil-½ tsp
- Dried oregano-½ tsp
- Chopped parsley-2 tbsps
- Olive oil-2 tbsps
- Seasoning-Salt and black pepper to the taste
- 5garlic cloves minced
- Butter-2 tbsps
- Grated parmesan-1/3 cup
- 3-lbs red potatoes; halved
- Dried thyme

DIRECTIONS

1. Combine and mix potato halves with parsley, garlic, basil, oregano, thyme, oil, butter, seasoned with salt and pepper in a bowl.
2. Toss the mixture really well and transfer to your air fryer's basket to cook.
3. Cover with lid and cook for 20 minutes with a temperature of 400°F, flipping them once and drizzle with parmesan on top.
4. Share potatoes between plates and serve.

831. Sweet Eggplant Dish with Garlic flavor

Preparation Time: 30 Minutes

Servings: 6

INGREDIENTS

- Onion powder-1 tsp
- Juice from ½ lemon
- 2bay leaves
- Garlic powder-1 tsp
- Olive oil-1 tbsps
- Cubed eggplant-1 ½-lbs
- Za'atar-2 tsp
- Sumac-1 tsp

DIRECTIONS

1. Combine and mixture eggplant cubes with oil, garlic powder, onion powder, sumac, za'atar, lemon juice, and bay leaves in your air fryer.
2. Toss well and cook for 20 minutes at a temp at a temperature of 370°F. Share among plates and serve.

832. Nice Cauliflower Healthy Dish

Preparation Time: 20 Minutes

Servings: 4

INGREDIENTS

- Turmeric powder-1/4 tsp
- Lemon juice-2 tsp
- Seasoning-Salt and black pepper to the taste
- Cooking spray
- Steamed florets-12 cauliflower
- White flour-3 tbsps
- Grated Ginger-1 tbsps
- Water - 2 tbsps
- Corn flour-½ tsp
- Red chili powder-1½ tsp

DIRECTIONS

1. Combine and mix chili powder with turmeric powder, ginger paste, salt, pepper, lemon juice, white flour, corn flour and water in a bowl, stir carefully.
2. Put cauliflower, toss well and transfer them to your air fryer's basket and Coat them with cooking spray.
3. Cook for 10 minutes at a temperature of 400°F. Share among plates and serve.

833. Sweet Cauliflower Rice Dish

Preparation Time: 50 Minutes

Servings: 8

INGREDIENTS

- 3garlic cloves; minced
- 1cauliflower head; riced
- 1Whisked egg
- Drained water chestnuts-9-ounce
- Peas-3/4 cup
- Grated Ginger-1 tbsps
- Juice from ½ lemon
- Soy sauce-4 tbsps
- Peanut oil-1 tbsps
- Sesame oil-1 tbsps
- Chopped mushrooms-15-ounce

DIRECTIONS

1. Combine and mix cauliflower rice with peanut oil, sesame oil, soy sauce, garlic, ginger and lemon juice in your air fryer; stir well.
2. Cover with lid and cook for 20 minutes at a temperature of 350°F.
3. Put chestnuts, peas, mushrooms, and egg; toss and cook for another 20 minutes at a temperature of 360°F.
4. Share among plates and serve for breakfast

834. Tasty Hassel-Back Potatoes

Preparation Time: 30 Minutes

Servings: 2

INGREDIENTS

- Sweet paprika-½ tsp
- Olive oil - 2 tbsps
- 2potatoes peeled and thinly sliced almost all the way horizontally
- Dried oregano-½ tsp
- Dried basil-½ tsp
- Minced Garlic-1 tsp
- Seasoning- Salt and black pepper to the taste

DIRECTIONS

1. Combine and mix oil with garlic, salt, pepper, oregano, basil, and paprika in a bowl and whisk really well
2. Grease potatoes with this mix, place them in your air fryer's basket and fry them for 20 minutes at a temperature of 360°F.
3. Share between plates and serve.

835. Easy Buttered-Mushroom Cakes

Preparation Time: 18 Minutes

Servings: 8

INGREDIENTS

- Flour-1 ½ tbsps
- Bread crumbs-1 tbsps
- Milk-14-ounces
- Chopped mushrooms-4-ounce
- 1yellow onion; chopped.
- Ground Nutmeg-½ tsp
- Olive oil-2 tbsps
- Butter-1 tbsps
- Seasoning-Salt and black pepper to the taste

DIRECTIONS:

1. With medium-high temperature, Heat up the butter in a pan, put onion and mushrooms; stir well, cook for 3 minutes, add flour then stir well again and put off the heat.
2. Put milk gradually, seasoned with salt, pepper, and nutmeg, stir carefully and set aside to cool down completely.
3. Mix oil with bread crumbs and whisk in a bowl.
4. A spoonful of the mushroom filling should be added to breadcrumbs mix, coat well, shape patties out of this mix.
5. Transfer them in your air fryer's basket and cook for 8 minutes at 400°F.
6. Share among plates and serve.

836. Delicious Beet Wedges Dish

Preparation Time: 25 Minutes

Servings: 4

INGREDIENTS

- 4beets washed, peeled and cut into large wedges
- Lemon juice-1 tsp
- Seasoning-Salt and black to the taste
- Olive oil-1 tbsps
- 2garlic cloves; minced

DIRECTIONS

1. Combine and mix beets with oil, salt, pepper, garlic and lemon juice in a bowl; toss well,
2. Place mixture in your air fryer's basket and cook for 15minutes at a temperature of 400°F.
3. Share beets wedges on plates and serve.

837. Tasty Roasted Peppers Dish

Preparation Time: 20 Minutes

Servings: 4

INGREDIENTS

- 1lettuce head; cut into strips
- Seasoning-Salt and black pepper to the taste
- Lemon juice-1 tbsps
- Greek yogurt-3 tbsps
- Olive oil-2 tbsps
- Yellow bell pepper-2 tbsps
- Red bell pepper – 1 Quantity
- Green bell pepper-1 Quantity
- Rocket leaves -1-ounce

DIRECTIONS

1. Transfer bell peppers in your air fryer's basket and cook for 10 minutes at a temperature of 400°F.
2. Transfer bell pepper into a bowl, set aside for 10 minutes, peel and discard seeds, cut them into strips, transfer to a larger bowl.
3. Add rocket leaves and lettuce strips and toss
4. In a separate bowl, combine and mix oil with lemon juice, yogurt, salt, and pepper, then whisk well. Put this over bell peppers mix, toss well to coat.
5. Share among plates and serve as a side salad.

838. Nice Vermouth-White Mushrooms Recipe

Preparation Time: 35 Minutes

Servings: 4

]

INGREDIENTS

- Olive oil-1 tbsps
- Herbs de Provence-2 tsp
- 2Minced garlic cloves.

- White mushrooms-2-lbs
- White vermouth-2 tbsps

DIRECTIONS

1. In your air fryer; Combine and mix oil with mushrooms, herbs de Provence and garlic in a bowl, then ensure its tossed well.
2. Cook for 20 minutes at a temperature of 350° F, add vermouth, toss and cook for another 5 minutes more.
3. Share among plates and serve as a side dish

839. Sweet Pumpkin Rice Dish

Preparation Time: 35 Minutes

Servings: 4

INGREDIENTS

- Allspice-½ tsp
- heavy cream-4-ounce
- Chicken stock-4 cups
- Pumpkin puree-6-ounce
- Olive oil-2 tbsps 2 garlic cloves; minced
- Nutmeg-½ tsp
- White rice-12-ounce
- Chopped thyme-1 tsp
- Grated ginger-½ tsp
- Cinnamon powder-½ tsp
- 1small yellow onion chopped

DIRECTIONS

1. Combine and mix oil with garlic, onion, stock, rice, pumpkin puree, nutmeg, ginger, thyme, cinnamon, allspice and cream in a dish that fits your air fryer, stir well.
2. Transfer dish in your air fryer's basket and cook for 30 minutes at 360°F.
3. Share among plates and serve.

Snack

840. Delicious Fried Creamy Cabbage

Preparation Time: 30 Minutes

Servings: 4

INGREDIENTS:

- 1green cabbage head chopped
- Whipped cream-1 cup
- 4bacon slices chopped.
- Seasoning-Salt and black pepper to the taste
- Cornstarch-2 tbsps
- 1yellow onion; chopped

DIRECTIONS

1. Put cabbage, bacon, and onion in your air fryer
2. Combine and mix cornstarch with cream, salt, and pepper in a bowl, stir well and add over cabbage. Toss carefully.
3. Cook for 20 minutes at a temperature of 400°F. Share among plates and serve.

841. Delicious Onion Rings Dish

Preparation Time: 20 Minutes

Servings: 3

INGREDIENTS

- White flour-1¼ cups
- Baking powder-1 tsp
- 1onion cut into medium slices and rings separated
- Egg- 1 quantity
- Milk-1 cup
- A pinch of salt
- Bread crumbs-3/4 cup

DIRECTIONS:

1. Combine and mix flour with salt and baking powder in a bowl, stir well.

2. Onion rings should be dredged in this mix and transfer them on a separate plate.
3. Put milk and egg to the flour mix and whisk well
4. Onion rings should be dipped in this mix, then they should be dredge in breadcrumbs, then place them in your air fryer's basket.
5. Cook for 10 minutes at a temperature of 360°F.
6. Share among plates and serve as a side dish for a steak

842. Pleasant Cajun Onion Wedges Dish

Preparation Time: 25 Minutes

Servings: 4

INGREDIENTS

- 2eggs
- Cajun seasoning -½ tsp
- Panko-1/3 cup
- A drizzle of olive oil
- Salt and black pepper to the taste
- 2big white onions; cut into wedges
- Milk-1/4 cup
- Paprika-1 ½ tsp
- Garlic powder-1 tsp

DIRECTIONS

1. Mix panko with Cajun seasoning and oil in a bowl and stir carefully.
2. In a separate bowl, Combine and mix the egg with milk, seasoned with salt and pepper then stir carefully again.
3. With paprika and garlic powder, drizzle onion wedges, dip them in egg mix, then in bread crumbs mix.
4. Place in your air fryer's basket, cook for 10 minutes at a temperature of 360°F. also, flip and cook for another 5 minutes.
5. Share among plates and serve as a side dish.

843. Sweet Tortilla Chips

Preparation Time: 16 Minutes

Servings: 4

INGREDIENTS

- A pinch of sweet paprika
- A pinch of garlic powder
- 8 corn tortillas; cut into triangles
- Olive oil-1 tbsps
- Salt and black pepper to the taste

DIRECTIONS

1. Combine and mix tortilla chips with oil, add salt, pepper, garlic powder, and paprika in a bowl, Carefully.
2. Transfer to your air fryer's basket and cook for 6 minutes at a temperature of 400°F.
3. Share among plates then Serve them as a side for a fish dish

844. Rice and Sausage Dish Recipe

Preparation Time: 30 Minutes
Servings: 4

INGREDIENTS

- Already Boiled White rice -2 cups
- Butter-1 tbsps
- 4garlic cloves; minced
- Grated cheddar cheese-3 tbsps
- 1pork sausage chopped
- Seasoning-Salt and black pepper to the taste
- Chopped carrot-2 tbsps
- Shredded mozzarella cheese-2 tbsps

DIRECTIONS

1. Ensure your air fryer is heated up to a temperature of 350°F, put butter, melt it, then add garlic, stir carefully and brown for 2 minutes.

2. Put the following ingredients; sausage, salt, pepper, carrots and rice; stir and also cook for 10 minutes at 350°F.
3. Lastly, put cheddar and mozzarella, toss well, then share among plates and serve as a side dish.

845. Coconut-Potatoes Recipes

Preparation Time: 30 Minutes
Servings: 4

INGREDIENTS
- 2Whisked eggs
- Grated cheddar cheese
- Coconut cream-4-ounce
- Seasoning-Salt and black pepper to the taste
- Flour-1 tbsps
- 2Sliced potatoes

DIRECTIONS
1. In your air fryer's basket, put potato slices and cook for 10 minutes at a temperature of 360°F.
2. In a clean bowl, Combine and mix eggs with coconut cream, salt, pepper, and flour.
3. Put potatoes in your air fryer's pan in an orderly manner, put coconut cream mix over them, then sprinkle cheese all over.
4. Transfer to air fryer's basket and cook for another 10 minutes at a temperature of 400°F.
5. Share among plates then serve.

846. Sweet Glazed Beets Recipe

Preparation Time: 50 Minutes
Servings: 8

INGREDIENTS
- Trimmed Small beets-3-lbss
- Duck fat-1 tbsps
- Maple syrup-4 tbsps

DIRECTIONS
1. Preheat your air fryer at a temperature of 360°F, put duck fat and heat up.
2. Put beets and maple syrup, then toss carefully.
3. Cook for 40 minutes, then share among plates and serve.

847. Veggie Rice Recipe

Preparation Time: 35 Minutes
Servings: 4

INGREDIENTS
- Cumin seeds-1 tbsps
- Butter-2 tbsps
- 1tsp cinnamon powder
- Sugar-1 tbsps
- Bay leaves-2 quantity
- Water-2 cups
- Minced Green chili-½ tsp
- Grated ginger-½ tsp
- Black peppercorns- 5 quantity
- 2whole cardamoms
- 3whole cloves
- 3garlic cloves minced
- Salt to the taste
- 1cup mixed carrots peas, corn, and green beans
- Basmati rice-2 cups

DIRECTIONS
1. In a heatproof dish that fits your air fryer, pour the water.
2. Put rice and the following ingredients; mixed veggies, green chili, grated ginger, garlic cloves, cinnamon, cloves, butter, cumin seeds, bay leaves, cardamoms, black peppercorns, seasoned with salt and sugar; stir carefully, then put in your air fryer's basket and cook for 25 minutes at a temperature of 370°F.
3. Share among plates and serve.

DESSERTS

848. Ginger Cookies Cheesecake

Preparation time: 15 minutes

Cooking time: 15 minutes

Servings: 6

INGREDIENTS

- 2cups water, for the pressure cooker
- 2teaspoons butter, melted
- ½ cup ginger cookies, crumbled
- 16ounces cream cheese, soft
- 2eggs
- ½ cup sugar

DIRECTIONS

1. Grease a cake pan with the butter, add cookie crumbs and spread them evenly.
2. In a bowl, beat cream cheese with a mixer.
3. Add eggs and sugar and stir very well.
4. Add the water to your pressure cooker, add steamer basket, add cake pan inside, cover and cook on High for 15 minutes.
5. Keep cheesecake in the fridge for a few hours before serving it.

NUTRITION: Calories 394, Fat 12, Fiber 3, Carbs 20, Protein

849. Winter Cherry Mix

Preparation time: 10 minutes

Cooking time: 5 minutes

Servings: 6

INGREDIENTS

- 16ounces cherries, pitted
- 2tablespoons water
- 2tablespoons lemon juice
- Sugar to the taste
- 2tablespoons cornstarch

DIRECTIONS

1. In your pressure cooker, mix cherries with sugar and lemon juice, stir, cover and cook on High for 3 minutes.
2. In a bowl, mix water with cornstarch, stir well, add to the pot, set the cooker on sauté mode, add the rest of the cherries, stir, cook for 2 minutes, divide into bowls and serve cold.

NUTRITION: Calories 161, Fat 4, Fiber 2, Carbs 8, Protein

850. Carrot Pudding and Rum Sauce

Preparation time: 10 minutes

Cooking time: 1 hour and 10 minutes

Servings: 2

INGREDIENTS

- 1and ½ cups water
- Cooking spray
- 2tablespoons brown sugar
- 1egg
- 2tablespoons molasses
- 2tablespoon flour
- A pinch of allspice
- A pinch of cinnamon powder
- A pinch of nutmeg, ground
- ¼ teaspoon baking soda
- 1/3 cup shortening, grated
- 3tablespoons pecans, chopped
- 3tablespoons carrots, grated
- 3tablespoons raisins
- ½ cup bread crumbs
- For the sauce:

- 1 and ½ tablespoons butter
- 2 tablespoons brown sugar
- 2 tablespoons heavy cream
- ½ tablespoons rum
- A pinch of cinnamon powder

DIRECTIONS

1. In a bowl, mix molasses with eggs and 2 tablespoons sugar, flour, shortening, carrots, nuts, raisins, bread crumbs, salt, a pinch of cinnamon, allspice, nutmeg and baking soda, stir everything, pour into a pudding pan greased with cooking spray and cover with tin foil. Add the water to your pressure cooker, add the steamer basket, add pudding inside, cover and cook on High 1 hour. Meanwhile, heat up a pan with the butter for the sauce over medium heat, add 2 tablespoons sugar, stir and cook for 2 minutes. Add cream, rum and a pinch of cinnamon, stir and simmer for 2 minutes more.
2. Divide pudding into 2 bowls, drizzle rum sauce all over and serve.

NUTRITION: Calories 261, Fat 6, Fiber 6, Carbs 10, Protein

851. Lemon Pudding

Preparation time: 30 minutes

Cooking time: 10 minutes

Servings: 2

INGREDIENTS

- ½ cup milk
- Zest from ½ lemon, grated
- 3 egg yolks
- ½ cup fresh cream
- 1 cup water
- 3 tablespoons sugar
- Blackberry syrup for serving

DIRECTIONS

1. Heat up a pan over medium heat, add milk, lemon zest and cream, stir, bring to a boil, take off heat and leave aside for 30 minutes.
2. In a bowl, mix egg yolks with sugar and cream mix, stir well, pour into your 2 greased ramekins and cover with tin foil.
3. Add the water to your pressure cooker, add the steamer basket, add ramekins, cover and cook on High for 10 minutes.
4. Serve with blackberry syrup on top.

NUTRITION: Calories 162, Fat 2, Fiber 2, Carbs 8, Protein

852. Strawberry and Chia Marmalade

Preparation time: 10 minutes

Cooking time: 4 minutes

Servings: 6

INGREDIENTS

- 2 tablespoons chia seeds
- 4 tablespoons sugar
- 2 pounds strawberries, halved
- ½ teaspoon vanilla extract
- Zest of 1 lemon, grated

DIRECTIONS

1. In your pressure cooker, mix sugar with strawberries, vanilla extract, lemon zest and chia seeds, stir, cover and cook on High for 4 minutes.
2. Stir again, divide into cups and serve cold

NUTRITION: Calories 110, Fat 2, Fiber 2, Carbs 2, Protein

853. Lemon and Maple Syrup Pudding

Preparation time: 10 minutes

Cooking time: 5 minutes

Servings: 7

INGREDIENTS

- 3cups milk
- Juice of 2 lemons
- Lemon zest from 2 lemons, grated
- ½ cup maple syrup
- 2tablespoons gelatin
- 1cup water, for the pressure cooker

DIRECTIONS

1. In your blender, mix milk with lemon juice, lemon zest, maple syrup and gelatin, pulse really well and divide into ramekins.
2. Add the water to your pressure cooker, add steamer basket, add ramekins inside, cover and cook on High for 5 minutes.
3. Serve puddings cold.

NUTRITION: Calories 151, Fat 3, Fiber 2, Carbs 18, Protein

854. Sweet Corn Pudding

Preparation time: 10 minutes

Cooking time: 30 minutes

Servings: 2

INGREDIENTS:

- 6ounces canned creamed corn
- 2cups water
- 1cup milk
- 1and ½ tablespoons sugar
- 1egg, whisked
- 1tablespoon flour
- ½ tablespoon butter
- Cooking spray

DIRECTIONS

1. Put the water in your pressure cooker, set on Simmer mode and bring to a boil.
2. In a bowl, mix corn with eggs, milk, butter, salt, flour and sugar, stir well, pour into a heat proof dish greased with cooking spray and cover with tin foil
3. Add the steamer basket into the pot, add the pan, cover and cook on High for 20 minutes.
4. Divide into 2 bowls and serve cold.

NUTRITION: Calories 162, Fat 3, Fiber 2, Carbs 8, Protein

855. Apricot Jam

Preparation time: 10 minutes

Cooking time: 14 minutes

Servings: 2

INGREDIENTS

- 1pound apricots, stones removed and halved
- ½ pound white sugar
- 1orange, peeled and sliced
- 1teaspoon orange zest, grated
- ½ tablespoon butter
- ¼ teaspoon almond extract

DIRECTIONS

1. Put apricots in your food processor, pulse really well, transfer to your pressure cooker, add sugar, orange slices and orange zest, stir, set the cooker on sauté mode and boil the jam for 6 minutes.
2. Add butter and almond extract, cover, cook on High for 8 minutes, divide into 2 jars and serve cold

NUTRITION: Calories 180, Fat 0, Fiber 3, Carbs 3, Protein

856. Banana Cake

Preparation time: 10 minutes

Cooking time: 1 hour

Servings: 4

INGREDIENTS

- 1cup water, for the pressure cooker
- 1and ½ cups sugar
- 2cups flour
- 4bananas, peeled and mashed
- 1teaspoon cinnamon powder
- 1teaspoon nutmeg powder

DIRECTIONS

1. In a bowl, mix sugar with flour, bananas, cinnamon and nutmeg, stir, pour into a greased cake pan and cover with tin foil.
2. Add the water to your pressure cooker, add steamer basket, add cake pan, cover and cook on High for 1 hour.
3. Slice, divide between plates and serve cold.

NUTRITION: Calories 300, Fat 10, Fiber 4, Carbs 45, Protein

857. Pineapple Pudding

Preparation time: 10 minutes

Cooking time: 5 minutes

Servings: 8

INGREDIENTS

- 1tablespoon avocado oil
- 1cup rice
- 14ounces milk
- Sugar to the taste
- 8ounces canned pineapple, chopped

DIRECTIONS

1. In your pressure cooker, mix oil, milk and rice, stir, cover and cook on High for 3 minutes.
2. Add sugar and pineapple, stir, cover and cook on High for 2 minutes more.
3. Divide into dessert bowls and serve.

NUTRITION: Calories 154, Fat 4, Fiber 1, Carbs 14, Protein

858. Blueberry Jam

Preparation time: 10 minutes

Cooking time: 11 minutes

Servings: 2

INGREDIENTS

- ½ pound blueberries
- 1/3 pound sugar
- Zest from ½ lemon, grated
- ½ tablespoon butter
- A pinch of cinnamon powder

DIRECTIONS

1. Put the blueberries in your blender, pulse them well, strain, transfer to your pressure cooker, add sugar, lemon zest and cinnamon, stir, cover and simmer on sauté mode for 3 minutes.
2. Add butter, stir, cover the cooker and cook on High for 8 minutes.
3. Transfer to a jar and serve.

NUTRITION: Calories 211, Fat 3, Fiber 3, Carbs 6, Protein

859. Bread Pudding

Preparation time: 10 minutes

Cooking time: 20 minutes

Servings: 4

INGREDIENTS:

- 2egg yolks
- 1and ½ cups brioche cubed
- 1cup half and half
- ¼ teaspoon vanilla extract
- ½ cup sugar
- 1tablespoon butter, soft
- ½ cup cranberries
- 2cups water
- 3tablespoons raisins
- Zest from 1 lime, grated

DIRECTIONS

1. In a bowl mix, egg yolks with half and half, cubed brioche, vanilla extract, sugar, cranberries, raisins and lime zest, stir, pour into a baking dish greased with the butter and leave aside for 10 minutes.
2. Add the water to your pressure cooker, add the steamer basket, add the dish, cover and cook on High for 20 minutes.
3. Serve this cold.

NUTRITION: Calories 162, Fat 6, Fiber 7, Carbs 9, Protein

860. Coconut Cream and Cinnamon Pudding

Preparation time: 10 minutes

Cooking time: 10 minutes

Servings: 6

INGREDIENTS

- 2cups coconut cream
- 1teaspoon cinnamon powder
- 6tablespoons flour
- 5tablespoons sugar
- Zest of 1 lemon, grated
- 2cups water, for the pressure cooker

DIRECTIONS:

1. Set your pressure cooker on sauté mode, add coconut cream, cinnamon and orange zest, stir, simmer for a couple of minutes, transfer to a bowl and leave aside.
2. Add flour and sugar, stir well and divide this into ramekins.
3. Add the water to your pressure cooker, add steamer basket, add ramekins, cover pot, cook on Low for 10 minutes and serve cold.

NUTRITION: Calories 170, Fat 5, Fiber 2, Carbs 8, Protein 10

861. Plum Jam

Preparation time: 20 minutes

Cooking time: 8 minutes

Servings: 12

INGREDIENTS

- 3pounds plums, stones removed and roughly chopped
- 2tablespoons lemon juice
- 2pounds sugar
- 1teaspoon vanilla extract
- 3ounces water

DIRECTIONS

1. In your pressure cooker, mix plums with sugar and vanilla extract, stir and leave aside for 20 minutes
2. Add lemon juice and water, stir, cover and cook on High for 8 minutes.
3. Divide into bowls and serve cold.

NUTRITION: Calories 191, Fat 3, Fiber 4, Carb 12, Protein

862. Cranberry Bread Pudding

Preparation time: 10 minutes

Cooking time: 15 minutes

Servings: 2

INGREDIENTS

- 2 egg yolks
- 1 and ½ cups bread, cubed
- 1 cup heavy cream
- Zest from ½ orange, grated
- Juice from ½ orange
- 2 teaspoons vanilla extract
- ½ cup sugar
- 2 cups water
- 1 tablespoon butter
- ½ cup cranberries

DIRECTIONS

1. In a bowl, mix egg yolks with bread, heavy cream, orange zest and juice, vanilla extract, sugar, butter and cranberries, stir and pour into a baking dish.
2. Add the water to your pressure cooker, add the steamer basket, add baking dish, cover cooker and cook on High for 15 minutes.
3. Divide between 2 plates and serve cold.

NUTRITION: Calories 189, Fat 3, Fiber 1, Carbs 4, Protein

863. Apples and Pears Salad

Preparation time: 10 minutes

Cooking time: 15 minutes

Servings: 2

INGREDIENTS:

- 1 quart water
- 1 tablespoon sugar
- ½ pound mixed apples, pears and cranberries
- 3 star anise
- A pinch of cloves, ground
- 1 cinnamon sticks
- Zest from ½ orange, grated
- Zest from ½ lemon, grated

DIRECTIONS

1. Put the water, sugar, apples, pears, cranberries, star anise, cinnamon, orange and lemon zest and cloves in your pressure cooker, cover and cook on High for 15 minutes.
2. Discard cinnamon stick. Divide salad into 2 bowls and serve cold.

NUTRITION: Calories 83, Fat 0, Fiber 0, Carbs 0, Protein

864. Blueberry and Coconut Sweet Bowls

Preparation time: 10 minutes

Cooking time: 6 minutes

Servings: 1

INGREDIENTS

- 1 cup coconut milk
- 1 cup coconut, unsweetened and flaked
- 1 cup vanilla yogurt
- 1 cup blueberries
- 2 teaspoons sugar
- 1 and ½ cups water, for the pressure cooker

DIRECTIONS

1. In a heatproof dish, combine milk with coconut, yogurt, blueberries and sugar, stir well and cover with tin foil.
2. Put the water in your pressure cooker, add trivet, add dish, cover and cook on High for 6 minutes.

3. Divide into bowls and serve cold.

NUTRITION: Calories 142, Fat 2, Fiber 3, Carbs 4, Protein

865. Coconut Pancake

Preparation time: 10 minutes

Cooking time: 40 minutes

Servings: 4

INGREDIENTS

- 2cups self-raising flour
- 2tablespoons sugar
- 2eggs
- 1and ½ cups coconut milk
- A drizzle of olive oil

DIRECTIONS

1. In a bowl, mix eggs with sugar, milk and flour and whisk until you obtain a batter.
2. Grease your pressure cooker with the oil, add the batter, spread into the pot, cover and cook on Low for 40 minutes.
3. Slice pancake, divide between plates and serve cold.

NUTRITION: Calories 162, Fat 3, Fiber 2, Carbs 7, Protein

866. Apples and Red Grape Juice

Preparation time: 10 minutes

Cooking time: 10 minutes

Servings: 2

INGREDIENTS

- 2apples
- ½ cup natural red grape juice
- 2tablespoons raisins
- 1teaspoon cinnamon powder
- ½ tablespoons sugar

DIRECTIONS:

1. Put the apples in your pressure cooker, add grape juice, raisins, cinnamon and stevia, toss a bit, cover and cook on High for 10 minutes.
2. Divide into 2 bowls and serve.

NUTRITION: Calories 110, Fat 1, Fiber 1, Carbs 3, Protein

867. Strawberry Shortcakes

Preparation time: 20 minutes

Cooking time: 25 minutes

Servings: 2

INGREDIENTS

- Cooking spray
- 3tablespoons sugar
- 1cup white flour
- 1cup water
- ½ teaspoon baking powder
- ¼ teaspoon baking soda
- 3tablespoons butter
- ½ cup buttermilk
- 1egg, whisked
- 1and ½ tablespoons sugar
- 1cups strawberries, sliced
- ½ tablespoon rum
- ½ tablespoon mint, chopped
- ½ teaspoon lime zest, grated

DIRECTIONS

1. In a bowl, mix flour with 2 tablespoons sugar, baking powder and baking soda and stir.
2. In another bowl, mix buttermilk with egg, stir, add to flour mixture and whisk everything.

3. Spoon this dough into 2 jars greased with cooking spray and cover with tin foil.
4. Add the water to your pressure cooker, add the steamer basket inside, add jars, cover cooker and cook on High for 25 minutes.
5. Meanwhile, in a bowl, mix strawberries with 1 tablespoon sugar, rum, mint and lime zest and toss to coat
6. Divide strawberry mix on shortcakes and serve.

868. Coconut and Avocado Pudding

Preparation time: 2 hours

Cooking time: 2 minutes

Servings: 3

INGREDIENTS

- ½ cup avocado oil
- 4 tablespoons sugar
- 1 tablespoon cocoa powder
- 14 ounces canned coconut milk
- 1 avocado, pitted, peeled and chopped

DIRECTIONS

1. In a bowl, mix oil with cocoa powder and half of the sugar, stir well, transfer to a lined container, keep in the fridge for 1 hour and chop into small pieces.
2. In your pressure cooker, mix coconut milk with avocado and the rest of the sugar, blend using an immersion blender, cover cooker and cook on High for 2 minutes.
3. Add chocolate chips, stir, divide pudding into bowls and keep in the fridge until you serve it.

NUTRITION: Calories 140, Fat 3, Fiber 2, Carbs 3, Protein

869. Cocoa and Milk Pudding

Preparation time: 50 minutes

Cooking time: 3 minutes

Servings: 4

INGREDIENTS

- 1 and ½ cups water, for the pressure cooker + 2 tablespoons
- 2 tablespoons gelatin
- 4 tablespoons sugar
- 4 tablespoons cocoa powder
- 2 cups coconut milk, hot
- ½ teaspoon cinnamon powder

DIRECTIONS

1. In a bowl, mix milk with sugar, cinnamon and cocoa powder and stir well.
2. In a bowl, mix gelatin with 2 tablespoons water, stir well, add to cocoa mix, stir and divide into ramekins.
3. Add the water to your pressure cooker, add the steamer basket, add ramekins inside, cover and cook on High for 4 minutes.
4. Serve puddings cold.

NUTRITION: Calories 120, Fat 2, Fiber 1, Carbs 4, Protein

870. Caramel Pudding

Preparation time: 20 minutes

Cooking time: 20 minutes

Servings: 2

INGREDIENTS

- Cooking spray
- ½ teaspoon baking powder

- ½ cup white flour
- 2 tablespoons white sugar
- ¼ teaspoon cinnamon
- 2 tablespoons butter
- 4 tablespoons milk
- 3 tablespoons pecans chopped
- 1 and ½ cups water
- 3 tablespoons raisins
- 3 tablespoons orange zest, grated
- 3 tablespoons brown sugar
- 3 tablespoons orange juice
- Caramel topping

DIRECTIONS

1. In a bowl, mix flour with white sugar, baking powder and cinnamon and stir.
2. Add half of butter and milk and stir again well.
3. Add pecans and raisins, stir and pour into a pudding pan greased with cooking spray.
4. Heat up a small pan over medium high heat, add ½ cup water, orange juice, orange zest, the rest of the butter and the brown sugar, stir, bring to a boil for 2 minutes and pour over pudding.
5. Add 1 cup water to your pressure cooker, add the steamer basket, add pudding pan inside, cover and cook on High for 20 minutes.
6. Divide into 2 bowls and serve with caramel topping on top.

NUTRITION: Calories 194, Fat 3, Fiber 2, Carbs 6, Protein

871. Black Tea Cake

Preparation time: 10 minutes

Cooking time: 30 minutes

Servings: 2

INGREDIENTS

- 2 tablespoons black tea powder
- ½ cup milk
- 1 tablespoon butter
- 1 cup sugar
- 2 eggs
- 1 teaspoons vanilla extract
- 3 tablespoons coconut oil
- 2 cups flour
- ¼ teaspoon baking soda
- 2 cups water
- 1 teaspoon baking powder
- For the cream:
- 1 and ½ tablespoons honey
- 1 and ½ cups sugar
- ¼ cup butter, soft

DIRECTIONS

1. Put the milk and tea in a pot, warm it up over medium heat, take off the stove and leave aside to cool down.
2. In a bowl, mix 1 tablespoon butter with 1 cup sugar, eggs, oil, vanilla extract, baking powder, baking soda and 2 cups flour, stir everything really well and pour into a greased pan.
3. Add the water to your pressure cooker, add the steamer basket, add the cake pan, cover and cook on High for 30 minutes.
4. Meanwhile, in a bowl, mix honey with 1 and ½ cups sugar and ¼ cup butter and whisk well.
5. Spread this over cake, leave aside to cool down, divide between 2 plates and serve.

NUTRITION: Calories 150, Fat 4, Fiber 4, Carbs 6, Protein

872. Cinnamon Rolls

Preparation time: 2 hours

Cooking time: 15 minutes

Servings: 8

INGREDIENTS

- 1pound vegan bread dough
- ¾ cup coconut sugar
- 1and ½ tablespoons cinnamon powder
- 2tablespoons vegetable oil

DIRECTIONS

1. Roll dough on a floured working surface, shape a rectangle and brush with the oil.
2. In a bowl, mix cinnamon with sugar, stir, sprinkle this over dough, roll into a log, seal well and cut into 8 pieces.
3. Leave rolls to rise for 2 hours, place them in your air fryer's basket, cook at 350 degrees F for 5 minutes, flip them, cook for 4 minutes more and transfer to a platter.
4. Enjoy!

NUTRITION: Calories 170, Fat 1, Fiber 1, Carbs 7, Protein 6

873. Vegan Donuts

Preparation time: 10 minutes

Cooking time: 15 minutes

Servings: 4

INGREDIENTS

- 8ounces whole wheat flour
- 2tablespoons coconut sugar
- 1tablespoon flax meal mixed with 2 tablespoons water
- 2and ½ tablespoons vegetable oil
- 4ounces almond milk
- 1teaspoon baking powder

DIRECTIONS

1. In a bowl, mix 1 tablespoon oil with sugar, baking powder and flour and stir.
2. In a second bowl, mix flax meal with 1 and ½ tablespoons oil and milk and stir well.
3. Combine the 2 mixtures, stir, shape donuts from this mix, place them in your air fryer's basket and cook at 360 degrees F for 15 minutes.
4. Serve them warm.
5. Enjoy!

NUTRITION: Calories 210, Fat 12, Fiber 1, Carbs 12, Protein 4

874. Apple Cake

Preparation time: 10 minutes

Cooking time: 40 minutes

Servings: 6

INGREDIENTS

- 3cups apples, cored and cubed
- 1cup coconut sugar
- 1tablespoon vanilla extract
- 2tablespoons flax meal combined with 3 tablespoons water
- 1tablespoon apple pie spice
- 2cups whole wheat flour
- 1tablespoon baking powder
- 2tablespoons vegetable oil

DIRECTIONS

1. In a bowl mix flax meal with oil, apple pie spice, apples, vanilla and sugar and stir using your mixer
2. In another bowl, mix baking powder with flour and stir.
3. Combine the 2 mixtures, stir and pour into a springform pan.
4. Put springform pan in your air fryer and cook at 320 degrees F for 40 minutes

5. Slice and serve.
6. Enjoy!

NUTRITION: Calories 202, Fat 6, Fiber 7, Carbs 14, Protein 7

875. Orange Lava Cake

Preparation time: 10 minutes

Cooking time: 20 minutes

Servings: 3

INGREDIENTS

- 1 tablespoon flax meal combined with 2 tablespoons water
- 4 tablespoons coconut sugar
- 2 tablespoons olive oil
- 4 tablespoons almond milk
- 4 tablespoons whole wheat flour
- 1 tablespoon cocoa powder
- ½ teaspoon baking powder
- ½ teaspoon orange zest, grated

DIRECTIONS

1. In a bowl, mix flax meal with sugar, oil, milk, flour, cocoa powder, baking powder and orange zest, stir very well and pour this into a greased ramekin that fits your air fryer.
2. Add ramekin to your air fryer, cook at 320 degrees F for 20 minutes and serve warm.
3. Enjoy!

NUTRITION: Calories 191, Fat 7, Fiber 8, Carbs 13, Protein 4

876. Cinnamon Apples

Preparation time: 10 minutes

Cooking time: 10 minutes

Servings: 4

INGREDIENTS

- 2 teaspoons cinnamon powder
- 5 apples, cored and cut into chunks
- ½ teaspoon nutmeg powder
- 1 tablespoon maple syrup
- ½ cup water
- 4 tablespoons vegetable oil
- ¼ cup whole wheat flour
- ¾ cup old-fashioned rolled oats
- ¼ cup coconut sugar

DIRECTIONS

1. Put the apples in a pan that fits your air fryer, add cinnamon, nutmeg, maple syrup and water.
2. Add oil mixed with oats, sugar and flour, stir, spread on top of the apples, introduce in your air fryer, cook at 350 degrees F for 10 minutes and serve them warm.
3. Enjoy!

NUTRITION: Calories 180, Fat 6, Fiber 8, Carbs 19, Protein 12

877. Carrot and Pineapple Cinnamon Bread

Preparation time: 10 minutes

Cooking time: 45 minutes

Servings: 6

INGREDIENTS

- 5 ounces whole wheat flour
- ¾ teaspoon baking powder
- ½ teaspoon baking soda
- ½ teaspoon cinnamon powder
- ¼ teaspoon nutmeg, ground
- 1 tablespoon flax meal combined with 2 tablespoons water
- 3 tablespoons coconut cream
- ½ cup sugar

- ¼ cup pineapple juice
- 4 tablespoons sunflower oil
- 1/3 cup carrots, grated
- 1/3 cup pecans, toasted and chopped
- 1/3 cup coconut flakes, shredded
- Cooking spray

DIRECTIONS:

1. In a bowl, mix flour with baking soda and powder, salt, cinnamon and nutmeg and stir.
2. In another bowl, mix flax meal with coconut cream, sugar, pineapple juice, oil, carrots, pecans and coconut flakes and stir well.
3. Combine the two mixtures and stir well, pour into a springform pan greased with cooking spray, transfer to your air fryer and cook on 320 degrees F for 45 minutes.
4. Leave the cake to cool down, cut and serve it.
5. Enjoy!

NUTRITION: Calories 180, Fat 6, Fiber 2, Carbs 12, Protein 4

878. Cocoa and Coconut Bars

Preparation time: 10 minutes

Cooking time: 14 minutes

Servings: 12

INGREDIENTS

- 6 ounces coconut oil, melted
- 3 tablespoons flax meal combined with 3 tablespoons water
- 3 ounces cocoa powder
- 2 teaspoons vanilla
- ½ teaspoon baking powder
- 4 ounces coconut cream
- 5 tablespoons coconut sugar

DIRECTIONS

1. In a blender, mix flax meal with oil, cocoa powder, baking powder, vanilla, cream and sugar and pulse.
2. Pour this into a lined baking dish that fits your air fryer, introduce in the fryer at 320 degrees F, bake for 14 minutes, slice into rectangles and serve.
3. Enjoy!

NUTRITION: Calories 178, Fat 14, Fiber 2, Carbs 12, Protein 5

879. Vanilla Cake

Preparation time: 10 minutes

Cooking time: 25 minutes

Servings: 12

INGREDIENTS

- 6 tablespoons black tea powder
- 2 cups almond milk, heated
- 2 cups coconut sugar
- 3 tablespoons flax meal combined with 3 tablespoons water
- 2 teaspoons vanilla extract
- ½ cup vegetable oil
- 3 and ½ cups whole wheat flour
- 1 teaspoon baking soda
- 3 teaspoons baking powder

DIRECTIONS

1. In a bowl, mix heated milk with tea powder, stir and leave aside for now.
2. In a larger bowl, mix the oil with sugar, flax meal, vanilla extract, baking powder, baking soda and flour and stir everything really well.
3. Add tea and milk mix, stir well and pour into a greased cake pan.
4. Introduce in the fryer, cook at 330 degrees F for 25 minutes, leave aside to cool down, slice and serve it.

5. Enjoy!

Nutrition: Calories 180, Fat 4, Fiber 4, Carbs 6, Protein 2

880. Sweet Apple Cupcakes

Preparation time: 10 minutes

Cooking time: 20 minutes

Servings: 4

INGREDIENTS

- 4 tablespoons vegetable oil
- 3 tablespoons flax meal combined with 3 tablespoons water
- ½ cup pure applesauce
- 2 teaspoons cinnamon powder
- 1 teaspoon vanilla extract
- 1 apple, cored and chopped
- 4 teaspoons maple syrup
- ¾ cup whole wheat flour
- ½ teaspoon baking powder

DIRECTIONS

1. Heat up a pan with the oil over medium heat, add applesauce, vanilla, flax meal and maple syrup, stir, take off heat and cool down.
2. Add flour, cinnamon, baking powder and apples, whisk, pour into a cupcake pan, introduce in your air fryer at 350 degrees F and bake for 20 minutes.
3. Transfer cupcakes to a platter and serve them warm.
4. Enjoy!

NUTRITION: Calories 200, Fat 3, Fiber 1, Carbs 5, Protein 4

881. Orange Bread with Almonds

Preparation time: 20 minutes

Cooking time: 40 minutes

Servings: 8

INGREDIENTS

- 1 orange, peeled and sliced
- Juice of 2 oranges
- 3 tablespoons vegetable oil
- 2 tablespoons flax meal combined with 2 tablespoons water
- ¾ cup coconut sugar + 2 tablespoons
- ¾ cup whole wheat flour
- ¾ cup almonds, ground

DIRECTIONS

1. Grease a loaf pan with some oil, sprinkle 2 tablespoons sugar and arrange orange slices on the bottom.
2. In a bowl, mix the oil with ¾ cup sugar, almonds, flour and orange juice, stir, spoon this over orange slices, place the pan in your air fryer and cook at 360 degrees F for 40 minutes.
3. Slice and serve the bread right away.
4. Enjoy!

NUTRITION: Calories 202, Fat 3, Fiber 2, Carbs 6, Protein 6

882. Tangerine Cake

Preparation time: 10 minutes

Cooking time: 20 minutes

Servings: 8

INGREDIENTS:

- ¾ cup coconut sugar
- 2 cups whole wheat flour
- ¼ cup olive oil
- ½ cup almond milk
- 1 teaspoon cider vinegar
- ½ teaspoon vanilla extract
- Juice and zest of 2 lemons
- Juice and zest of 1 tangerine

DIRECTIONS

1. In a bowl, mix flour with sugar and stir.
2. In another bowl, mix oil with milk, vinegar, vanilla extract, lemon juice and zest, tangerine zest and flour, whisk very well, pour this into a cake pan that fits your air fryer, introduce in the fryer and cook at 360 degrees F for 20 minutes.
3. Serve right away.
4. Enjoy!

NUTRITION: Calories 210, Fat 1, Fiber 1, Carbs 6, Protein 4

883. Maple Tomato Bread

Preparation time: 10 minutes

Cooking time: 30 minutes

Servings: 4

INGREDIENTS

- 1 and ½ cups whole wheat flour
- 1 teaspoon cinnamon powder
- 1 teaspoon baking powder
- 1 teaspoon baking soda
- ¾ cup maple syrup
- 1 cup tomatoes, chopped
- ½ cup olive oil
- 2 tablespoon apple cider vinegar

DIRECTIONS

1. In a bowl, mix flour with baking powder, baking soda, cinnamon and maple syrup and stir well.
2. In another bowl, mix tomatoes with olive oil and vinegar and stir well.
3. Combine the 2 mixtures, stir well, pour into a greased loaf pan that fits your air fryer, introduce in the fryer and cook at 360 degrees F for 30 minutes.
4. Leave the cake to cool down, slice and serve.
5. Enjoy!

NUTRITION: Calories 203, Fat 2, Fiber 1, Carbs 12, Protein 4

884. Lemon Squares

Preparation time: 10 minutes

Cooking time: 30 minutes

Servings: 6

INGREDIENTS

- 1 cup whole wheat flour
- ½ cup vegetable oil
- 1 and ¼ cups coconut sugar
- 1 medium banana
- 2 teaspoons lemon peel, grated
- 2 tablespoons lemon juice
- 2 tablespoons flax meal combined with 2 tablespoons water
- ½ teaspoon baking powder

DIRECTIONS:

1. In a bowl, mix flour with ¼ cup sugar and oil, stir well, press on the bottom of a pan that fits your air fryer, introduce in the fryer and bake at 350 degrees F for 14 minutes.
2. In another bowl, mix the rest of the sugar with lemon juice, lemon peel, banana, and baking powder, stir using your mixer and spread over baked crust.
3. Bake for 15 minutes more, leave aside to cool down, cut into medium squares and serve cold.
4. Enjoy!

NUTRITION: Calories 140, Fat 4, Fiber 1, Carbs 12, Protein 1

885. Dates and Cashew Sticks

Preparation time: 10 minutes

Cooking time: 15 minutes

Servings: 6

INGREDIENTS

- 1/3 cup stevia
- ¼ cup almond meal
- 1 tablespoon almond butter
- 1 and ½ cups cashews, chopped
- 4 dates, chopped
- ¾ cup coconut, shredded
- 1 tablespoon chia seeds

DIRECTIONS

1. In a bowl, mix stevia with almond meal, almond butter, cashews, coconut, dates and chia seeds and stir well again.
2. Spread this on a lined baking sheet that fits your air fryer, press well, introduce in the fryer and cook at 300 degrees F for 15 minutes.
3. Leave mix to cool down, cut into medium sticks and serve.
4. Enjoy!

NUTRITION: Calories 162, Fat 4, Fiber 7, Carbs 5, Protein 6

886. Grape Pudding

Preparation time: 10 minutes

Cooking time: 40 minutes

Servings: 6

INGREDIENTS:

- 1 cup grapes curd
- 3 cups grapes
- 3 and ½ ounces maple syrup
- 3 tablespoons flax meal combined with 3 tablespoons water
- 2 ounces coconut butter, melted
- 3 and ½ ounces almond milk
- ½ cup almond flour
- ½ teaspoon baking powder

DIRECTIONS

1. In a bowl, mix the half of the fruit curd with the grapes stir and divide into 6 heatproof ramekins.
2. In a bowl, mix flax meal with maple syrup, melted coconut butter, the rest of the curd, baking powder, milk and flour and stir well.
3. Divide this into the ramekins as well, introduce in the fryer and cook at 200 degrees F for 40 minutes.
4. Leave puddings to cool down and serve!
5. Enjoy!

NUTRITION: Calories 230, Fat 22, Fiber 3, Carbs 17, Protein 8

887. Coconut and Pumpkin Seeds Bars

Preparation time: 10 minutes

Cooking time: 35 minutes

Servings: 4

INGREDIENTS:

- 1 cup coconut, shredded
- ½ cup almonds
- ½ cup pecans, chopped
- 2 tablespoons coconut sugar
- ½ cup pumpkin seeds
- ½ cup sunflower seeds
- 2 tablespoons sunflower oil
- 1 teaspoon nutmeg, ground
- 1 teaspoon pumpkin pie spice

DIRECTIONS

1. In a bowl, mix almonds and pecans with pumpkin seeds, sunflower seeds, coconut, nutmeg and pie spice and stir well.
2. Heat up a pan with the oil over medium heat, add sugar, stir well, pour this over nuts and coconut mix and stir well.

3. Spread this on a lined baking sheet that fits your air fryer, introduce in your air fryer and cook at 300 degrees F and bake for 25 minutes.
4. Leave the mix aside to cool down, cut and serve.
5. Enjoy!

NUTRITION: Calories 252, Fat 7, Fiber 8, Carbs 12, Protein 7

888. Chocolate Cookies

Preparation time: 10 minutes

Cooking time: 25 minutes

Servings: 12

INGREDIENTS

- 1 teaspoon vanilla extract
- ½ cup coconut butter, melted
- 1 tablespoon flax meal combined with 2 tablespoons water
- 4 tablespoons coconut sugar
- 2 cups flour
- ½ cup unsweetened vegan chocolate chips

DIRECTIONS

1. In a bowl, mix flax meal with vanilla extract and sugar and stir well.
2. Add melted butter, flour and half of the chocolate chips and stir everything.
3. Transfer this to a pan that fits your air fryer, spread the rest of the chocolate chips on top, introduce in the fryer at 330 degrees F and bake for 25 minutes.
4. Slice when it's cold and serve.
5. Enjoy!

NUTRITION: Calories 230, Fat 12, Fiber 2, Carbs 13, Protein 5

889. Cinnamon Bananas

Preparation time: 10 minutes

Cooking time: 15 minutes

Servings: 4

INGREDIENTS

- 3 tablespoons coconut butter
- 2 tablespoons flax meal combined with 2 tablespoons water
- 8 bananas, peeled and halved
- ½ cup corn flour
- 3 tablespoons cinnamon powder
- 1 cup vegan breadcrumbs

DIRECTIONS

1. Heat up a pan with the butter over medium-high heat, add breadcrumbs, stir and cook for 4 minutes and then transfer to a bowl.
2. Roll each banana in flour, flax meal and breadcrumbs mix.
3. Arrange bananas in your air fryer's basket, dust with cinnamon sugar and cook at 280 degrees F for 10 minutes.
4. Transfer to plates and serve.
5. Enjoy!

NUTRITION: Calories 214, Fat 1, Fiber 4, Carbs 12, Protein 4

890. Coffee Pudding

Preparation time: 10 minutes

Cooking time: 10 minutes

Servings: 4

INGREDIENTS

- 4 ounces coconut butter
- 4 ounces dark vegan chocolate, chopped

- Juice of ½ orange
- 1 teaspoon baking powder
- 2 ounces whole wheat flour
- ½ teaspoon instant coffee
- 2 tablespoons flax meal combined with 2 tablespoons water
- 2 ounces coconut sugar

DIRECTIONS

1. Heat up a pan with the coconut butter over medium heat, add chocolate and orange juice, stir well and take off heat.
2. In a bowl, mix sugar with instant coffee and flax meal, beat using your mixer, add chocolate mix, flour, salt and baking powder and stir well.
3. Pour this into a greased pan, introduce in your air fryer, cook at 360 degrees F for 10 minutes, divide between plates and serve.
4. Enjoy!

NUTRITION: Calories 189, Fat 6, Fiber 4, Carbs 14, Protein 3

891. Almond and Cocoa Cake

Preparation time: 10 minutes

Cooking time: 30 minutes

Servings: 8

INGREDIENTS:

- 1 and ½ cup stevia
- 1 cup flour
- ¼ cup cocoa powder + 2 tablespoons
- ½ cup chocolate almond milk
- 2 teaspoons baking powder
- 2 tablespoons canola oil
- 1 teaspoon vanilla extract
- 1 and ½ cups hot water
- Cooking spray

DIRECTIONS

1. In a bowl, mix flour with 2 tablespoons cocoa, baking powder, almond milk, oil and vanilla extract, whisk well and spread on the bottom of a cake pan greased with cooking spray.
2. In a separate bowl, mix stevia with the rest of the cocoa and the water, whisk well and spread over the batter in the pan.
3. Introduce in the fryer and cook at 350 degrees F for 30 minutes.
4. Leave the cake to cool down, slice and serve.
5. Enjoy!

NUTRITION: Calories 250, Fat 4, Fiber 3, Carbs 10, Protein 2

892. Blueberry Cake

Preparation time: 10 minutes

Cooking time: 30 minutes

Servings: 6

INGREDIENTS

- ½ cup whole wheat flour
- ¼ teaspoon baking powder
- ¼ teaspoon stevia
- ¼ cup blueberries
- 1/3 cup almond milk
- 1 teaspoon olive oil
- 1 teaspoon flaxseed, ground
- ½ teaspoon lemon zest, grated
- ¼ teaspoon vanilla extract
- ¼ teaspoon lemon extract
- Cooking spray

DIRECTIONS

1. In a bowl, mix flour with baking powder, stevia, blueberries, milk, oil, flaxseeds, lemon zest, vanilla extract and lemon extract and whisk well.

2. Spray a cake pan with cooking spray, line it with parchment paper, pour cake batter, introduce in the fryer and cook at 350 degrees F for 30 minutes.
3. Leave the cake to cool down, slice and serve.
4. Enjoy!

NUTRITION: Calories 210, Fat 4, Fiber 4, Carbs 10, Protein 4

893. Peach Cinnamon Cobbler

Preparation time: 10 minutes

Cooking time: 30 minutes

Servings: 4

INGREDIENTS

- 4cups peaches, peeled and sliced
- ¼ cup coconut sugar
- ½ teaspoon cinnamon powder
- 1and ½ cups vegan crackers, crushed
- ¼ cup stevia
- ¼ teaspoon nutmeg, ground
- ½ cup almond milk
- 1teaspoon vanilla extract
- Cooking spray

DIRECTIONS

1. In a bowl, mix peaches with coconut sugar and cinnamon and stir.
2. In a separate bowl, mix crackers with stevia, nutmeg, almond milk and vanilla extract and stir.
3. Spray a pie pan that fits your air fryer with cooking spray and spread peaches on the bottom.
4. Add crackers mix, spread, introduce into the fryer and cook at 350 degrees F for 30 minutes
5. Divide the cobbler between plates and serve.
6. Enjoy!

NUTRITION: Calories 201, Fat 4, Fiber 4, Carbs 7, Protein 3

894. Easy Pears Dessert

Preparation time: 10 minutes

Cooking time: 25 minutes

Servings: 12

INGREDIENTS

- 6big pears, cored and chopped
- ½ cup raisins
- 1teaspoon ginger powder
- ¼ cup coconut sugar
- 1teaspoon lemon zest, grated

DIRECTIONS

1. In a pan that fits your air fryer, mix pears with raisins, ginger, sugar and lemon zest, stir, introduce in the fryer and cook at 350 degrees F for 25 minutes.
2. Divide into bowls and serve cold.
3. Enjoy!

NUTRITION: Calories 200, Fat 3, Fiber 4, Carbs 6, Protein 6

895. Strawberry Cheesecake

Preparation time: 10 minutes

Cooking time: 20 minutes

Servings: 4

INGREDIENTS

- 2cups cream cheese, soft
- 1cup strawberries, chopped
- ½ teaspoon almond extract
- 2eggs, whisked
- 4tablespoons sugar
- 1cup graham cookies, crushed
- 2tablespoons butter, melted

DIRECTIONS

1. In a bowl, mix the cookies with the butter and press this on the bottom of a lined cake pan.
2. In a bowl, mix the cream cheese with the rest of the ingredients, whisk, spread this over the crust and cook your cheesecake in your air fryer at 310 degrees F for 20 minutes.
3. Cool the cheesecake down and keep in the fridge for a few hours before serving.

NUTRITION: Calories 195, Fat 12, Fiber 4, Carbs 20, Protein 7

896. Cherries and Rhubarb Bowls

Preparation time: 10 minutes

Cooking time: 25 minutes

Servings: 4

INGREDIENTS

- 2cups cherries, pitted and halved
- 1cup rhubarb, sliced
- 1cup apple juice
- 2tablespoons sugar
- ½ cup raisins.

DIRECTIONS

1. In a pan that fits your air fryer, combine the cherries with the rhubarb and the other ingredients, toss, cook at 330 degrees F for 35 minutes, divide into bowls, cool down and serve.

NUTRITION: Calories 212, Fat 8, Fiber 2, Carbs 13, Protein 7

897. Chocolate Chips Cream

Preparation time: 10 minutes

Cooking time: 15 minutes

Servings: 4

INGREDIENTS

- 1cup coconut cream
- 2tablespoons sugar
- 1tablespoon cocoa powder
- 1teaspoon cinnamon powder
- 1cup heavy cream
- 1cup chocolate chips

DIRECTIONS:

1. In a bowl, mix the cream with the sugar and the other ingredients, whisk and divide into 4 ramekins.
2. Put the ramekins in the air fryer, cook at 340 degrees F for 15 minutes and serve cold.

NUTRITION: Calories 190, Fat 2, Fiber 1, Carbs 6, Protein 3

898. Cinnamon Cream

Preparation time: 10 minutes

Cooking time: 20 minutes

Servings: 4

INGREDIENTS:

- 1cup cream cheese, soft
- 1cup coconut cream
- ½ cup heavy cream
- 3tablespoons sugar
- 1and ½ tablespoons cinnamon powder
- 2eggs, whisked

DIRECTIONS

1. In the air fryer's pan, combine the cream cheese with the cream and the other ingredients, whisk well, cook at 350 degrees F for 20 minutes, divide into bowls and serve warm.

NUTRITION: Calories 200, Fat 11, Fiber 2, Carbs 15, Protein 4

899. Pumpkin Bowls

Preparation time: 10 minutes

Cooking time: 15 minutes

Servings: 4

INGREDIENTS

- 2cups pumpkin flesh, cubed
- 1cup heavy cream
- 1teaspoon cinnamon powder
- 3tablespoons sugar
- 1teaspoon nutmeg, ground

DIRECTIONS

1. In a pan that fits your air fryer, combine the pumpkin with the cream and the other ingredients, introduce in the fryer and cook at 360 degrees F for 15 minutes.
2. Divide into bowls and serve.

NUTRITION: Calories 212, Fat 5, Fiber 2, Carbs 15, Protein 7

900. Mango and Pears Bowls

Preparation time: 10 minutes

Cooking time: 15 minutes

Servings: 4

INGREDIENTS

- 2pears, cored and cut into wedges
- 1cup mango, peeled and roughly cubed
- 1cup apple juice
- 1teaspoon nutmeg, ground
- ½ teaspoon cinnamon powder
- 2tablespoons sugar

DIRECTIONS

1. In the air fryer's pan, mix the pears with the mango and the other ingredients, put the pan in the machine and cook at 320 degrees F for 15 minutes.
2. Divide into bowls and serve warm.

NUTRITION: Calories 210, Fat 2, Fiber 1, Carbs 12, Protein 3

901. Plums and Pineapple Cookies

Preparation time: 10 minutes

Cooking time: 20 minutes

Servings: 4

INGREDIENTS

- 1cup almond flour
- ½ cup plums, pitted and chopped
- ½ cup pineapple, peeled and chopped
- ½ cup coconut cream
- 1tablespoon brown sugar
- 2eggs, whisked
- 2tablespoons butter, melted
- 1teaspoon baking powder

DIRECTIONS

1. In a bowl, mix the almond flour with the plums and the other ingredients and whisk.
2. Shape balls from this mix, flatten them a bit, place them in your air fryer's basket and cook at 360 degrees F for 20 minutes.
3. Serve the cookies warm.

NUTRITION: Calories 190, Fat 8, Fiber 1, Carbs 14, Protein 3

902. Apple Jam

Preparation time: 10 minutes

Cooking time: 25 minutes

Servings: 4

INGREDIENTS

- 1cup water
- ½ cup sugar
- 1pound apples, cored, peeled and chopped
- ½ teaspoon nutmeg, ground

DIRECTIONS

1. In a pan that fits your air fryer, mix the apples with the water and the other ingredients, toss, introduce the pan in the fryer and cook at 370 degrees F for 25 minutes.
2. Blend a bit using an immersion blender, divide into jars and serve.

NUTRITION: Calories 204, Fat 3, Fiber 4, Carbs 12, Protein 4

903. Pears Cake

Preparation time: 10 minutes

Cooking time: 25 minutes

Servings: 6

INGREDIENTS

- 1cup pears, peeled, cored and cubed
- 1cup almond flour
- 3eggs, whisked
- ½ cup heavy cream
- 3tablespoons sugar
- 1tablespoon lemon juice
- 1teaspoon vanilla extract

DIRECTIONS:

1. In a bowl, mix the pears with the flour and the other ingredients, stir, pour into a greased cake pan, introduce in the fryer and cook at 360 degrees F for 25 minutes.
2. Cool cake down, slice and serve.

NUTRITION: Calories 220, Fat 11, Fiber 3, Carbs 15, Protein 7

904. Yogurt and Pumpkin Cream

Preparation time: 10 minutes

Cooking time: 30 minutes

Servings: 4

INGREDIENTS

- 1cup yogurt
- 1cup pumpkin puree
- 2eggs, whisked
- 2tablespoons sugar
- ½ teaspoon vanilla extract

DIRECTIONS:

1. In a bowl, mix the yogurt with the pumpkin puree and the other ingredients, whisk well, pour into 4 ramekins, put them in the air fryer and cook at 370 degrees F for 30 minutes.
2. Cool down and serve.

NUTRITION: Calories 192, Fat 7, Fiber 7, Carbs 12, Protein 4

905. Raisins Rice Mix

Preparation time: 10 minutes

Cooking time: 25 minutes

Servings: 6

INGREDIENTS

- 1cup white rice
- 2cups coconut milk
- 3tablespoons sugar
- 1teaspoon vanilla extract
- ½ cup raisins

DIRECTIONS:

1. In the air fryer's pan, combine the rice with the milk and the other ingredients, introduce the pan in the fryer and cook at 320 degrees F for 25 minutes.
2. Divide into bowls and serve warm.

NUTRITION: Calories 132, Fat 6, Fiber 7, Carbs 11, Protein 7

906. Zucchini Bread

Preparation time: 10 minutes

Cooking time: 40 minutes

Servings: 8

INGREDIENTS

- 3tablespoons butter, melted
- 2tablespoons sugar
- 1teaspoon vanilla extract
- 1cup zucchinis, grated
- 2eggs, whisked
- 1teaspoon baking soda
- 2cups almond flour
- 1cup almond milk
- 1teaspoon almond extract

DIRECTIONS

1. In a bowl, mix the melted butter with the sugar and the other ingredients, stir, pour into a lined loaf pan, place the pan in the air fryer and cook at 340 degrees F for 40 minutes
2. Cool down, slice and serve.

NUTRITION: Calories 222, Fat 7, Fiber 8, Carbs 14, Protein 4

907. Orange Bowls

Preparation time: 10 minutes

Cooking time: 10 minutes

Servings: 4

INGREDIENTS

- 1cup oranges, peeled and cut into segments
- 1cup cherries, pitted and halved
- 1cup mango, peeled and cubed
- 1cup orange juice
- 2tablespoon sugar

DIRECTIONS

1. In the air fryer's pan, mix the oranges with the cherries and the other ingredients, toss and cook at 320 degrees F for 10 minutes.
2. Divide into bowls and serve cold.

NUTRITION: Calories 191, Fat 7, Fiber 3, Carbs 14, Protein 4

908. Maple Pears Mix

Preparation time: 10 minutes

Cooking time: 15 minutes

Servings: 4

INGREDIENTS

- 1pound pears, cored and cut into wedges
- 1teaspoon cinnamon powder
- ½ cup coconut cream
- ½ teaspoon nutmeg powder
- 1tablespoon maple syrup
- 2tablespoon sugar
- 1tablespoon coconut oil, melted

DIRECTIONS

1. In a pan that fits your air fryer, mix the pears with the cream and the other ingredients, toss, introduce the pan in the fryer and cook at 360 degrees F for 15 minutes.
2. Divide into bowls and serve.

NUTRITION: Calories 180, Fat 6, Fiber 8, Carbs 19, Protein 12

909. Carrot and Zucchini Cake

Preparation time: 10 minutes

Cooking time: 40 minutes

Servings: 6

INGREDIENTS

- 1 and ½ cups almond flour
- ½ cup carrots, peeled and grated
- ½ cup zucchinis, grated
- ½ teaspoon baking soda
- 2 eggs, whisked
- 3 tablespoons butter, melted
- 3 tablespoons sugar
- ½ cup coconut cream
- Cooking spray

DIRECTIONS

1. In a bowl, mix the flour with the zucchinis, carrots and the other ingredients except the cooking spray and whisk well.
2. Pour this into a cake pan that fits your air fryer greased with cooking spray, transfer to your air fryer, cook at 320 degrees F for 40 minutes, cool down, cut and serve it.

NUTRITION: Calories 200, Fat 6, Fiber 7, Carbs 12, Protein 4

910. Apples Cheesecake

Preparation time: 10 minutes

Cooking time: 25 minutes

Servings: 6

INGREDIENTS

- 2 tablespoons butter, melted
- 1 cup graham cookies, crumbled
- 1 cup apples, cored and cubed
- 1 cup cream cheese, soft
- 2 tablespoon sugar
- ½ teaspoon almond extract
- ½ teaspoon vanilla extract

DIRECTIONS

1. In a bowl, mix the melted butter with the graham cookies, stir and press on the bottom of a cake pan that fits the air fryer.
2. In a bowl, mix the rest of the ingredients, whisk, spread over the cookie crust, introduce in your air fryer and cook at 340 degrees F for 25 minutes.
3. Serve the cheesecake really cold.

NUTRITION: Calories 212, Fat 12, Fiber 6, Carbs 12, Protein 7

911. Strawberry Jam

Preparation time: 10 minutes

Cooking time: 25 minutes

Servings: 8

INGREDIENTS

- 1 pound strawberries, chopped
- 1 tablespoon lemon zest, grated
- 1 and ½ cups water
- ½ cup sugar
- ½ tablespoon lemon juice

DIRECTIONS

1. In the air fryer's pan, mix the berries with the water and the other ingredients, stir, introduce the pan in your air fryer and cook at 330 degrees F for 25 minutes.
2. Divide into bowls and serve cold.

NUTRITION: Calories 202, Fat 8, Fiber 2, Carbs 6, Protein 7

912. Caramel Cream

Preparation time: 10 minutes

Cooking time: 15 minutes

Servings: 4

INGREDIENTS

- 1cup heavy cream
- 3tablespoons caramel syrup
- ½ cup coconut cream
- 1tablespoon sugar
- ½ teaspoon cinnamon powder

DIRECTIONS

1. In a bowl, mix the cream with the caramel syrup and the other ingredients, whisk, divide into small ramekins, introduce in the fryer and cook at 320 degrees F and bake for 15 minutes.
2. Divide into bowls and serve cold.

NUTRITION: Calories 234, Fat 13, Fiber 4, Carbs 11, Protein 5

913. Cherry Squares

Preparation time: 10 minutes

Cooking time: 25 minutes

Servings: 12

INGREDIENTS:

- 4eggs, whisked
- 1cup cherries, pitted and chopped
- 1cup almond flour
- ½ cup cream cheese
- ½ cup coconut cream
- 1tablespoon sugar
- 2tablespoons cocoa powder
- 2teaspoons vanilla extract
- ½ teaspoon baking powder

DIRECTIONS

1. In a bowl, mix the eggs with the cherries and the other ingredients, whisk well, pour this into a lined baking dish that fits your air fryer, introduce in the fryer at 320 degrees F, bake for 25 minutes, cool down, cut into squares and serve.

NUTRITION: Calories 178, Fat 11, Fiber 3, Carbs 3, Protein 5

914. Sweet Walnut Mix

Preparation time: 10 minutes

Cooking time: 15 minutes

Servings: 4

INGREDIENTS

- 2cups walnuts
- 2tablespoons sugar
- ½ cup coconut cream
- 4tablespoons butter, melted
- ½ teaspoon vanilla extract
- ½ teaspoon cinnamon powder

DIRECTIONS

1. In your air fryer's pan, mix the walnuts with the cream and the other ingredients, toss, introduce in the fryer and cook at 320 degrees F and bake for 15 minutes.
2. Divide into bowls and serve.

NUTRITION: Calories 203, Fat 12, Fiber 1, Carbs 13, Protein 6

915. Creamy Blueberry Mix

Preparation time: 10 minutes

Cooking time: 15 minutes

Servings: 6

INGREDIENTS:

- 2cups blueberries
- 1teaspoon vanilla extract
- ½ cup heavy cream
- 3tablespoons sugar
- 2teaspoons almond extract

DIRECTIONS

1. In the air fryer's pan, mix the blueberries with the cream and the other ingredients, introduce it in the fryer and cook at 320 degrees F for 15 minutes.
2. Divide into bowls and serve cold.

NUTRITION: Calories 230, Fat 2, Fiber 2, Carbs 14, Protein 7

916. Butter Brownies

Preparation time: 10 minutes

Cooking time: 25 minutes

Servings: 10

INGREDIENTS

- 1cup butter, melted
- 2eggs, whisked
- ½ cup heavy cream
- 4tablespoons sugar
- 2cups almond flour
- ½ tablespoon cocoa powder

DIRECTIONS

1. In a bowl, mix the melted butter with the eggs and the other ingredients, whisk, spread this into a pan that fits your air fryer, introduce in the fryer and cook at 360 degrees F and bake for 25 minutes.

2. Cool down, cut into bars and serve.

NUTRITION: Calories 230, Fat 12, Fiber 2, Carbs 12, Protein 5

917. Mandarin Cake

Preparation time: 10 minutes

Cooking time: 35 minutes

Servings: 10

INGREDIENTS

- 6eggs, whisked
- 1cup mandarin, peeled and chopped
- 1teaspoon vanilla extract
- 1teaspoon baking soda
- 1and ½ cups almond flour
- 3tablespoons sugar
- 1cup heavy cream
- 1cup coconut cream

DIRECTIONS

1. In a bowl, mix the eggs with the mandarin and the other ingredients, whisk and pour into a cake pan lined with parchment paper.
2. Put the pan in the air fryer, cook at 360 degrees F for 35 minutes, cool down, slice and serve.

NUTRITION: Calories 231, Fat 13, Fiber 2, Carbs 11, Protein 5

918. White Chocolate Ramekins

Preparation time: 10 minutes

Cooking time: 20 minutes

Servings: 4

INGREDIENTS

- 1cup cream cheese, soft
- 3tablespoons sugar
- 3eggs, whisked

- ½ teaspoon vanilla extract
- ½ cup heavy cream
- 1 cup white chocolate, melted

DIRECTIONS

1. In a bowl, mix the cream cheese with the sugar and the other ingredients, whisk and divide into 4 ramekins.
2. Put them in the fryer, cook at 320 degrees F for 20 minutes, cool down and serve.

NUTRITION: Calories 261, Fat 12, Fiber 6, Carbs 12, Protein 6

919. Rhubarb Jam

Preparation time: 10 minutes

Cooking time: 25 minutes

Servings: 4

INGREDIENTS

- 1 pound rhubarb, sliced
- 1 and ½ cups water
- 1 cup sugar
- 1 teaspoon vanilla extract
- ½ teaspoon almond extract

DIRECTIONS:

1. In the air fryer's pan, mix the rhubarb with the water and the other ingredients, toss, introduce the pan in the air fryer and cook at 330 degrees F for 25 minutes.

2. Cool the jam down, divide into bowls and serve.

NUTRITION: Calories 214, Fat 9, Fiber 3, Carbs 14, Protein 8

920. Banana Cream

Preparation time: 10 minutes

Cooking time: 20 minutes

Servings: 4

INGREDIENTS

- 4 bananas, peeled and mashed
- 1 cup heavy cream
- 1 teaspoon almond extract
- 2 tablespoons sugar
- 2 tablespoons butter, melted

DIRECTIONS

1. In a bowl, mix the bananas with the cream and the other ingredients, whisk, divide into 4 ramekins, introduce them in the air fryer and cook at 340 degrees F for 20 minutes.
2. Cool the cream down and serve.

NUTRITION: Calories 200, Fat 5, Fiber 3, Carbs 13, Protein 7

921. Banana and Rice Bowls

Preparation time: 10 minutes

Cooking time: 25 minutes

Servings: 4

INGREDIENTS

- 1 cup white rice
- 2 cups coconut milk
- 2 bananas, peeled and mashed
- 1 teaspoon vanilla extract
- 1 teaspoon cinnamon powder
- 3 tablespoons sugar

DIRECTIONS

1. In the air fryer's pan, mix the rice with the milk and the other ingredients, introduce the pan in the air fryer and cook at 360 degrees F for 25 minutes.
2. Divide into bowls and serve.

NUTRITION: Calories 211, Fat 4, Fiber 6, Carbs 14, Protein 6

922. Lemon Mango Bowls

Preparation time: 10 minutes

Cooking time: 20 minutes

Servings: 4

INGREDIENTS

- 2 cups mango, peeled and roughly cubed
- Juice of 1 lemon
- ½ cup heavy cream
- 2 tablespoon sugar
- 1 tablespoon ginger, grated
- 1 teaspoon lemon zest, grated

DIRECTIONS

1. In the air fryer's pan, mix the mango with the lemon juice and the other ingredients, put the pan in the air fryer and cook at 320 degrees F for 20 minutes.
2. Divide into bowls and serve cold.

NUTRITION: Calories 213, Fat 5, Fiber 5, Carbs 15, Protein 6

923. Pear Stew

Preparation time: 10 minutes

Cooking time: 20 minutes

Servings: 4

INGREDIENTS

- 1 pound pears, cored and roughly cut into cubes
- 2 tablespoons sugar
- 1 cup apple juice
- 1 teaspoon almond extract

DIRECTIONS

1. In a pan that fits your air fryer, mix the pears with the sugar and the other ingredients, introduce the pan in the air fryer and cook at 300 degrees F for 20 minutes.
2. Divide into bowls and serve cold.

NUTRITION: Calories 200, Fat 3, Fiber 4, Carbs 16, Protein 4

924. Orange Jam

Preparation time: 10 minutes

Cooking time: 20 minutes

Servings: 6

INGREDIENTS

- 1 pound oranges, peeled and cut into segments
- 1 and ¼ cups white sugar
- 1 and ½ cups water
- 1 teaspoon vanilla extract

DIRECTIONS:

1. In a pan that fits your air fryer, mix the oranges with the sugar and the other ingredients, whisk, introduce in the fryer and cook at 320 degrees F for 20 minutes.
2. Divide the jam into bowls and serve cold.

NUTRITION: Calories 171, Fat 1, Fiber 4, Carbs 8, Protein 2

925. Baked Apples and Pears

Preparation time: 10 minutes

Cooking time: 20 minutes

Servings: 4

Desserts

INGREDIENTS

- ½ pound pears, cored and cut into wedges
- ½ pound apples, cored and cut into wedges
- 1cup apple juice
- 1teaspoon nutmeg, ground
- 1teaspoon cinnamon powder
- 2tablespoons sugar

DIRECTIONS

1. In a pan that fits your air fryer, mix the apples with the pears and the other ingredients, toss, introduce the pan in the fryer and cook at 340 degrees F for 20 minutes.
2. Divide into bowls and serve.

NUTRITION: Calories 200, Fat 1, Fiber 4, Carbs 12, Protein 3

926. Apricots Cream

Preparation time: 10 minutes

Cooking time: 15 minutes

Servings: 4

INGREDIENTS

- 1cup apricots, chopped
- 1cup heavy cream
- 2tablespoons sugar
- 1teaspoon ginger, grated

DIRECTIONS

1. In the air fryer's pan, mix the apricots with the cream and the other ingredients, whisk, introduce the pan in the air fryer and cook at 380 degrees F for 15 minutes.
2. Divide into bowls and serve.

NUTRITION: Calories 200, Fat 3, Fiber 4, Carbs 11, Protein 3

927. Ginger Cake

Preparation time: 10 minutes

Cooking time: 30 minutes

Servings: 4

INGREDIENTS

- 1cup almond flour
- 2tablespoons ginger, grated
- 1cup heavy cream
- 1teaspoon baking powder
- 3tablespoons sugar
- ½ cup coconut cream
- 1teaspoon cinnamon powder
- 3tablespoons butter, melted
- 4eggs, whisked

DIRECTIONS

1. In a bowl, mix the flour with the ginger, cream and the other ingredients, stir well, pour this into a lined cake pan, introduce the pan in the fryer and cook at 370 degrees F for 30 minutes.
2. Leave the cake to cool down, slice and serve.

NUTRITION: Calories 213, Fat 3, Fiber 6, Carbs 15, Protein 4

928. Nutmeg Banana and Chia Bowls

Preparation time: 10 minutes

Cooking time: 25 minutes

Serving: 4

INGREDIENTS

- 1cup banana, peeled and sliced
- 2tablespoons chia seeds
- 1teaspoon nutmeg, ground
- 1cup heavy cream
- ½ cup coconut cream

- 3 tablespoons sugar
- 1 teaspoon cinnamon powder

DIRECTIONS

1. In the air fryer's pan, mix the bananas with the chia seeds and the other ingredients, toss, put the pan in the air fryer and cook at 340 degrees F for 25 minutes.
2. Divide into bowls and serve.

NUTRITION: Calories 200, Fat 4, Fiber 6, Carbs 15, Protein 4

929. Chicken Dip

Preparation time: 5 minutes

Cooking time: 20 minutes

Servings: 4

INGREDIENTS

- 1 pound chicken breast, skinless, boneless, ground and browned
- 1 cup cheddar cheese, shredded
- 1 red bell pepper, chopped
- 1 green bell pepper, chopped
- 1 red onion, chopped
- Salt and black pepper to the taste
- A drizzle of olive oil
- 1 tablespoon chives, chopped

DIRECTIONS

1. In the air fryer's pan, mix the meat with the peppers and the other ingredients except the cheese and toss.
2. Sprinkle the cheese on top, introduce the pan in the machine and cook at 370 degrees F for 20 minutes.
3. Divide between plates and serve as an appetizer.

NUTRITION: Calories 202, Fat 12, Fiber 2, Carbs 4, Protein 7

930. Beet Salsa

Preparation time: 5 minutes

Cooking time: 20 minutes

Servings: 4

INGREDIENTS

- 2 cups beets, peeled and cubed
- 1 cup kalamata olives, pitted and halved
- 1 cup cherry tomatoes, halved
- 1 tablespoon olive oil
- A pinch of salt and black pepper
- 1 tablespoon balsamic vinegar
- ¼ teaspoon sweet paprika

DIRECTIONS

1. In the air fryer's pan, mix the beets with the olives and the other ingredients, toss, put the pan in the machine and cook at 370 degrees F for 20 minutes.
2. Transfer to bowls and serve.

NUTRITION: Calories 170, Fat 2, Fiber 3, Carbs 4, Protein 6

931. Carrot Chips

Preparation time: 5 minutes

Cooking time: 15 minutes

Servings: 4

INGREDIENTS

- 1 pound carrots, peeled and sliced
- 1 tablespoon olive oil
- A pinch of salt and black pepper
- 1 teaspoon sweet paprika

DIRECTIONS

1. In the air fryer's pan, mix the carrot chips with the other ingredients, toss and cook at 400 degrees F for 15 minutes.
2. Cool the chips down and serve.

NUTRITION: Calories 150, Fat 4, Fiber 3, Carbs 4, Protein 6

932. Zucchini Cakes

Preparation time: 5 minutes

Cooking time: 16 minutes

Servings: 6

INGREDIENTS:

- Cooking spray
- 1pound zucchinis, grated
- ½ cup coconut flour
- 1teaspoon turmeric powder
- 2eggs, whisked
- 2garlic cloves, minced
- Salt and black pepper to the taste
- 3spring onions, chopped

DIRECTIONS

1. In a bowl, mix all the zucchinis with the flour and the other ingredients except the cooking spray, stir well and shape medium cakes out of this mixture.
2. Place the cakes in your air fryer's basket, grease them with cooking spray and cook at 380 degrees F for 8 minutes on each side.
3. Serve them as an appetizer.

NUTRITION: Calories 165, Fat 5, Fiber 2, Carbs 3, Protein 7

933. Rosemary Mushroom and Beets Salsa

Preparation time: 5 minutes

Cooking time: 15 minutes

Servings: 4

INGREDIENTS

- 1pound wild mushrooms, halved
- 1cup red beets, peeled and cubed
- 1cup kalamata olives, pitted and halved
- 1tablespoon rosemary, chopped
- 2tablespoons olive oil
- Juice of 1 lime
- 2garlic clove, minced

DIRECTIONS

1. In the air fryer's pan, mix the mushrooms with the beets and the other ingredients, put the pan in the machine and cook at 380 degrees F for 15 minutes.
2. Serve as an appetizer.

NUTRITION: Calories 151, Fat 2, Fiber 1, Carbs 3, Protein 6

934. Mushroom Cakes

Preparation time: 5 minutes

Cooking time: 15 minutes

Servings: 6

INGREDIENTS

- 1pound white mushrooms, chopped
- 1cup almond flour
- 2eggs, whisked
- 1tablespoon chives, chopped
- 1teaspoon chili powder
- Cooking spray
- Salt and black pepper to the taste

DIRECTIONS

1. In a bowl, mix the mushrooms with the flour and the other ingredients except the

cooking spray, stir and shape medium meatballs out of this mix.
2. Arrange the cakes in your air fryer's basket, grease them with the cooking spray, cook at 350 degrees F for 15 minutes and serve.

NUTRITION: Calories 120, Fat 4, Fiber 2, Carbs 3, Protein 5

935. Avocado Salsa

Preparation time: 5 minutes

Cooking time: 8 minutes

Servings: 4

INGREDIENTS

- 2avocados, peeled, pitted and cubed
- 1cup cherry tomatoes, halved
- 1cup cucumbers, cubed
- Juice of 1 lime
- 1tablespoon basil, chopped
- 1tablespoon chives, chopped
- A pinch of salt and black pepper
- 1tablespoon balsamic vinegar

DIRECTIONS

1. In the air fryer's pan, mix the avocado with the tomatoes and the other ingredients, put the pan in the machine and cook at 360 degrees F for 8 minutes.
2. Divide into bowls and serve as an appetizer.

NUTRITION: Calories 161, Fat 4, Fiber 2, Carbs 4, Protein 6

936. Carrot Wraps

Preparation time: 5 minutes

Cooking time: 20 minutes

Servings: 12

INGREDIENTS

- 12bacon strips
- 12carrot sliced
- A pinch of salt and black pepper
- 1teaspoon sweet paprika
- A drizzle of olive oil

DIRECTIONS

1. Wrap each carrot slice in a bacon strip, season with salt, pepper and paprika, brush them with the oil, put them in your air fryer's basket and cook at 370 degrees F for 20 minutes.
2. Arrange on a platter and serve as an appetizer.

NUTRITION: Calories 140, Fat 5, Fiber 2, Carbs 4, Protein 4

937. Bacon Corn Mix

Preparation time: 5 minutes

Cooking time: 12 minutes

Servings: 4

INGREDIENTS

- ½ cup bacon, cooked and chopped
- 2cups corn
- 1cup heavy cream
- A pinch of salt and black pepper

DIRECTIONS

1. In the air fryer's pan, mix the bacon with the corn and the other ingredients, toss, put the pan in the machine and cook at 350 degrees F for 12 minutes.
2. Serve as a party dip.

NUTRITION: Calories 151, Fat 4, Fiber 2, Carbs 4, Protein 8

938. Mayo Corn Spread

Preparation time: 5 minutes

Cooking time: 20 minutes

Servings: 4

INGREDIENTS

- ½ cup mayonnaise
- 1 cup corn
- 1 cup avocado, peeled, pitted and cubed
- 1 cup heavy cream
- A pinch of salt and black pepper
- 1 teaspoon turmeric powder

DIRECTIONS

1. In the air fryer's pan, mix the corn with the mayonnaise and the other ingredients, put the pan in the machine and cook at 380 degrees F for 20 minutes.
2. Blend using an immersion blender, divide into bowls and serve as an appetizer.

NUTRITION: Calories 100, Fat 4, Fiber 2, Carbs 3, Protein 4

939. Avocado Cakes

Preparation time: 5 minutes

Cooking time: 8 minutes

Servings: 4

INGREDIENTS

- 1 cup avocado, peeled, pitted and mashed
- 1 tablespoon basil, chopped
- 1 tablespoon oregano, chopped
- 3 tablespoons almond flour
- 2 garlic cloves, minced
- 1 tablespoon lime juice
- A pinch of salt and black pepper
- 2 eggs, whisked
- Cooking spray

DIRECTIONS

1. In a bowl, mix all the avocado with the basil, oregano and the other ingredients except the cooking spray, stir well and shape medium cakes out of this mix.
2. Place them in your air fryer's basket, grease with cooking spray and cook at 370 degrees F for 8 minutes.
3. Serve as an appetizer.

NUTRITION: Calories 160, Fat 6, Fiber 3, Carbs 4, Protein 6

940. Shrimp and Avocado Bowls

Preparation time: 5 minutes

Cooking time: 15 minutes

Servings: 4

INGREDIENTS

- 1 pound shrimp, peeled and deveined
- 1 cup avocado, peeled, pitted and cubed
- 1 cup cherry tomatoes, halved
- Juice of 1 lime
- 1 tablespoon olive oil
- A pinch of salt and black pepper
- 1 tablespoon cilantro, chopped

DIRECTIONS

1. In the air fryer's pan, mix the shrimp with the avocado and the other ingredients, toss, put the pan in the machine, cook at 350 degrees F for 15 minutes, divide into bowls and serve as an appetizer.

NUTRITION: Calories 184, Fat 5, Fiber 2, Carbs 4, Protein 7

941. Cashew Dip

Preparation time: 5 minutes

Cooking time: 12 minutes

Servings: 6

INGREDIENTS

- 1cup cashews, soaked in water for 4 hours and drained
- 1cup heavy cream
- 1tablespoon lemon zest, grated
- 1tablespoon lemon juice
- A pinch of salt and black pepper
- 1tablespoon chives, chopped

DIRECTIONS

1. In a blender, combine all the ingredients, pulse well and transfer to a ramekin.
2. Put the ramekin in your air fryer's basket and cook at 350 degrees F for 12 minutes.
3. Serve as a party dip.

NUTRITION: Calories 144, Fat 2, Fiber 1, Carbs 3, Protein 4

942. Smoked Salmon Salad

Preparation time: 5 minutes

Cooking time: 10 minutes

Servings: 4

INGREDIENTS:

- 4ounces smoked salmon, skinless, boneless and cubed
- 1cup kalamata olives, pitted and halved
- 1cup corn
- 1cup baby spinach
- 2tablespoons lemon juice
- 1teaspoon avocado oil
- 1tablespoon chives, chopped
- A pinch of salt and black pepper

DIRECTIONS

1. In the air fryer's pan, mix the salmon with the olives and the other ingredients, put the pan in the machine and cook at 350 degrees F for 10 minutes.
2. Divide into bowls and serve as an appetizer.

NUTRITION: Calories 100, Fat 2, Fiber 1, Carbs 2, Protein 2

943. Salmon Meatballs

Preparation time: 5 minutes

Cooking time: 20 minutes

Servings: 6

INGREDIENTS

- 1pound salmon fillets, boneless, skinless and ground
- 2eggs, whisked
- ¼ cup almond flour
- ½ teaspoon sweet paprika
- 1teaspoon garlic powder
- A pinch of salt and black pepper
- 1tablespoon parsley, chopped
- Cooking spray

DIRECTIONS

1. In a bowl, mix the salmon with the eggs and the other ingredients except the cooking spray, stir well and shape medium meatballs out of this mix.
2. Pace them in your lined air fryer's basket, grease with cooking spray and cook at 360 degrees F for 20 minutes.
3. Serve as an appetizer.

NUTRITION: Calories 180, Fat 5, Fiber 2, Carbs 5, Protein 7

944. Chicken Meatballs

Preparation time: 5 minutes

Cooking time: 20 minutes

Servings: 8

INGREDIENTS

- 1 and ½ pounds chicken breast, skinless, boneless and ground
- 2 eggs, whisked
- 1 tablespoon oregano, chopped
- 1 tablespoon chives, chopped
- ¼ cup almond flour
- A pinch of salt and black pepper
- 2 garlic cloves, minced
- 2 spring onions, chopped
- Cooking spray

DIRECTIONS

1. In a bowl, mix the meat with the eggs and the other ingredients except the cooking spray, stir well and shape medium meatballs out of this mix.
2. Arrange the meatballs in your air fryer's basket, grease them with cooking spray and cook at 360 degrees F for 20 minutes.
3. Serve as an appetizer.

NUTRITION: Calories 257, Fat 14, Fiber 1, Carbs 3, Protein 17

945. Ginger Dip

Preparation time: 5 minutes

Cooking time: 20 minutes

Servings: 6

INGREDIENTS

- 1 cup Greek yogurt
- ½ cup heavy cream
- 2 tablespoons ginger, grated
- 2 shallots, chopped
- 1 tablespoon chives, chopped
- A pinch of salt and black pepper
- Cooking spray

DIRECTIONS:

1. In the air fryer's pan, mix the cream with the yogurt and the other ingredients, put the pan in the machine and cook at 380 degrees F for 20 minutes.
2. Serve as a party dip.

NUTRITION: Calories 200, Fat 12, Fiber 2, Carbs 3, Protein 14

946. Asparagus and Olives Bowls

Preparation time: 5 minutes

Cooking time: 15 minutes

Servings: 8

INGREDIENTS

- ½ pound asparagus, roughly chopped
- 1 cup black olives, pitted and halved
- 1 cup kalamata olives, pitted and halved
- 1 cup baby spinach
- Juice of 1 lime
- 2 tablespoons olive oil
- A pinch of salt and black pepper

DIRECTIONS

1. In the air fryer's pan, mix the asparagus with the olives and the other ingredients, put the pan in the machine and cook at 390 degrees F for 15 minutes.
2. Divide into bowls and serve as an appetizer.

NUTRITION: Calories 173, Fat 4, Fiber 2, Carbs 3, Protein 6

947. Walnuts and Radish Bites

Preparation time: 5 minutes

Cooking time: 15 minutes

Servings: 4

INGREDIENTS

- 1 pound radishes, halved
- 1 cup walnuts
- 1 teaspoon chili powder
- 1 teaspoon sweet paprika
- A pinch of salt and black pepper
- 2 tablespoons avocado oil

DIRECTIONS:

1. In the air fryer's basket, mix the radishes with the walnuts and the other ingredients, toss and cook at 400 degrees F for 15 minutes.
2. Serve as a snack.

NUTRITION: Calories 174, Fat 5, Fiber 1, Carbs 3, Protein 6

948. Olives Spread

Preparation time: 5 minutes

Cooking time: 5 minutes

Servings: 6

INGREDIENTS

- 1 cup black olives, pitted and chopped
- 1 cup kalamata olives, pitted and chopped
- 1 cup green olives, pitted and chopped
- 1 cup Greek yogurt
- 1 tablespoon olive oil
- 3 tablespoons lemon juice
- 1 cup basil, chopped
- A pinch of salt and black pepper

DIRECTIONS

1. In a blender, combine the olives with the yogurt and the other ingredients, pulse well and transfer to a ramekin.
2. Place the ramekin in your air fryer's basket and cook at 350 degrees F for 5 minutes.
3. Serve as a party spread.

NUTRITION: Calories 120, Fat 5, Fiber 2, Carbs 3, Protein 7

949. Melon Salsa

Preparation time: 5 minutes

Cooking time: 5 minutes

Servings: 4

INGREDIENTS:

- 1 cup watermelon, peeled and cubed
- 1 cup cherry tomatoes, halved
- 1 cup corn
- 1 cup baby spinach
- 2 spring onions, chopped
- 2 tablespoons lime juice
- 1 tablespoon avocado oil
- 2 teaspoons parsley, chopped
- Cooking spray

DIRECTIONS

1. In the air fryer's pan, mix the watermelon with the tomatoes and the other ingredients and toss.
2. Introduce the pan in the machine and cook at 360 degrees F for 5 minutes.
3. Divide into bowls and serve as an appetizer.

NUTRITION: Calories 148, Fat 1, Fiber 2, Carbs 3, Protein 5

950. Shrimp Spread

Preparation time: 5 minutes

Cooking time: 6 minutes

Servings: 4

INGREDIENTS

- 1cup cream cheese, soft
- Juice of 1 lime
- Zest of 1 lime, grated
- 1pound shrimp, peeled, deveined and minced
- A pinch of salt and black pepper
- 1tablespoon chives, chopped

DIRECTIONS

1. In a bowl, mix all the ingredients, whisk them really well, transfer the mix to a ramekin, place it in your air fryer's basket and cook at 370 degrees F for 6 minutes.
2. Serve as a party spread.

NUTRITION: Calories 180, Fat 7, Fiber 1, Carbs 5, Protein 7

951. Pork Dip

Preparation time: 10 minutes

Cooking time: 20 minutes

Servings: 4

INGREDIENTS

- 1pound pork stew meat, ground
- 1tablespoon olive oil
- 1red onion, chopped
- ¼ teaspoon rosemary, dried
- ½ teaspoon coriander, ground
- 1cup heavy cream
- 1tablespoon cilantro, chopped
- 2garlic cloves, minced
- A pinch of salt and black pepper

DIRECTIONS

1. Preheat the air fryer with the oil at 370 degrees F, add the meat and cook for 5 minutes.
2. Add the rest of the ingredients, cook for 15 minutes more, divide into bowls and serve as a party dip.

NUTRITION: Calories 249, Fat 16, Fiber 2, Carbs 3, Protein 17

952. Spinach Dip

Preparation time: 6 minutes

Cooking time: 20 minutes

Servings: 6

INGREDIENTS

- 1cup cream cheese, soft
- 1cup mozzarella, shredded
- 2cups baby spinach
- 1cup heavy cream
- A pinch of salt and black pepper
- 2tablespoons butter, melted

DIRECTIONS

1. In the air fryer's pan, mix the cream cheese with the mozzarella and the other ingredients, put the pan in the machine and cook at 360 degrees F for 20 minutes.
2. Serve as a party dip.

NUTRITION: Calories 210, Fat 8, Fiber 1, Carbs 3, Protein 8

953. Pork and Spinach Bowls

Preparation time: 10 minutes

Cooking time: 20 minutes

Servings: 6

INGREDIENTS

- 1pound pork stew meat, cut into strips
- 1cup baby spinach
- 1cup cherry tomatoes, halved
- 1tablespoon balsamic vinegar
- 2tablespoons olive oil
- 1teaspoon sweet paprika
- A pinch of salt and black pepper
- 1tablespoon chives, chopped

DIRECTIONS

1. In the air fryer's pan, mix the meat with the spinach and the other ingredients, put the pan in the machine and cook at 360 degrees F for 20 minutes.
2. Divide into bowls and serve as a snack.

NUTRITION: Calories 251, Fat 14, Fiber 3, Carbs 5, Protein 18

954. Tomato and Radish Bowls

Preparation time: 5 minutes

Cooking time: 20 minutes

Servings: 6

INGREDIENTS

- 1pound cherry tomatoes, halved
- 2cups radishes, halved
- 1cup baby kale
- 1cup carrots, peeled and grated
- 1tablespoon olive oil
- Juice of 1 lime
- 2ounces watercress
- A pinch of salt and black pepper
- 1tablespoon chives, chopped

DIRECTIONS

1. In the air fryer's pan, mix the tomatoes with the radishes and the other ingredients, put the pan in the machine and cook at 360 degrees F for 20 minutes.
2. Divide into bowls and serve.

NUTRITION: Calories 131, Fat 7, Fiber 2, Carbs 4, Protein 7

955. Green Beans Bites

Preparation time: 5 minutes

Cooking time: 15 minutes

Servings: 4

INGREDIENTS

- 12ounces green beans, trimmed and halved
- 1teaspoon sweet paprika
- A drizzle of olive oil
- ½ teaspoon coriander, ground
- 1egg, whisked
- A pinch of salt and black pepper

DIRECTIONS

1. In a bowl, mix the green beans with the other ingredients except the egg and toss.
2. Put the egg in a separate bowl,
3. Dredge the green beans in the egg mix, arrange the green beans in your air fryer's basket and cook at 380 degrees F for 12 minutes.
4. Serve as a snack.

NUTRITION: Calories 112, Fat 6, Fiber 1, Carbs 2, Protein 9

956. Rosemary Shrimp Platter

Preparation time: 5 minutes

Cooking time: 10 minutes

Servings: 4

INGREDIENTS

- 1 pound shrimp, peeled and deveined
- 2 tablespoons avocado oil
- 1 tablespoon rosemary, chopped
- Juice of ½ lemon
- A pinch of salt and black pepper

DIRECTIONS

1. In a pan that fits your air fryer, mix the shrimp with the oil and the other ingredients, toss, introduce in the fryer and cook at 370 degrees F for 10 minutes.
2. Serve as an appetizer.

NUTRITION: Calories 242, Fat 14, Fiber 2, Carbs 3, Protein 17

957. Chocolate Cake

Preparation time: 30 minutes

Cooking time: 30 minutes

Servings: 12

INGREDIENTS

- 2½ cups almond flour
- ¼ cup coconut flour
- ¼ cup chocolate protein powder
- ½ tsp salt
- ¼ cup unsweetened cocoa powder
- 1 Tbsp baking powder
- 2/3 cup granulated erythritol
- ½ cup butter
- ¾ cup whole milk
- 1 tsp vanilla
- 4 whole eggs

DIRECTIONS:

1. Preheat your air fryer to 325 degrees F and grease and 8" cake pan.
2. Place the butter in a mixing bowl along with the erythritol and beat until fluffy.
3. In a separate bowl, mix the eggs, milk and vanilla together.
4. In a third bowl, combine the remaining dry ingredients.
5. Add half of the wet mixture to the bowl with the fluffy butter and beat together slowly.
6. Add half of the dry mix to the bowl and beat again until smooth.
7. Add the remaining wet ingredients, mix and add the remaining dry ingredients and blend until a smooth batter forms.
8. Pour the cake batter into the prepared pan and place in the air fryer to cook for 30 minutes. The cake will be golden brown and a toothpick will come out cleanly when inserted into the center of the cake.
9. Remove from the air fryer and cool in the pan for 20 minutes. Flip the cake out of the pan, slice and enjoy! You can also frost the cake however you'd like with a tasty keto frosting.

NUTRITION: Calories 348, Total Fat 36g, Saturated Fat 16g, Total Carbs 9g, Net Carbs 4g, Protein 11g, Sugar 4g, Fiber 5g, Sodium 321mg, Potassium 63g

958. Peanut Butter Cake

Preparation time: 30 minutes

Cooking time: 30 minutes

Servings: 12

INGREDIENTS

- 2½ cups almond flour
- ¼ cup coconut flour
- ¼ cup vanilla protein powder
- ½ tsp salt
- 1 Tbsp baking powder
- 2/3 cup granulated erythritol
- ¼ cup butter

- ¼ cup peanut butter
- ¾ cup whole milk
- 1tsp vanilla
- 4whole eggs

DIRECTIONS:

1. Preheat your air fryer to 325 degrees F and grease and 8" cake pan.
2. Place the butter and peanut butter in a mixing bowl along with the erythritol and beat until fluffy.
3. In a separate bowl, mix the eggs, milk and vanilla together.
4. In a third bowl, combine the remaining dry ingredients.
5. Add half of the wet mixture to the bowl with the fluffy butter and beat together slowly.
6. Add half of the dry mix to the bowl and beat again until smooth.
7. Add the remaining wet ingredients, mix and add the remaining dry ingredients and blend until a smooth batter forms.
8. Pour the cake batter into the prepared pan and place in the air fryer to cook for 30 minutes. The cake will be golden brown and a toothpick will come out cleanly when inserted into the center of the cake.
9. Remove from the air fryer and cool in the pan for 20 minutes. Flip the cake out of the pan, slice and enjoy!

NUTRITION: Calories 351, Total Fat 36g, Saturated Fat 19g, Total Carbs 10g, Net Carbs 6g, Protein 10g, Sugar 5g, Fiber 4g, Sodium 483mg, Potassium 89g

959. Hazelnut Cake

Preparation time: 30 minutes

Cooking time: 30 minutes

Servings: 12

INGREDIENTS

- 2cups almond flour
- ¾ cup hazelnut flour
- ¼ cup vanilla protein powder
- ½ tsp salt
- 1Tbsp baking powder
- 2/3 cup granulated erythritol
- ¼ cup butter
- ¼ cup hazelnut butter
- ¾ cup whole milk
- 1tsp vanilla
- 4whole eggs

DIRECTIONS:

1. Preheat your air fryer to 325 degrees F and grease and 8" cake pan.
2. Place the butter and hazelnut butter in a mixing bowl along with the erythritol and beat until fluffy.
3. In a separate bowl, mix the eggs, milk and vanilla together.
4. In a third bowl, combine the remaining dry ingredients.
5. Add half of the wet mixture to the bowl with the fluffy butter and beat together slowly.
6. Add half of the dry mix to the bowl and beat again until smooth.
7. Add the remaining wet ingredients, mix and add the remaining dry ingredients and blend until a smooth batter forms.
8. Pour the cake batter into the prepared pan and place in the air fryer to cook for 30 minutes. The cake will be golden brown and a toothpick will come out cleanly when inserted into the center of the cake.
9. Remove from the air fryer and cool in the pan for 20 minutes. Flip the cake out of the pan, slice and enjoy!

NUTRITION: Calories 429, Total Fat 43g, Saturated Fat 24g, Total Carbs 14g, Net Carbs 9g, Protein 10g, Sugar 5g, Fiber 5g, Sodium 477mg, Potassium 97g

960. Walnut Cake

Preparation time: 30 minutes

Cooking time: 30 minutes

Servings: 12

INGREDIENTS

- 2 cups almond flour
- ¾ cup walnut flour
- ¼ cup vanilla protein powder
- ½ tsp salt
- 1 Tbsp baking powder
- 2/3 cup granulated erythritol
- ½ cup butter
- ¾ cup whole milk
- 1 tsp vanilla
- 4 whole eggs

DIRECTIONS:

1. Preheat your air fryer to 325 degrees F and grease and 8" cake pan.
2. Place the butter and in a mixing bowl along with the erythritol and beat until fluffy.
3. In a separate bowl, mix the eggs, milk and vanilla together.
4. In a third bowl, combine the remaining dry ingredients.
5. Add half of the wet mixture to the bowl with the fluffy butter and beat together slowly.
6. Add half of the dry mix to the bowl and beat again until smooth.
7. Add the remaining wet ingredients, mix and add the remaining dry ingredients and blend until a smooth batter forms.
8. Pour the cake batter into the prepared pan and place in the air fryer to cook for 30 minutes. The cake will be golden brown and a toothpick will come out cleanly when inserted into the center of the cake.
9. Remove from the air fryer and cool in the pan for 20 minutes. Flip the cake out of the pan, slice and enjoy!

NUTRITION: Calories 357, Total Fat 38g, Saturated Fat 21g, Total Carbs 11g, Net Carbs 6g, Protein 11g, Sugar 5g, Fiber 5g, Sodium 483mg, Potassium 102g

961. NY Keto Cheesecake

Preparation time: 15 minutes

Cooking time: 1 hour 15 minutes

Servings: 12

INGREDIENTS

- 1½ pounds cream cheese
- 5 Tbsp butter
- 1 cup powdered erythritol
- 3 eggs
- 1½ tsp vanilla extract
- ¾ cup sour cream

DIRECTIONS:

1. Preheat your air fryer to 275 degrees F and grease an 8" spring form cake pan. Place a piece of parchment in the bottom of the pan as well.
2. Place the cream cheese and butter in a large bowl and beat until combined.
3. Add the powdered erythritol and beat again until smooth.
4. Add the eggs, one at a time, allowing them to fully mix in after each addition.
5. Add the sour cream and vanilla extract and stir one last time, making sure the batter is smooth and all the ingredients are well blended.
6. Pour the batter into the prepared cake pan and then place the pan on a larger tray with high sides that will fit in the air fryer. Fill the pan with water, creating a water bath for the cheese cake.

7. Place in the pre heated air fryer and bake for an hour and 15 minutes. The cheesecake will be mostly set but may have a very slight jiggle in the center.
8. Allow the cheesecake to cool for 3 hours in the fridge before removing from the pan and serving.

NUTRITION: Calories 287, Total Fat 26g, Saturated Fat 14g, Total Carbs 3g, Net Carbs 1g, Protein 5g, Sugar 1g, Fiber 2g, Sodium 192mg, Potassium 80g

962. Strawberry Cheesecake

Preparation time: 15 minutes

Cooking time: 1 hour 15 minutes

Servings: 12

INGREDIENTS

- 1½ pounds cream cheese
- 5Tbsp butter
- 1cup powdered erythritol
- 3eggs
- 1½ tsp vanilla extract
- ¾ cup sour cream
- ¾ cup chopped, fresh strawberries

DIRECTIONS:

1. Preheat your air fryer to 275 degrees F and grease an 8" spring form cake pan. Place a piece of parchment in the bottom of the pan as well.
2. Place the cream cheese and butter in a large bowl and beat until combined.
3. Add the powdered erythritol and beat again until smooth.
4. Add the eggs, one at a time, allowing them to fully mix in after each addition.
5. Add the sour cream and vanilla extract and stir one last time, making sure the batter is smooth and all the ingredients are well blended.
6. Fold in the chopped strawberries
7. Pour the batter into the prepared cake pan and then place the pan on a larger tray with high sides that will fit in the air fryer. Fill the pan with water, creating a water bath for the cheese cake.
8. Place in the pre heated air fryer and bake for an hour and 15 minutes. The cheesecake will be mostly set but may have a very slight jiggle in the center.
9. Allow the cheesecake to cool for 3 hours in the fridge before removing from the pan and serving.

NUTRITION: Calories 315, Total Fat 26g, Saturated Fat 14g, Total Carbs 8g, Net Carbs 6g, Protein 5g, Sugar 5g, Fiber 2g, Sodium 192mg, Potassium 110g

963. Blueberry Cheesecake

Preparation time: 15 minutes

Cooking time: 1 hour 15 minutes

Servings: 12

INGREDIENTS

- 1½ pounds cream cheese
- 5Tbsp butter
- 1cup powdered erythritol
- 3eggs
- 1½ tsp vanilla extract
- ¾ cup sour cream
- 1cup fresh blueberries

DIRECTIONS:

1. Preheat your air fryer to 275 degrees F and grease an 8" spring form cake pan. Place a piece of parchment in the bottom of the pan as well.
2. Place the cream cheese and butter in a large bowl and beat until combined.
3. Add the powdered erythritol and beat again until smooth.

4. Add the eggs, one at a time, allowing them to fully mix in after each addition.
5. Add the sour cream and vanilla extract and stir one last time, making sure the batter is smooth and all the ingredients are well blended.
6. Fold in the blueberries gently.
7. Pour the batter into the prepared cake pan and then place the pan on a larger tray with high sides that will fit in the air fryer. Fill the pan with water, creating a water bath for the cheese cake.
8. Place in the pre heated air fryer and bake for an hour and 15 minutes. The cheesecake will be mostly set but may have a very slight jiggle in the center.
9. Allow the cheesecake to cool for 3 hours in the fridge before removing from the pan and serving.

NUTRITION: Calories 322, Total Fat 26g, Saturated Fat 14g, Total Carbs 9g, Net Carbs 7g, Protein 5g, Sugar 6g, Fiber 2g, Sodium 192mg, Potassium 125g

964. Raspberry Cheesecake

Preparation time: 15 minutes

Cooking time: 1 hour 15 minutes

Servings: 12

INGREDIENTS:

- 1½ pounds cream cheese
- 5Tbsp butter
- 1cup powdered erythritol
- 3eggs
- 1½ tsp vanilla extract
- ¾ cup sour cream
- 1cup fresh raspberries

DIRECTIONS:

1. Preheat your air fryer to 275 degrees F and grease an 8" spring form cake pan. Place a piece of parchment in the bottom of the pan as well.
2. Place the cream cheese and butter in a large bowl and beat until combined.
3. Add the powdered erythritol and beat again until smooth.
4. Add the eggs, one at a time, allowing them to fully mix in after each addition.
5. Add the sour cream and vanilla extract and stir one last time, making sure the batter is smooth and all the ingredients are well blended.
6. Fold in the raspberries gently.
7. Pour the batter into the prepared cake pan and then place the pan on a larger tray with high sides that will fit in the air fryer. Fill the pan with water, creating a water bath for the cheese cake.
8. Place in the pre heated air fryer and bake for an hour and 15 minutes. The cheesecake will be mostly set but may have a very slight jiggle in the center.
9. Allow the cheesecake to cool for 3 hours in the fridge before removing from the pan and serving.

NUTRITION: Calories 319, Total Fat 26g, Saturated Fat 14g, Total Carbs 9g, Net Carbs 7g, Protein 5g, Sugar 6g, Fiber 2g, Sodium 192mg, Potassium 121g

965. Cinnamon Cheesecake

Preparation time: 15 minutes

Cooking time: 1 hour 15 minutes

Servings: 12

INGREDIENTS

- 1½ pounds cream cheese
- 5Tbsp butter
- 1cup powdered erythritol
- 1tsp ground cinnamon
- 3eggs
- 1½ tsp vanilla extract
- ¾ cup sour cream

DIRECTIONS:

1. Preheat your air fryer to 275 degrees F and grease an 8" spring form cake pan. Place a piece of parchment in the bottom of the pan as well.
2. Place the cream cheese and butter in a large bowl and beat until combined.
3. Add the powdered erythritol, cinnamon and beat again until smooth.
4. Add the eggs, one at a time, allowing them to fully mix in after each addition.
5. Add the sour cream and vanilla extract and stir one last time, making sure the batter is smooth and all the ingredients are well blended.
6. Pour the batter into the prepared cake pan and then place the pan on a larger tray with high sides that will fit in the air fryer. Fill the pan with water, creating a water bath for the cheese cake.
7. Place in the pre heated air fryer and bake for an hour and 15 minutes. The cheesecake will be mostly set but may have a very slight jiggle in the center.
8. Allow the cheesecake to cool for 3 hours in the fridge before removing from the pan and serving.

NUTRITION: Calories 292, Total Fat 26g, Saturated Fat 14g, Total Carbs 3g, Net Carbs 1g, Protein 5g, Sugar 1g, Fiber 2g, Sodium 192mg, Potassium 80g

966. Chocolate Keto Cheesecake

Preparation time: 15 minutes

Cooking time: 1 hour 15 minutes

Servings: 12

INGREDIENTS

- 1½ pounds cream cheese
- 5 Tbsp butter
- 1 cup powdered erythritol
- ¼ cup unsweetened cocoa powder
- 3 eggs
- 1½ tsp vanilla extract
- ¾ cup sour cream

DIRECTIONS:

1. Preheat your air fryer to 275 degrees F and grease an 8" spring form cake pan. Place a piece of parchment in the bottom of the pan as well.
2. Place the cream cheese and butter in a large bowl and beat until combined.
3. Add the powdered erythritol, cocoa powder and beat again until smooth.
4. Add the eggs, one at a time, allowing them to fully mix in after each addition.
5. Add the sour cream and vanilla extract and stir one last time, making sure the batter is smooth and all the ingredients are well blended.
6. Pour the batter into the prepared cake pan and then place the pan on a larger tray with high sides that will fit in the air fryer. Fill the pan with water, creating a water bath for the cheese cake.
7. Place in the pre heated air fryer and bake for an hour and 15 minutes. The cheesecake will be mostly set but may have a very slight jiggle in the center.
8. Allow the cheesecake to cool for 3 hours in the fridge before removing from the pan and serving.

NUTRITION: Calories 302, Total Fat 34g, Saturated Fat 18g, Total Carbs 4g, Net Carbs 2g, Protein 5g, Sugar 2g, Fiber 2g, Sodium 192mg, Potassium 80g

967. Chocolate Chip Cheesecake

Preparation time: 15 minutes

Cooking time: 1 hour 15 minutes

Servings: 12

INGREDIENTS

- 1½ pounds cream cheese
- 5 Tbsp butter
- 1 cup powdered erythritol
- 3 eggs
- 1½ tsp vanilla extract
- ¾ cup sour cream
- 1 cup dark chocolate chips

DIRECTIONS:

1. Preheat your air fryer to 275 degrees F and grease an 8" spring form cake pan. Place a piece of parchment in the bottom of the pan as well.
2. Place the cream cheese and butter in a large bowl and beat until combined.
3. Add the powdered erythritol and beat again until smooth.
4. Add the eggs, one at a time, allowing them to fully mix in after each addition.
5. Add the sour cream and vanilla extract and stir one last time, making sure the batter is smooth and all the ingredients are well blended.
6. Fold in the dark chocolate chips.
7. Pour the batter into the prepared cake pan and then place the pan on a larger tray with high sides that will fit in the air fryer. Fill the pan with water, creating a water bath for the cheesecake.
8. Place in the pre heated air fryer and bake for an hour and 15 minutes. The cheesecake will be mostly set but may have a very slight jiggle in the center.
9. Allow the cheesecake to cool for 3 hours in the fridge before removing from the pan and serving.

NUTRITION: Calories 364, Total Fat 36g, Saturated Fat 20g, Total Carbs 8g, Net Carbs 6g, Protein 5g, Sugar 3g, Fiber 2g, Sodium 190mg, Potassium 102g

968. Pumpkin Spice Cheesecake

Preparation time: 15 minutes

Cooking time: 1 hour 15 minutes

Servings: 12

INGREDIENTS

- 1½ pounds cream cheese
- 5 Tbsp butter
- 1 cup powdered erythritol
- 2 tsp pumpkin spice
- 3 eggs
- 1½ tsp vanilla extract
- ¾ cup sour cream

DIRECTIONS:

1. Preheat your air fryer to 275 degrees F and grease an 8" spring form cake pan. Place a piece of parchment in the bottom of the pan as well.
2. Place the cream cheese and butter in a large bowl and beat until combined.
3. Add the powdered erythritol and pumpkin spice and beat again until smooth.
4. Add the eggs, one at a time, allowing them to fully mix in after each addition.
5. Add the sour cream and vanilla extract and stir one last time, making sure the batter is smooth and all the ingredients are well blended.
6. Pour the batter into the prepared cake pan and then place the pan on a larger tray with high sides that will fit in the air fryer. Fill the pan with water, creating a water bath for the cheese cake.
7. Place in the pre heated air fryer and bake for an hour and 15 minutes. The cheesecake will be mostly set but may have a very slight jiggle in the center.
8. Allow the cheesecake to cool for 3 hours in the fridge before removing from the pan and serving.

NUTRITION: Calories 293, Total Fat 26g, Saturated Fat 14g, Total Carbs 3g, Net Carbs 1g, Protein 5g, Sugar 1g, Fiber 2g, Sodium 195mg, Potassium 83g

969. Lemon Cheesecake

Preparation time: 15 minutes

Cooking time: 1 hour 15 minutes

Servings: 12

INGREDIENTS

- 1½ pounds cream cheese
- 5 Tbsp butter
- 1 cup powdered erythritol
- 3 eggs
- 1½ tsp vanilla extract
- ¾ cup sour cream
- 1 tsp lemon zest

DIRECTIONS:

1. Preheat your air fryer to 275 degrees F and grease an 8" spring form cake pan. Place a piece of parchment in the bottom of the pan as well.
2. Place the cream cheese and butter in a large bowl and beat until combined.
3. Add the powdered erythritol and beat again until smooth.
4. Add the eggs, one at a time, allowing them to fully mix in after each addition.
5. Add the sour cream, lemon zest and vanilla extract and stir one last time, making sure the batter is smooth and all the ingredients are well blended.
6. Pour the batter into the prepared cake pan and then place the pan on a larger tray with high sides that will fit in the air fryer. Fill the pan with water, creating a water bath for the cheese cake.
7. Place in the pre heated air fryer and bake for an hour and 15 minutes. The cheesecake will be mostly set but may have a very slight jiggle in the center.
8. Allow the cheesecake to cool for 3 hours in the fridge before removing from the pan and serving.

Nutrition: Calories 294, Total Fat 27g, Saturated Fat 14g, Total Carbs 5g, Net Carbs 1g, Protein 5g, Sugar 3g, Fiber 2g, Sodium 198mg, Potassium 87g

970. Gingerbread Cheesecake

Preparation time: 15 minutes

Cooking time: 1 hour 15 minutes

Servings: 12

INGREDIENTS

- 1½ pounds cream cheese
- 5 Tbsp butter
- 1 cup powdered erythritol
- ½ tsp ground ginger
- ¼ tsp ground cinnamon
- 3 eggs
- 1½ tsp vanilla extract
- ¾ cup sour cream

DIRECTIONS:

1. Preheat your air fryer to 275 degrees F and grease an 8" spring form cake pan. Place a piece of parchment in the bottom of the pan as well.
2. Place the cream cheese and butter in a large bowl and beat until combined.
3. Add the powdered erythritol, cinnamon, ginger and beat again until smooth.
4. Add the eggs, one at a time, allowing them to fully mix in after each addition.
5. Add the sour cream and vanilla extract and stir one last time, making sure the batter is smooth and all the ingredients are well blended.
6. Pour the batter into the prepared cake pan and then place the pan on a larger tray with high sides that will fit in the air fryer. Fill the pan with water, creating a water bath for the cheesecake.
7. Place in the pre heated air fryer and bake for an hour and 15 minutes. The

cheesecake will be mostly set but may have a very slight jiggle in the center.
8. Allow the cheesecake to cool for 3 hours in the fridge before removing from the pan and serving.

NUTRITION: Calories 293, Total Fat 26g, Saturated Fat 14g, Total Carbs 3g, Net Carbs 1g, Protein 5g, Sugar 1g, Fiber 2g, Sodium 195mg, Potassium 82g

971. Mascarpone Cheesecake

Preparation time: 15 minutes

Cooking time: 1 hour 15 minutes

Servings: 12

INGREDIENTS

- 1pound cream cheese
- ½ pound mascarpone cheese
- 5Tbsp butter
- 1cup powdered erythritol
- 3eggs
- 1½ tsp vanilla extract
- ¾ cup sour cream

DIRECTIONS:

1. Preheat your air fryer to 275 degrees F and grease an 8" spring form cake pan. Place a piece of parchment in the bottom of the pan as well.
2. Place the cream cheese, mascarpone and butter in a large bowl and beat until combined.
3. Add the powdered erythritol and beat again until smooth.
4. Add the eggs, one at a time, allowing them to fully mix in after each addition.
5. Add the sour cream and vanilla extract and stir one last time, making sure the batter is smooth and all the ingredients are well blended.
6. Pour the batter into the prepared cake pan and then place the pan on a larger tray with high sides that will fit in the air fryer. Fill the pan with water, creating a water bath for the cheese cake.
7. Place in the pre heated air fryer and bake for an hour and 15 minutes. The cheesecake will be mostly set but may have a very slight jiggle in the center.
8. Allow the cheesecake to cool for 3 hours in the fridge before removing from the pan and serving.

NUTRITION: Calories 295, Total Fat 31g, Saturated Fat 19g, Total Carbs 4g, Net Carbs 2g, Protein 5g, Sugar 2g, Fiber 2g, Sodium 198mg, Potassium 86g

972. Coconut Cheesecake

Preparation time: 15 minutes

Cooking time: 1 hour 15 minutes

Servings: 12

INGREDIENTS

- 1½ pounds cream cheese
- 5Tbsp butter
- 1cup powdered erythritol
- 3eggs
- 1½ tsp coconut extract
- ¾ cup sour cream
- ½ cup unsweetened coconut flakes

DIRECTIONS:

1. Preheat your air fryer to 275 degrees F and grease an 8" spring form cake pan. Place a piece of parchment in the bottom of the pan as well.
2. Place the cream cheese and butter in a large bowl and beat until combined.
3. Add the powdered erythritol and beat again until smooth.
4. Add the eggs, one at a time, allowing them to fully mix in after each addition.
5. Add the sour cream and coconut extract and stir one last time, making sure the

batter is smooth and all the ingredients are well blended.
6. Fold in the unsweetened coconut flakes
7. Pour the batter into the prepared cake pan and then place the pan on a larger tray with high sides that will fit in the air fryer. Fill the pan with water, creating a water bath for the cheese cake.
8. Place in the pre heated air fryer and bake for an hour and 15 minutes. The cheesecake will be mostly set but may have a very slight jiggle in the center.
9. Allow the cheesecake to cool for 3 hours in the fridge before removing from the pan and serving.

NUTRITION: Calories 311, Total Fat 29g, Saturated Fat 17g, Total Carbs 6g, Net Carbs 4g, Protein 5g, Sugar 3g, Fiber 2g, Sodium 192mg, Potassium 80g

973. Fudge Brownies

Preparation time: 15 minutes

Cooking time: 20 minutes

Servings: 16

INGREDIENTS

- ½ cup melted butter
- 2/3 cup swerve
- ½ tsp vanilla extract
- 3 room temperature eggs
- ½ cup almond flour
- 1/3 cup unsweetened cocoa powder
- 1 Tbsp plain, unsweetened gelatin
- ½ tsp salt
- ½ tsp baking powder
- ¼ cup water

DIRECTIONS:

1. Preheat your air fryer to 325 degrees F and grease an 8x8 inch square baking pan.
2. Combine the eggs, vanilla extract, swerve, and melted butter in a bowl and whisk together well.
3. Add the cocoa powder, almond flour, baking powder, gelatin, and salt and whisk again until smooth.
4. Add the water and stir again.
5. Pour the batter into the greased baking pan and place in the preheated air fryer. Bake for 15 minutes. The center will seem a little wet while the edges will be more firm- this is perfect.
6. Let the brownies cool in the pan before slicing and serving.

NUTRITION: Calories 110, Total Fat 10g, Saturated Fat 4g, Total Carbs 4g, Net Carbs 1g, Protein 3g, Sugar 1g, Fiber 3g, Sodium 283mg, Potassium 316g

974. Double Chocolate Brownies

Preparation time: 15 minutes

Cooking time: 20 minutes

Servings: 16

INGREDIENTS

- ½ cup melted butter
- 2/3 cup swerve
- ½ tsp vanilla extract
- 3 room temperature eggs
- ½ cup almond flour
- 1/3 cup unsweetened cocoa powder
- 1 Tbsp plain, unsweetened gelatin
- ½ tsp salt
- ½ tsp baking powder
- ¼ cup water
- ½ cup dark chocolate chips, unsweetened

DIRECTIONS:

1. Preheat your air fryer to 325 degrees F and grease an 8x8 inch square baking pan.
2. Combine the eggs, vanilla extract, swerve, and melted butter in a bowl and whisk together well.
3. Add the cocoa powder, almond flour, baking powder, gelatin, and salt and whisk again until smooth.
4. Add the water and stir again.
5. Fold in the chocolate chips.
6. Pour the batter into the greased baking pan and place in the preheated air fryer. Bake for 15 minutes. The center will seem a little wet while the edges will be more firm- this is perfect.
7. Let the brownies cool in the pan before slicing and serving.

NUTRITION: Calories 193, Total Fat 10g, Saturated Fat 4g, Total Carbs 6g, Net Carbs 3g, Protein 3g, Sugar 3g, Fiber 3g, Sodium 299mg, Potassium 322g

975. Chocolate Walnuts Brownies

Preparation time: 15 minutes

Cooking time: 20 minutes

Servings: 16

INGREDIENTS

- ½ cup melted butter
- 2/3 cup swerve
- ½ tsp vanilla extract
- 3 room temperature eggs
- ½ cup almond flour
- 1/3 cup unsweetened cocoa powder
- 1 Tbsp plain, unsweetened gelatin
- ½ tsp salt
- ½ tsp baking powder
- ¼ cup water
- ½ cup chopped walnuts

DIRECTIONS:

1. Preheat your air fryer to 325 degrees F and grease an 8x8 inch square baking pan.
2. Combine the eggs, vanilla extract, swerve, and melted butter in a bowl and whisk together well.
3. Add the cocoa powder, almond flour, baking powder, gelatin, and salt and whisk again until smooth.
4. Add the water and stir again.
5. Fold in walnuts.
6. Pour the batter into the greased baking pan and place in the preheated air fryer. Bake for 15 minutes. The center will seem a little wet while the edges will be more firm- this is perfect.
7. Let the brownies cool in the pan before slicing and serving.

NUTRITION: Calories 178, Total Fat 19g, Saturated Fat 5g, Total Carbs 8g, Net Carbs 4g, Protein 3g, Sugar 2g, Fiber 4g, Sodium 283mg, Potassium 322g

976. Peanut Butter Brownies

Preparation time: 15 minutes

Cooking time: 20 minutes

Servings: 16

INGREDIENTS

- ½ cup peanut butter
- 2/3 cup swerve
- ½ tsp vanilla extract
- 3 room temperature eggs
- ½ cup almond flour
- 1/3 cup unsweetened cocoa powder
- 1 Tbsp plain, unsweetened gelatin
- ½ tsp salt
- ½ tsp baking powder
- ¼ cup water

DIRECTIONS:

1. Preheat your air fryer to 325 degrees F and grease an 8x8 inch square baking pan.
2. Combine the peanut butter, vanilla extract, swerve, and eggs in a bowl and whisk together well.
3. Add the cocoa powder, almond flour, baking powder, gelatin, and salt and whisk again until smooth.
4. Add the water and stir again.
5. Pour the batter into the greased baking pan and place in the preheated air fryer. Bake for 15 minutes. The center will seem a little wet while the edges will be more firm- this is perfect.
6. Let the brownies cool in the pan before slicing and serving.

NUTRITION: Calories 131, Total Fat 11g, Saturated Fat 5g, Total Carbs 6g, Net Carbs 3g, Protein 6g, Sugar 4g, Fiber 3g, Sodium 283mg, Potassium 324g

977. Almond Brownies

Preparation time: 15 minutes

Cooking time: 20 minutes

Servings: 16

INGREDIENTS

- ½ cup melted butter
- 2/3 cup swerve
- ½ tsp almond extract
- 3 room temperature eggs
- ½ cup almond flour
- 1/3 cup unsweetened cocoa powder
- 1 Tbsp plain, unsweetened gelatin
- ½ tsp salt
- ½ tsp baking powder
- ¼ cup water

DIRECTIONS:

1. Preheat your air fryer to 325 degrees F and grease an 8x8 inch square baking pan.
2. Combine the eggs, almond extract, swerve, and melted butter in a bowl and whisk together well.
3. Add the cocoa powder, almond flour, baking powder, gelatin, and salt and whisk again until smooth.
4. Add the water and stir again.
5. Pour the batter into the greased baking pan and place in the preheated air fryer. Bake for 15 minutes. The center will seem a little wet while the edges will be more firm- this is perfect.
6. Let the brownies cool in the pan before slicing and serving.

NUTRITION: Calories 110, Total Fat 10g, Saturated Fat 4g, Total Carbs 4g, Net Carbs 1g, Protein 3g, Sugar 1g, Fiber 3g, Sodium 283mg, Potassium 316g

978. Chocolate Coconut Brownies

Preparation time: 15 minutes

Cooking time: 20 minutes

Servings: 16

INGREDIENTS

- ½ cup melted butter
- 2/3 cup swerve
- ½ tsp vanilla extract
- 3 room temperature eggs
- ½ cup almond flour
- 1/3 cup unsweetened cocoa powder
- 1 Tbsp plain, unsweetened gelatin
- ½ tsp salt
- ½ tsp baking powder
- ¼ cup water
- ½ cup unsweetened shredded coconut

Desserts

DIRECTIONS:

1. Preheat your air fryer to 325 degrees F and grease an 8x8 inch square baking pan.
2. Combine the eggs, vanilla extract, swerve, and melted butter in a bowl and whisk together well.
3. Add the cocoa powder, almond flour, baking powder, gelatin, and salt and whisk again until smooth.
4. Add the water and stir again.
5. Fold in the shredded coconut.
6. Pour the batter into the greased baking pan and place in the preheated air fryer. Bake for 15 minutes. The center will seem a little wet while the edges will be more firm- this is perfect.
7. Let the brownies cool in the pan before slicing and serving.

NUTRITION: Calories 218, Total Fat 22g, Saturated Fat 8g, Total Carbs 9g, Net Carbs 5g, Protein 3g, Sugar 3g, Fiber 4g, Sodium 283mg, Potassium 389g

979. Chocolate Mint Brownies

Preparation time: 15 minutes

Cooking time: 20 minutes

Servings: 16

INGREDIENTS

- ½ cup melted butter
- 2/3 cup swerve
- ½ tsp peppermint extract
- 3 room temperature eggs
- ½ cup almond flour
- 1/3 cup unsweetened cocoa powder
- 1 Tbsp plain, unsweetened gelatin
- ½ tsp salt
- ½ tsp baking powder
- ¼ cup water

DIRECTIONS:

1. Preheat your air fryer to 325 degrees F and grease an 8x8 inch square baking pan.
2. Combine the eggs, peppermint extract, swerve, and melted butter in a bowl and whisk together well.
3. Add the cocoa powder, almond flour, baking powder, gelatin, and salt and whisk again until smooth.
4. Add the water and stir again.
5. Pour the batter into the greased baking pan and place in the preheated air fryer. Bake for 15 minutes. The center will seem a little wet while the edges will be more firm- this is perfect.
6. Let the brownies cool in the pan before slicing and serving.

NUTRITION: Calories 110, Total Fat 10g, Saturated Fat 4g, Total Carbs 4g, Net Carbs 1g, Protein 3g, Sugar 1g, Fiber 3g, Sodium 283mg, Potassium 316g

980. Hazelnut Brownies

Preparation time: 15 minutes

Cooking time: 20 minutes

Servings: 16

INGREDIENTS

- ½ cup melted butter
- 2/3 cup swerve
- ½ tsp vanilla extract
- 3 room temperature eggs
- ½ cup almond flour
- 1/3 cup unsweetened cocoa powder
- 1 Tbsp plain, unsweetened gelatin
- ½ tsp salt
- ½ tsp baking powder
- ¼ cup water
- ½ cup chopped hazelnuts

DIRECTIONS:

1. Preheat your air fryer to 325 degrees F and grease an 8x8 inch square baking pan.
2. Combine the eggs, vanilla extract, swerve, and melted butter in a bowl and whisk together well.
3. Add the cocoa powder, almond flour, baking powder, gelatin, and salt and whisk again until smooth.
4. Add the water and stir again.
5. Pour the batter into the greased baking pan, sprinkle with the chopped hazelnuts and place in the preheated air fryer. Bake for 15 minutes. The center will seem a little wet while the edges will be more firm- this is perfect.
6. Let the brownies cool in the pan before slicing and serving.

NUTRITION: Calories 152, Total Fat 23g, Saturated Fat 6g, Total Carbs 8g, Net Carbs 2g, Protein 3g, Sugar 1g, Fiber 6g, Sodium 292mg, Potassium 489g

981. Espresso Brownies

Preparation time: 15 minutes

Cooking time: 20 minutes

Servings: 16

INGREDIENTS

- ½ cup melted butter
- 2/3 cup swerve
- ½ tsp vanilla extract
- 3 room temperature eggs
- ½ cup almond flour
- 1/3 cup unsweetened cocoa powder
- 1 Tbsp plain, unsweetened gelatin
- ½ tsp salt
- ½ tsp baking powder
- ¼ cup brewed espresso

DIRECTIONS:

1. Preheat your air fryer to 325 degrees F and grease an 8x8 inch square baking pan.
2. Combine the eggs, vanilla extract, swerve, and melted butter in a bowl and whisk together well.
3. Add the cocoa powder, almond flour, baking powder, gelatin, and salt and whisk again until smooth.
4. Add the brewed espresso and stir again.
5. Pour the batter into the greased baking pan and place in the preheated air fryer. Bake for 15 minutes. The center will seem a little wet while the edges will be more firm- this is perfect.
6. Let the brownies cool in the pan before slicing and serving.

NUTRITION: Calories 116, Total Fat 10g, Saturated Fat 4g, Total Carbs 4g, Net Carbs 1g, Protein 3g, Sugar 1g, Fiber 3g, Sodium 283mg, Potassium 316g

982. Caramel Fudge Brownies

Preparation time: 15 minutes

Cooking time: 20 minutes

Servings: 16

INGREDIENTS

- ½ cup melted butter
- 2/3 cup swerve
- ½ tsp vanilla extract
- 3 room temperature eggs
- ½ cup almond flour
- 1/3 cup unsweetened cocoa powder
- 1 Tbsp plain, unsweetened gelatin
- ½ tsp salt
- ½ tsp baking powder
- ¼ cup water
- ½ cup keto caramel sauce

DIRECTIONS:

1. Preheat your air fryer to 325 degrees F and grease an 8x8 inch square baking pan.
2. Combine the eggs, vanilla extract, swerve, and melted butter in a bowl and whisk together well.
3. Add the cocoa powder, almond flour, baking powder, gelatin, and salt and whisk again until smooth.
4. Add the water and stir again.
5. Pour the batter into the greased baking pan and swirl in the caramel sauce.
6. Place the pan in the preheated air fryer. Bake for 15 minutes. The center will seem a little wet while the edges will be more firm- this is perfect.
7. Let the brownies cool in the pan before slicing and serving.

NUTRITION: Calories 208, Total Fat 11g, Saturated Fat 4g, Total Carbs 10g, Net Carbs 7g, Protein 3g, Sugar 5g, Fiber 3g, Sodium 383mg, Potassium 316g

DIRECTIONS:

1. Preheat your air fryer to 325 degrees F and grease an 8x8 inch square baking pan.
2. Combine the eggs, vanilla extract, swerve, and melted butter in a bowl and whisk together well.
3. Add the cocoa powder, almond flour, baking powder, gelatin, and salt and whisk again until smooth.
4. Add the water and stir again.
5. Fold in the fresh raspberries.
6. Pour the batter into the greased baking pan and place in the preheated air fryer. Bake for 15 minutes. The center will seem a little wet while the edges will be more firm- this is perfect.
7. Let the brownies cool in the pan before slicing and serving.

NUTRITION: Calories 170, Total Fat 10g, Saturated Fat 4g, Total Carbs 9g, Net Carbs 3g, Protein 3g, Sugar 3g, Fiber 6g, Sodium 283mg, Potassium 368g

983. Raspberry Brownies

Preparation time: 15 minutes

Cooking time: 20 minutes

Servings: 16

INGREDIENTS

- ½ cup melted butter
- 2/3 cup swerve
- ½ tsp vanilla extract
- 3 room temperature eggs
- ½ cup almond flour
- 1/3 cup unsweetened cocoa powder
- 1 Tbsp plain, unsweetened gelatin
- ½ tsp salt
- ½ tsp baking powder
- ¼ cup water
- ½ cup fresh raspberries, cut in half

984. Cauliflower Rice and Plum Pudding

Preparation Time: 30 minutes

Servings: 4

INGREDIENTS

- 4 plums, pitted and roughly chopped.
- 1½ cups cauliflower rice
- 2 cups coconut milk
- 2 tbsp. ghee; melted
- 3 tbsp. stevia

DIRECTIONS

1. Take a bowl and mix all the ingredients, toss, divide into ramekins, put them in the air fryer and cook at 340°F for 25 minutes. Cool down and serve

NUTRITION: Calories: 221; Fat: 4g; Fiber: 1g; Carbs: 3g; Protein: 3g

985. Creamy Chia Seeds Pudding

Preparation Time: 35 minutes

Servings: 6

INGREDIENTS

- 2cups coconut cream
- ¼ cup chia seeds
- 6egg yolks, whisked
- 1tbsp. ghee; melted
- 2tbsp. stevia
- 2tsp. cinnamon powder

DIRECTIONS:

1. Take a bowl and mix all the ingredients, whisk, divide into 6 ramekins, place them all in your air fryer and cook at 340°F for 25 minutes. Cool the puddings down and serve

NUTRITION: Calories: 180; Fat: 4g; Fiber: 2 carbs 5g; Protein: 7g

986. Ginger Cookies

Preparation Time: 25 minutes

Servings: 12

INGREDIENTS

- ¼ cup butter; melted
- 2cups almond flour
- 1cup swerve
- 1egg
- ¼ tsp. nutmeg, ground
- ¼ tsp. cinnamon powder
- 2tsp. ginger, grated
- 1tsp. vanilla extract

DIRECTIONS

1. Take a bowl and mix all the ingredients and whisk well.
2. Spoon small balls out of this mix on a lined baking sheet that fits the air fryer lined with parchment paper and flatten them
3. Put the sheet in the fryer and cook at 360°F for 15 minutes
4. Cool the cookies down and serve.

NUTRITION: Calories: 220; Fat: 13g; Fiber: 2g; Carbs: 4g; Protein: 3g

987. Spiced Avocado Pudding

Preparation Time: 30 minutes

Servings: 6

INGREDIENTS

- 4small avocados, peeled, pitted and mashed
- 2eggs, whisked
- ¾ cup swerve
- 1cup coconut milk
- 1tsp. cinnamon powder
- ½ tsp. ginger powder

DIRECTIONS:

1. Take a bowl and mix all the ingredients and whisk well.
2. Pour into a pudding mould, put it in the air fryer and cook at 350°F for 25 minutes
3. Servings warm

NUTRITION: Calories: 192; Fat: 8g; Fiber: 2g; Carbs: 5g; Protein: 4g

988. Coconut Bars

Preparation Time: 45 minutes

Servings: 12

INGREDIENTS

- 1¼ cups almond flour
- ½ cup coconut cream
- 1½ cups coconut, flaked
- 1 egg yolk
- ¾ cup walnuts; chopped.
- 1 cup swerve
- 1 cup butter; melted
- ½ tsp. vanilla extract

DIRECTIONS

1. Take a bowl and mix the flour with half of the swerve and half of the butter, stir well and press this on the bottom of a baking pan that fits the air fryer.
2. Introduce this in the air fryer and cook at 350°F for 15 minutes
3. Meanwhile, heat up a pan with the rest of the butter over medium heat, add the remaining swerve and the rest of the ingredients, whisk, cook for 1-2 minutes, take off the heat and cool down
4. Spread this well over the crust, put the pan in the air fryer again and cook at 350°F for 25 minutes. Cool down; cut into bars and serve.

NUTRITION: Calories: 182; Fat: 12g; Fiber: 2g; Carbs: 4g; Protein: 4g

989. Plum Cream

Preparation Time: 25 minutes

Servings: 4

INGREDIENTS

- 1 lb. plums, pitted and chopped.
- 1½ cups heavy cream
- ¼ cup swerve
- 1 tbsp. lemon juice

DIRECTIONS

1. Take a bowl and mix all the ingredients and whisk really well.
2. Divide this into 4 ramekins, put them in the air fryer and cook at 340°F for 20 minutes
3. Servings cold

NUTRITION: Calories: 171; Fat: 4g; Fiber: 2g; Carbs: 4g; Protein: 4g

990. Raspberry Muffins

Preparation Time: 30 minutes

Servings: 8

INGREDIENTS

- ¾ cup raspberries
- ½ cup swerve
- ¼ cup coconut flour
- ¼ cup ghee; melted
- 1 egg
- 3 tbsp. cream cheese
- 2 tbsp. almond meal
- ½ tsp. baking soda
- ½ tsp. baking powder
- 1 tsp. cinnamon powder
- Cooking spray

DIRECTIONS

1. Take a bowl and mix all the ingredients except the cooking spray and whisk well.
2. Grease a muffin pan that fits the air fryer with the cooking spray
3. Pour the raspberry mix, put the pan in the machine and cook at 350°F for 20 minutes
   Servings the muffins cold

NUTRITION: Calories: 223; Fat: 7g; Fiber: 2g; Carbs: 4g; Protein: 5g

991. Cinnamon Plums

Preparation Time: 25 minutes

Servings: 4

INGREDIENTS

- 4plums; halved
- 3tbsp. swerve
- 4tbsp. butter; melted
- 2tsp. cinnamon powder

DIRECTIONS

1. In a pan that fits your air fryer, mix the plums with the rest of the ingredients, toss, put the pan in the air fryer and cook at 300°F for 20 minutes
2. Divide into cups and serve cold.

NUTRITION: Calories: 162; Fat: 3g; Fiber: 2g; Carbs: 4g; Protein: 5g

992. Strawberry Cake

Preparation Time: 45 minutes

Servings: 6

INGREDIENTS

- 1lb. strawberries; chopped.
- 1egg, whisked
- 1cup almond flour
- ¼ cup swerve
- 1cup cream cheese, soft
- 3tbsp. coconut oil; melted
- 1tbsp. lime juice
- 1tsp. vanilla extract
- 2tsp. baking powder

DIRECTIONS

1. Take a bowl and mix all the ingredients, stir well and pour this into a cake pan lined with parchment paper.
2. Put the pan in the air fryer, cook at 350°F for 35 minutes, cool down, slice and serve

NUTRITION: Calories: 200; Fat: 6g; Fiber: 2g; Carbs: 4g; Protein: 6g

993. Chocolate Pudding

Preparation Time: 30 minutes

Servings: 6

INGREDIENTS

- 24oz. cream cheese, soft
- 12oz. dark chocolate; melted
- ½ cup heavy cream
- ¼ cup erythritol
- 3eggs, whisked
- 1tbsp. vanilla extract
- 2tbsp. almond meal

DIRECTIONS

1. In a bowl mix all the ingredients and whisk well.
2. Divide this into 6 ramekins, put them in your air fryer and cook at 320°F for 20 minutes.
3. Keep in the fridge for 1 hour before serving

NUTRITION: Calories: 200; Fat: 7g; Fiber: 2g; Carbs: 4g; Protein: 6g

994. Cream Cheese Brownies

Preparation Time: 35 minutes

Servings: 6

INGREDIENTS

- 3eggs, whisked
- ¼ cup almond flour
- ¼ cup coconut flour
- ½ cup almond milk
- 2tbsp. cocoa powder

- 3tbsp. swerve
- 6tbsp. cream cheese, soft
- 3tbsp. coconut oil; melted
- 1tsp. vanilla extract
- ¼ tsp. baking soda
- Cooking spray

DIRECTIONS

1. Grease a cake pan that fits the air fryer with the cooking spray.
2. Take a bowl and mix rest of the ingredients, whisk well and pour into the pan
3. Put the pan in your air fryer, cook at 370°F for 25 minutes, cool the brownies down, slice and serve.

NUTRITION: Calories: 182; Fat: 12g; Fiber: 2g; Carbs: 4g; Protein: 6g

995. Lemon Coconut Pie

Preparation Time: 45 minutes

Servings: 8

INGREDIENTS

- 4oz. coconut, shredded
- 2eggs, whisked
- ¼ cup coconut flour
- ¾ cup swerve
- 2tbsp. butter; melted
- 1tsp. lemon zest, grated
- 1tsp. baking powder
- 1tsp. vanilla extract
- ½ tsp. lemon extract
- Cooking spray

DIRECTIONS

1. In a bowl, combine all the ingredients except the cooking spray and stir well.
2. Grease a pie pan that fits the air fryer with the cooking spray

3. Pour the mixture inside, put the pan in the air fryer and cook at 360°F for 35 minutes. Slice and serve warm.

NUTRITION: Calories: 212; Fat: 15g; Fiber: 2g; Carbs: 6g; Protein: 4g

996. Almond Butter Cookies

Preparation Time: 17 minutes

Servings: 12

INGREDIENTS

- 1cup almond butter, soft
- 1egg
- 2tbsp. erythritol
- 1tsp. vanilla extract

DIRECTIONS

1. Take a bowl and mix all the ingredients and whisk really well.
2. Spread this on a cookie sheet that fits the air fryer lined with parchment paper, introduce in the fryer and cook at 350°F and bake for 12 minutes. Cool down and serve

NUTRITION: Calories: 130; Fat: 12g; Fiber: 1g; Carbs: 3g; Protein: 5g

997. Avocado Granola

Preparation Time: 12 minutes

Servings: 6

INGREDIENTS

- 1cup avocado, peeled, pitted and cubed
- ¼ cup walnuts; chopped.
- ¼ cup almonds; chopped.
- ½ cup coconut flakes
- 2tbsp. stevia
- 2tbsp. ghee; melted

DIRECTIONS

1. In a pan that fits your air fryer, mix all the ingredients, toss, put the pan in the fryer and cook at 320°F for 8 minutes
2. Divide into bowls and serve right away.

NUTRITION: Calories: 170; Fat: 3g; Fiber: 2g; Carbs: 4g; Protein: 3g

998. Blackberry Chia Jam

Preparation Time: 40 minutes

Servings: 12

INGREDIENTS

- ¼ cup swerve
- 3 cups blackberries
- 4 tbsp. chia seeds
- 4 tbsp. lemon juice

DIRECTIONS

1. In a pan that fits the air fryer, combine all the ingredients and toss.
2. Put the pan in the machine and cook at 300°F for 30 minutes. Divide into cups and serve cold

NUTRITION: Calories: 100; Fat: 2g; Fiber: 1g; Carbs: 3g; Protein: 1g

999. Lemon Bars

Preparation Time: 45 minutes

Servings: 8

INGREDIENTS

- 1¾ cups almond flour
- 3 eggs, whisked
- ½ cup butter; melted
- 1 cup erythritol
- Zest of 1 lemon, grated
- Juice of 3 lemons

DIRECTIONS

1. Take a bowl and mix 1 cup flour with half of the erythritol and the butter, stir well and press into a baking dish that fits the air fryer lined with parchment paper
2. Put the dish in your air fryer and cook at 350°F for 10 minutes.
3. Meanwhile, in a bowl, mix the rest of the flour with the remaining erythritol and the other ingredients and whisk well
4. Spread this over the crust, put the dish in the air fryer once more and cook at 350°F for 25 minutes
5. Cool down; cut into bars and serve.

NUTRITION: Calories: 210; Fat: 12g; Fiber: 1g; Carbs: 4g; Protein: 8g

1000. Strawberries Stew

Preparation Time: 30 minutes

Servings: 4

INGREDIENTS

- 1 lb. strawberries; halved
- 1½ cups water
- 1 tbsp. lemon juice
- 4 tbsp. stevia

DIRECTIONS

1. In a pan that fits your air fryer, mix all the ingredients, toss, put it in the fryer and cook at 340°F for 20 minutes
2. Divide the stew into cups and serve cold.

NUTRITION: Calories: 176; Fat: 2g; Fiber: 1g; Carbs: 3g; Protein: 5g

1001. Blueberries and Chocolate Cream

Preparation Time: 25 minutes

Servings: 4

INGREDIENTS

- 2cups blueberries
- 3tbsp. cream cheese, soft
- 4tbsp. erythritol
- 3tbsp. chocolate; melted

DIRECTIONS

1. In a pan that fits the air fryer, combine all the ingredients, whisk.
2. Put the pan in the fryer and cook at 340°F for 20 minutes
3. Divide into bowls and serve cold.

NUTRITION: Calories: 200; Fat: 6g; Fiber: 2g; Carbs: 4g; Protein: 5g

1002. Cocoa Cake

Preparation Time: 25 minutes

Servings: 8

INGREDIENTS

- 2egg
- ¼ cup coconut milk
- 4tbsp. almond flour
- 1tbsp. cocoa powder
- 3tbsp. swerve
- 3tbsp. coconut oil; melted
- ½ tsp. baking powder

DIRECTIONS

1. Take a bowl and mix all the ingredients and stir well.
2. Pour this into a cake pan that fits the air fryer, put the pan in the machine and cook at 340°F for 20 minutes

NUTRITION: Calories: 191; Fat: 12g; Fiber: 2g; Carbs: 4g; Protein: 6g

1003. Mini Lava Cakes

Preparation Time: 30 minutes

Servings: 4

INGREDIENTS

- 3oz. dark chocolate; melted
- 2eggs, whisked
- ¼ cup coconut oil; melted
- 1tbsp. almond flour
- 2tbsp. swerve
- ¼ tsp. vanilla extract
- Cooking spray

DIRECTIONS

1. In bowl, combine all the ingredients except the cooking spray and whisk really well.
2. Divide this into 4 ramekins greased with cooking spray, put them in the fryer and cook at 360°F for 20 minutes

NUTRITION: Calories: 161; Fat: 12g; Fiber: 1g; Carbs: 4g; Protein: 7g

1004. Avocado Brownies

Preparation Time: 40 minutes

Servings: 12

INGREDIENTS

- 1cup avocado; peeled and mashed
- 2eggs, whisked
- ½ cup dark chocolate, unsweetened and melted
- ¾ cup almond flour
- 3tbsp. coconut oil; melted
- 4tbsp. cocoa powder
- 1tsp. baking powder
- 1tsp. stevia
- ½ tsp. vanilla extract
- ¼ tsp. baking soda

DIRECTIONS

1. Take a bowl and mix the flour with stevia, baking powder and soda and stir.
2. Add the rest of the ingredients gradually, whisk and pour into a cake pan that fits the air fryer after you lined it with parchment paper
3. Put the pan in your air fryer and cook at 350°F for 30 minutes. Cut into squares and serve cold.

NUTRITION: Calories: 155; Fat: 6g; Fiber: 2g; Carbs: 6g; Protein: 4g

1005. Baked Plums

Preparation Time: 25 minutes

Servings: 6

INGREDIENTS

- 6plums; cut into wedges
- 10drops stevia
- Zest of 1 lemon, grated
- 2tbsp. water
- 1tsp. ginger, ground
- ½ tsp. cinnamon powder

DIRECTIONS

1. In a pan that fits the air fryer, combine the plums with the rest of the ingredients, toss gently.
2. Put the pan in the air fryer and cook at 360°F for 20 minutes
3. Servings cold

NUTRITION: Calories: 170; Fat: 5g; Fiber: 1g; Carbs: 3g; Protein: 5g

1006. Lime Berry Pudding

Preparation Time: 20 minutes

Servings: 6

INGREDIENTS

- 1/3 cup blueberries
- 2cups coconut cream
- 1/3 cup blackberries
- Zest of 1 lime, grated
- 3tbsp. swerve

DIRECTIONS

1. In a blender, combine all the ingredients and pulse well.
2. Divide this into 6 small ramekins, put them in your air fryer and cook at 340°F for 15 minutes
3. Servings cold

NUTRITION: Calories: 173; Fat: 3g; Fiber: 1g; Carbs: 4g; Protein: 4g

1007. Currant Pudding

Preparation Time: 25 minutes

Servings: 6

INGREDIENTS:

- 1cup red currants, blended
- 1cup coconut cream
- 1cup black currants, blended
- 3tbsp. stevia

DIRECTIONS

1. In a bowl, combine all the ingredients and stir well.
2. Divide into ramekins, put them in the fryer and cook at 340°F for 20 minutes
3. Serve the pudding cold.

NUTRITION: Calories: 200; Fat: 4g; Fiber: 2g; Carbs: 4g; Protein: 6g

1008. Cocoa and Nuts Bombs

Preparation Time: 13 minutes

Servings: 12

INGREDIENTS

- 2cups macadamia nuts; chopped.
- ¼ cup cocoa powder
- 1/3 cup swerve
- 4tbsp. coconut oil; melted
- 1tsp. vanilla extract

DIRECTIONS

1. Take a bowl and mix all the ingredients and whisk well.
2. Shape medium balls out of this mix, place them in your air fryer and cook at 300°F for 8 minutes Servings cold

NUTRITION: Calories: 120; Fat: 12g; Fiber: 1g; Carbs: 2g; Protein: 1g

1009. Blueberry Cream

Preparation Time: 24 minutes

Servings: 6

INGREDIENTS

- 2cups blueberries
- 2tbsp. swerve
- 2tbsp. water
- 1tsp. vanilla extract
- Juice of ½ lemon

DIRECTIONS

1. Take a bowl and mix all the ingredients and whisk well.
2. Divide this into 6 ramekins, put them in the air fryer and cook at 340°F for 20 minutes.
3. Cool down and serve

NUTRITION: Calories: 123; Fat: 2g; Fiber: 2g; Carbs: 4g; Protein: 3g

1010. Strawberry Jam

Preparation Time: 30 minutes

Servings: 12

INGREDIENTS

- 8oz. strawberries; sliced
- ¼ cup swerve
- ¼ cup water
- 1tbsp. lemon juice

DIRECTIONS

1. In a pan that fits the air fryer, combine all the ingredients.
2. Put the pan in the machine and cook at 380°F for 20 minutes
3. Divide the mix into cups, cool down and serve.

NUTRITION: Calories: 100; Fat: 1g; Fiber: 0g; Carbs: 1g; Protein: 1g

1011. Butter Cookies

Preparation Time: 30 minutes

Servings: 12

INGREDIENTS

- 2eggs, whisked
- 2¾ cup almond flour
- ¼ cup swerve
- ½ cup butter; melted
- 1tbsp. heavy cream
- 2tsp. vanilla extract
- Cooking spray

DIRECTIONS

1. Take a bowl and mix all the ingredients except the cooking spray and stir well.
2. Shape 12 balls out of this mix, put them on a baking sheet that fits the air fryer greased with cooking spray and flatten them

3. Put the baking sheet in the air fryer and cook at 350°F for 20 minutes
4. Serve the cookies cold.

NUTRITION: Calories: 234; Fat: 13g; Fiber: 2g; Carbs: 4g; Protein: 7g

1012. Cream Cheese and Zucchinis Bars

Preparation Time: 25 minutes

Servings: 12

INGREDIENTS

- 3oz. zucchini, shredded
- 4oz. cream cheese
- 6eggs
- 2tbsp. erythritol
- 3tbsp. coconut oil; melted
- 2tsp. vanilla extract
- ½ tsp. baking powder

DIRECTIONS

1. In a bowl, combine all the ingredients and whisk well.
2. pour this into a baking dish that fits your air fryer lined with parchment paper, introduce in the fryer and cook at 320°F, bake for 15 minutes. Slice and serve cold

NUTRITION: Calories: 178; Fat: 8g; Fiber: 3g; Carbs: 4g; Protein: 5g

1013. Coconut Cookies

Preparation Time: 20 minutes

Servings: 8

INGREDIENTS

- 1½ cups coconut, shredded
- 2eggs, whisked
- 2tbsp. erythritol
- ¼ tsp. almond extract
- ½ tsp. baking powder

DIRECTIONS

1. Take a bowl and mix all the ingredients and whisk well.
2. Scoop 8 servings of this mix on a baking sheet that fits the air fryer which you've lined with parchment paper.
3. Put the baking sheet in your air fryer and cook at 350°F for 15 minutes
4. Servings cold

NUTRITION: Calories: 125; Fat: 7g; Fiber: 1g; Carbs: 5g; Protein: 4g

1014. Lemon Cookies

Preparation Time: 30 minutes

Servings: 12

INGREDIENTS

- ¼ cup cashew butter, soft
- 1egg, whisked
- ¾ cup swerve
- 1cup coconut cream
- Juice of 1 lemon
- 1tsp. baking powder
- 1tsp. lemon peel, grated

DIRECTIONS

1. In a bowl, combine all the ingredients gradually and stir well.
2. Spoon balls this on a cookie sheet lined with parchment paper and flatten them.
3. Put the cookie sheet in the fryer and cook at 350°F for 20 minutes
4. Servings the cookies cold

NUTRITION: Calories: 121; Fat: 5g; Fiber: 1g; Carbs: 4g; Protein: 2g

1015. Delicious cheesecake

Preparation Time: 25 Minutes

Servings: 15

INGREDIENTS

- Cream cheese: 1 lb
- Vanilla extract: ½ tbsp
- Graham crackers: 1 cup crumbled
- Butter: 2 tbsp
- Eggs: 2
- Sugar: 4 tbsp

DIRECTIONS

1. Mix crackers and butter in a bowl
2. Press the mix on a lined cake pan
3. Preheat your fryer to 350 °F
4. Place the pan the air fryer. Cook for 4 minutes
5. In another bowl, mix sugar, cream cheese, eggs and vanilla while stirring
6. Spread them onto the crackers. Cook at 310 °F for 15 minutes.
7. Cool it in the fridge for 15 minutes
8. Servings

NUTRITION: Calories: 245; Fat: 12; Protein: 3; Carbohydrates: 20; Fiber: 1

1016. Macaroons

Preparation Time: 18 Minutes

Servings: 20

INGREDIENTS

- Sugar 2 tbsp
- Coconut: 2 cups shredded
- Egg whites: 2
- Vanilla extract: 1 tbsp

DIRECTIONS

1. Beat egg whites with stevia in a bowl
2. While stirring, add coconut and vanilla extract
3. Shape them into balls
4. Place them in the air fryer. Cook until 340 °F and let it cook at this temperature for 8 minutes

Servings

NUTRITION: Calories: 55; Fat: 6; Protein: 1; Carbohydrates: 2; Fiber: 1

1017. Orange cake

Preparation Time: 42 Minutes

Servings: 12

INGREDIENTS

- Orange: 1 peeled and cut to quarters
- Vanilla extract: 1 tbsp
- Eggs: 6
- Orange zest: 2 tbsp
- Cream cheese: 4 oz.
- Baking powder: 1 tbsp
- Flour: 9 oz.
- Sugar: 2 oz. and 2 tbsp
- Yogurt: 4 oz.

DIRECTIONS

1. Pulse the orange in a food processor
2. Pour in the flour, 2 tbsp sugar, baking powder, eggs and vanilla extract. Pulse it again
3. Place it in 2 spring-form pans.
4. Place it in the air fryer then heat it to 330 °F after which let it cook for 16 minutes.
5. In another bowl, mix cream cheese, orange zest, yogurt and the remaining sugar while stirring
6. Sandwich half of the contents of the bowl between the two cake layers from each spring pan. Spread the half that remained on top of the cake. Serve.

NUTRITION: Calories: 200; Fat: 13; Protein: 8; Carbohydrates: 9; Fiber: 2

1018. Amaretto and bread dough

Preparation Time: 22 Minutes

Servings: 12

INGREDIENTS

- Bread dough: 1 lb
- Heavy cream: 1 cup
- Chocolate chips: 12 oz.
- Sugar: 1 cup
- Butter: 1 cup melted
- Amaretto liqueur: 2 tbsp

DIRECTIONS

1. Roll the dough on a working surface. Cut it into 20 slices. Further cut the 20 slices into halves
2. Brush each dough piece with butter then sprinkle sugar on it
3. Brush the air fryer with some butter
4. Place the dough pieces in the pan. Cook at 350 °F for 5 minutes.
5. Flip them and let them cook for 3 minutes
6. Place the heavy cream in a pan. Heat over medium meat.
7. Carefully add the chocolate chips and let them melt.
8. Add liqueur, stir then transfer them to a bowl. Serve.

NUTRITION: Calories: 200; Fat: 1; Protein: 6; Carbohydrates: 6; Fiber: 0

1019. Carrot cake

Preparation Time: 55 Minutes

Servings: 6

INGREDIENTS

- Flour: 5 oz.
- Baking powder: ¾ tbsp
- Nutmeg: ¼ tbsp
- Cinnamon powder: ½ tbsp
- Sugar: ½ cup
- Carrots: 1/3 cup grated
- Pecans: 1/3 cup toasted and chopped
- Pineapple juice: ¼ cup
- Allspice: ½ tbsp
- Egg: 1
- Yogurt: 3 tbsp
- Sunflower oil
- Coconut flakes: 1/3 cup shredded
- Cooking spray

DIRECTIONS

1. Mix flour, allspice, baking powder, baking soda, salt, cinnamon and nutmeg in a bowl A then stir
2. In another bowl B mix egg, yogurt, sugar, pineapple juice, oil, carrots, pecans and coconut flakes while stirring
3. While stirring, mix bowl A and bowl B
4. Pour contents in bowl C into a greased pan. Cook them for 45 minutes at 320°F
5. Let it cool. Serve.

NUTRITION: Calories: 200; Fat: 6; Protein: 4; Carbohydrates: 22; Fiber: 20

1020. Banana bread

Preparation Time: 50 Minutes

Servings: 6

INGREDIENTS

- Sugar: ¾ cup
- Butter: 1/3 cup
- Milk: 1/3 cup
- Vanilla extract: 1 tbsp
- Egg: 1
- Baking powder: 1 tbsp
- Flour: 1 ½ cups
- Baking soda: ½ tbsp
- Cream of tartar: 1 ½ tbsp
- Cooking spray

DIRECTIONS

1. While stirring, mix milk, cream of tartar, sugar, butter, egg, vanilla and bananas in a bowl A
2. In another bowl B mix flour, baking powder and baking soda
3. Combine bowl B and bowl A while stirring
4. Place it in a greased pan
5. Place it in an air fryer and cook for 40 minutes at 320 °F
6. Let it cool then serve.

NUTRITION: Calories: 292; Fat: 7; Protein: 4; Carbohydrates: 28; Fiber: 8

1021. Granola

Preparation Time: 45 Minutes

Servings: 4

INGREDIENTS

- Coconut: 1 cup shredded
- Almonds: ½ cup
- Pecans: ½ cup chopped
- Sugar: 2 tbsp
- Pumpkin seeds: ½ cup
- Sunflower seeds: ½ cup
- Sunflower oil: 2 tbsp
- Nutmeg: 1 tbsp ground
- Apple pie spice mix: 1 tbsp

DIRECTIONS

1. While stirring, mix almonds, pecans, pumpkin seeds, sunflower seeds, coconut, nutmeg and apple pie spice in a bowl
2. Heat a greased pan over medium heat
3. Add sugar and stir
4. Pour the bowl mixture in the pan and stir. Let it sit for a few minutes
5. Gently spread it on a baking sheet that has been lined
6. Place the baking sheet in the air fryer and bake for 25 minutes at 300 °F
7. Let it cool then serve.

NUTRITION: Calories: 322; Fat: 7; Protein: 7; Carbohydrates: 12; Fiber: 8

1022. Espresso cream and pears

Preparation Time: 40 Minutes

Servings: 4

INGREDIENTS

- Pears: 4 halved and cored
- Water: 2 tbsp
- Lemon juice: 2 tbsp
- Sugar: 1 tbsp
- Butter: 2 tbsp
- Cream Ingredients:
- Whipping cream: 1 cup
- Cold espresso: 1 tbsp
- Mascarpone: 1 cup
- Sugar: 1/3 cup

DIRECTIONS

1. Mix pears halves, lemon juice, 1 tbsp. sugar, butter and water in a bowl then toss well
2. Place them in an air fryer and cook for 30 minutes at 360 °F
3. Mix whipping cream, mascarpone, ⅓ cup sugar and espresso in a bowl A and whisk them well
4. Place bowl A in the fridge until the food in the air dryer is cooked. Serve.

NUTRITION: Calories: 211; Fat: 5; Protein: 7; Carbohydrates: 8; Fiber: 7

1023. Banana cake

Preparation Time: 40 Minutes

Servings: 4

INGREDIENTS

- Soft butter: 1tbsp
- Brown sugar: 1/3 cup

- Egg: 1
- Baking powder: 1 tbsp
- Cooking spray

DIRECTIONS

1. Grease a cake pan
2. Mix butter, sugar, banana, honey, egg, cinnamon, baking powder and flour in a bowl and whisk
3. Pour them in the pan and cook for 30 minutes in the air fryer at 350 °F
4. Let it cool then serve.

NUTRITION: Calories: 232; Fat: 4; Protein: 4; Carbohydrates: 34; Fiber: 1

1024. Fried banana

Preparation Time: 25 Minutes

Servings: 4

INGREDIENTS:

- Butter: 3 tbsp
- Cinnamon sugar: 3 tbsp
- Panko: 1 cup
- Eggs: 2
- Bananas: 8 peeled and halved
- Corn flour: ½ cup

DIRECTIONS:

1. Heat a greased pan over medium heat
2. Add panko in the pan then stir
3. Mix flour, eggs and panko
4. Roll the mixture and dust it with cinnamon
5. Place the rolls in the air fryer and cook for 10 minutes at 280 °F. Serve

NUTRITION: Calories: 164; Fat: 1; Protein: 4; Carbohydrates: 32; Fiber: 4

1025. Coffee cheesecakes

Preparation Time: 30 Minutes

Servings: 6

INGREDIENTS

- Butter: 2 tbsp
- Eggs: 3
- Sugar: 1/3 cup
- Cream cheese: 8 oz.
- Coffee: 3 tbsp
- Caramel syrup: 1 tbsp
- Frosting Ingredients:
- Caramel syrup: 3 tbsp
- Soft mascarpone cheese: 8 oz.
- Butter: 3 tbsp
- Sugar: 2 tbsp

DIRECTIONS

1. Mix cream cheese, eggs, 2 tbsp. butter, coffee, 1 tbsp. caramel syrup and ⅓ cup sugar in a blender then pulse
2. Spoon it into cupcake pans and cook them for 20 minutes at 320 °F
3. After it cools down, place it in the freezer for 3 hours
4. Mix 3 tbsp. butter, 3 tbsp. caramel syrup, 2 tbsp. sugar and mascarpone in a bowl and blend
5. Spread this mixture over the cheesecakes. Then serve.

NUTRITION: Calories: 254; Fat: 23; Protein: 5; Carbohydrates: 21; Fiber: 0

1026. Cinnamon rolls served with Cream cheese

Preparation Time: 2 hours 15 Minutes

Servings: 8

INGREDIENTS

- Bread.dough.1.1b
- Brown sugar 3/4
- melted butter 1/4
- cinnamon 1 ½ tbsp. ground

- Cream cheese ingredients
- Butter 2 tbsp
- Sugar 1. ¼ tbsp
- Vanilla ½ tbsp
- Cream Cheese 4 oz

DIRECTIONS

1. On a working surface, roll the dough and shape it rectangular

2. Brush the dough with ¼ tbsp butter

3. In a bowl, mix cinnamon and sugar and stir

4. Sprinkle contents of the bowl over the dough

5. Roll the dough into a log then seal it and cut it to 8 pieces. Leave them aside for 2 hours to rise

6. Place them in the air fryer then cook them for 4 minutes at 350 °F. Flip them and let them cook for 4 minutes

7. Mix cream cheese, butter, sugar and vanilla in a bowl then whisk them well. Serve it with the cinnamon rolls.

NUTRITION: Calories: 200; Fat: 1; Protein: 6; Carbohydrates: 5; Fiber: 0

1027. Pumpkin cookies

Preparation Time: 25 Minutes

Servings: 24

INGREDIENTS

A. Flour: 2 ½ cups

B. Baking soda: ½ tbsp

C. Butter: 2 tbsp

D. Vanilla extract: 1 tbsp

E. Flax seed: 1tbsp ground

F. Water: 3 tbsp

G. Pumpkin flesh: 1/2 cup mashed

H. Honey: ¼ cup

I. Dark chocolate chips: ½ cup

DIRECTIONS

1. In a bowl A, mix flax seed and water then stir. Leave it aside for a few minutes.

2. Take a bowl B and mix flour, salt and baking powder

3. Mix honey, pumpkin puree, butter, vanilla extract and flax-seed in another bowl C

4. Mix contents in bowl B, A and bowl C to form cookie dough

5. Take 1 tbsp of cookie dough and arrange them in the air fryer. Cook them for 15 minutes at 350 °F

6. Let it cool then serve

NUTRITION: Calories: 140; Fat: 2; Protein: 10; Carbohydrates: 7; Fiber: 2

1028. Apple bread

Preparation Time: 50 Minutes

Servings: 6

INGREDIENTS

A. Apples: 3 cups cored and cubed

B. Sugar: 1 tbsp

C. Baking powder: 1 tbsp

D. Butter: 1 stick

E. Vanilla: 1 tbsp

F. Eggs: 2

G. Apple pie spice: 1 tbsp

H. White flour: 2 cups

I. Water: 1 cup

DIRECTIONS

1. Mix egg, 1 butter stick, apple pie spice and sugar in a bowl A then stir using your mixer

2. While stirring, add apples

3. Mix baking powder and flour in another bowl B

4. Combine contents in bowl A and bowl B then stir

5. Pour them into a pan in such a way that they make a spring shape. Cook it in the air fryer for 40 minutes at 320°F then serve.

NUTRITION: Calories: 192; Fat: 6; Protein: 7; Carbohydrates: 14; Fiber: 7

1029. Strawberry pie

Preparation Time: 30 Minutes

Servings: 12

INGREDIENTS

1. Coconut: 1 cup shredded

2. Butter: ¼ cup

3. Sunflower seeds: 1 cup

4. Filling Ingredients:

5. Gelatin: 1 tbsp

6. Cream cheese: 8 oz.

7. Lemon juice: ½ tbsp

8. Ste-via: ¼ tbsp

9. Strawberries: 4 oz.

10. Water: 4 tbsp

11. Heavy cream: ½ cup

12. Strawberries: 8 oz. chopped for serving

DIRECTIONS

A. Mix sunflower seeds, coconut, a pinch of salt and butter in a food processor then pulse it

B. Press it on the bottom of your cake pan then heat the pan over medium heat

C. Slowly add gelatin and stir. Cook for a few minutes then leave it aside to cool

D. Place it to your food processor, and 4 oz. strawberries, cream cheese, lemon juice and Ste via. Blend it

E. Add heavy cream and stir.

F. Spread it over the crust top it with 4 oz. strawberries and cook in the air fryer for 15 minutes at 330 ° F

G. Keep it in the fridge, then serve when needed.

NUTRITION: Calories: 234; Fat: 23; Protein: 7; Carbohydrates: 6; Fiber: 2

1030. Bread pudding

Preparation Time: 1 hour 10 Minutes

Servings: 4

INGREDIENTS

1. Glazed doughnuts: 6 crumbled
2. Cherries: 1 cup
3. Egg yolks: 4
4. Sugar: ¼ tbsp
5. Chocolate chips: ½ cup.
6. Whipping cream: 1 ½ cups
7. Raisins: ½ cup

DIRECTIONS

A. Mix cherries, egg yolks and whipping cream in a bowl A then stir well.
B. Mix raisins, sugar, chocolate chips and doughnuts in another bowl B and stir
C. Combine the contents of bowl A and bowl B
D. Place them in a greased pan and cook for 1 hour at 310 ° F let it cool then serve.

NUTRITION: Calories: 302; Fat: 8; Protein: 10; Carbohydrates: 23; Fiber: 2

1031. Pomegranate and chocolate bars

Preparation Time: 2 hours 10 Minutes

Servings: 6

INGREDIENTS

1. Milk: ½ cup
2. Almonds: ½ cup chopped
3. Vanilla extract: 1 tbsp
4. Dark chocolate: 1 ½ cup chopped
5. Pomegranate seeds: ½ cup

DIRECTIONS

A. Pour milk in a pan. Heat it over medium heat
B Add chocolate and stir for 5 minutes then turn off the heat
C Add vanilla extract, half of the pomegranate seeds and half of the nuts then stir
D Pour it into a lined baking pan
E. Add a pinch of salt, the rest of the pomegranate and the rest of the nuts. Cook it for 4 minutes at 300°F in the air fryer
F. Place it in the fridge for 2 hours then serve.

NUTRITION: Calories: 68; Fat: 1; Protein: 1; Carbohydrates: 6; Fiber: 4

1032. Crisp apples

Preparation Time: 20 Minutes

Servings: 4

HINGREDIENTS

1. 1Cinnamon powder: 2 tbsp
2. Apples: 5 cored and cut into chunks
3. Butter: 4 tbsp
4. Flour: ¼ cup
5. Old fashioned rolled oats: ¾ cup
6. Nutmeg powder: ½ tbsp
7. Maple syrup: 1 tbsp

8. Water: ½ cup

9. Brown sugar: ¼ cup

DIRECTIONS

    A. Place the apples in a pa

    B. Add cinnamon, nutmeg, maple syrup and water

    C. Mix butter, oats, sugar, salt and flour in bowl and stir

    D. Place 3 spoonfuls of the bowl contents on the apples. Cook for 10 minutes at 350 °F in the air fryer. Serve while hot or warm.

NUTRITION: Calories: 200; Fat: 6; Protein: 12; Carbohydrates: 29; Fiber: 8

1033. Chocolate cookies

Preparation Time: 35 Minutes

Servings: 12

INGREDIENTS:

1. Vanilla extract: 1 tbsp

2. Flour: 2 cups

3. Butter: 1/2 cup

4. Egg: 1

5. Sugar: 4 tbsp

7. Unsweetened chocolate chips: ½ cup

DIRECTIONS

    A. Place butter in a pan and heat it over medium heat

    B. Mix egg, vanilla extract and sugar in a bowl while stirring

    C. Add melted butter, flour and half f the chocolate chips. Stir it well

    D. Transfer them to the air fryer, add the remaining chocolate chips and bake for 25 minutes at 330 °F. Serve when cold.

Nutrition: Calories: 230; Fat: 12; Protein: 5; Carbohydrates: 4; Fiber: 2

31-DAY MEAL PLAN

DAY	BREAKFAST	MAINS	DESSERTS
1.	Stuffed Portobello Mushrooms with Ground Beef	Indian Chickpeas	Butter Cookies
2.	Basil-Spinach Quiche	White Beans with Rosemary	Cream Cheese and Zucchinis Bars
3.	Stuffed Chicken Roll with Mushrooms	Squash Bowls	Coconut Cookies
4.	Eggs on Avocado Burgers	Cauliflower Stew with Tomatoes and Green Chilies	Lemon Cookies
5.	Applesauce Mash with Sweet Potato	Simple Quinoa Stew	Delicious cheesecake
6.	Bacon and Kale Breakfast Salad	Green Beans with Carrot	Macaroons
7.	Fish Fritatta	Chickpeas and Lentils Mix	Amaretto and bread dough
8.	Spinach Frittata	Garlic Pork Chops	Orange cake
9.	Kale Quiche with Eggs	Honey Ginger Salmon Steaks	Apple bread
10.	Olives Rice Mix	Mustard Pork Balls	Strawberry pie
11.	Sweet Quinoa Mix	Beef Meatballs in Tomato Sauce	Bread pudding
12.	Creamy Almond Rice	Green Stuffed Peppers	Pomegranate and chocolate bars
13.	Chives Quinoa Bowls	Sweet & Sour Chicken Skewer	Crisp apples
14.	Potato Casserole	Lamb Meatballs	Cocoa cookies
15.	Turkey and Peppers Bowls	Spiced Green Beans with Veggies	Strawberry shortcakes
16.	Turkey Tortillas	Chipotle Green Beans	Lentils and dates brownies
17.	Avocado Eggs Mix	Tomato and Cranberry Beans Pasta	Chocolate cookies
18.	Maple Apple Quinoa	Mexican Casserole	Mini lava cakes
19.	Chopped Kale with Ground Beef	Spicy Herb Chicken Wings	Banana bread
20.	Bacon Wrapped Chicken Fillet	Roasted Cauliflower with Nuts & Raisins	Granola
21.	Egg Whites with Sliced Tomatoes	Red Potatoes with Green Beans and Chutney	Tomato cake

22.	Beef Balls with Sesame and Dill	Simple Italian Veggie Salad	Chocolate cake
23.	Zucchini Rounds with Ground Chicken	Spiced Brown Rice with Mung Beans	Coffee cheesecakes
24.	Meatball Breakfast Salad	Eggplant and Tomato Sauce	Fried banana
25.	Tomatoes with Chicken	Lemony Endive Mix	Banana cake
26.	Cherry Tomatoes Fritatta	Lentils and Spinach Casserole	Espresso cream and pears
27.	Whisked Eggs with Ground Chicken	Scallions and Endives with Rice	Lime cheesecakes Wrapped Pears
28.	Breakfast Bacon Hash	Cabbage and Tomatoes	Strawberry cobbler
29.	Eggplant and Sweet Potato Hash	Lemon Halibut	Almond and cocoa bars
30.	Eggs in Avocado	Medium-Rare Beef Steak	Ginger cheesecake
31.	Spaghetti Squash Casserole Cups	Fried Cod & Spring Onion	Plum cake

CONCLUSION

I hope this book was able to help you to understand the benefits of an Air Fryer and the basics on how to use it. The next step is to plan your meals and gather the ingredients. This appliance is easy to use and you will eventually get the hang of the process. Once you have tried several recipes, you can already start tweaking the ingredients to create variations or start making your own.

Enjoy the process of preparing your meals in a healthier way using this innovation when it comes to cooking.

CPSIA information can be obtained
at www.ICGtesting.com
Printed in the USA
LVHW101313251020
669765LV00010B/526